Helen McGuinness

anatomy &
physiology

therapy basics

fourth edition

HODDER
EDUCATION
AN HACHETTE UK COMPANY

Every effort has been made to trace the copyright holders of material reproduced here. The authors and publishers would like to thank the following for permission to reproduce copyright illustrations:

p. 47, top to bottom, © Science Photo Library, © Dr Jeremy Burgess/Science Photo Library; p. 48, © Wellcome Photo Library; p. 56, © Photodisc/Getty Images; p. 57, all © Photodisc/Getty Images; p. 58, © Medical-On-Line/Alamy; p. 59, © Dr H. C. Robinson/Science Photo Library; p. 60, © Dr P. Marazzi/Science Photo Library; p. 62, © Dr P. Marazzi/Science Photo Library; p. 63, © Dr P. Marazzi/Science Photo Library; p. 64, top to bottom, © Dr P. Marazzi/Science Photo Library, © Wellcome Photo Library; p. 65, clockwise from top left, © Dr H. C. Robinson/Science Photo Library, © Dr Chris Hale/Science Photo Library, © Sue Ford/Science Photo Library, © Dr P. Marazzi/Science Photo Library; p. 66, top to bottom, © CNRI/Science Photo Library, © Biophoto Associates/Science Photo Library; p. 67, clockwise from top left, © CNRI/Science Photo Library, © Dr P. Marazzi/Science Photo Library, © BSIP/Science Photo Library; p. 68, both © Dr P. Marazzi/Science Photo Library; p. 69, © Wellcome Photo Library; p. 70, left to right, © Dr P. Marazzi/Science Photo Library, © J. F. Wilson/Science Photo Library; p. 71, © Dr P. Marazzi/Science Photo Library; p. 72, both © Dr P. Marazzi/Science Photo Library; p. 73, clockwise from top left, © Dr P. Marazzi/Science Photo Library, © CNRI/Science Photo Library, © Dr P. Marazzi/Science Photo Library; p. 74, © Dr P. Marazzi/Science Photo Library.

Orders: please contact Bookpoint Ltd, 130 Milton Park, Abingdon, Oxon OX14 4SB. Telephone: (44) 01235 827720. Fax: (44) 01235 400454. Lines are open from 9.00 - 5.00, Monday to Saturday, with a 24-hour message answering service. You can also order through our website www.hoddereducation.co.uk

If you have any comments to make about this, or any of our other titles, please send them to educationenquiries@hodder.co.uk

British Library Cataloguing in Publication Data
A catalogue record for this title is available from the British Library

ISBN: 978 1 444 109 238

First Edition published 1995
Second Edition published 2002
Third Edition published 2006
This Edition published 2010

Impression number   10 9 8 7 6 5 4 3
Year   2014, 2013, 2012

Cover photo from Ralph Mercer/Stone/Getty Images
Illustrations by Kate Nardoni/Cactus Design and Illustration Ltd
Typeset by MPS Limited, a Macmillan Company
Printed and bound in Dubai
338 Euston Road, London NW1 3BH

Contents

Acknowledgements

When I was preparing the original text of this book back in the early 1990s, I never dreamed it would be in circulation for more than 14 years and now be in its fourth networkable edition.

I would therefore like to extend my most significant thanks to my husband, Mark, for his love, support and understanding, constructive comments and his help in organisation of the files.

To my Mum (who sadly passed away earlier this year) and Dad for their love and words of encouragement and belief in my abilities.

To my dear friend Dee Chase for her constant love, support and encouragement throughout the revision of this book.

To Dr Nathan Moss for his original help in checking the accuracy of the text in the third edition.

I will always be greatly indebted to Deirdre Moynihan for her professional help and contributions throughout the preparation of the original text back in 1995.

To all the students, colleges and lecturers who've used this book over the past 14 years and who've been most encouraging and supportive of my work.

This book is devoted to our beautiful daughter Grace.

Guide to students

Dear Colleague,

This book has been designed for those studying beauty therapy, complementary therapies or any subject that requires a sound foundation knowledge of anatomy and physiology.

This book has been completely revised to include new interactive features that can be accessed through Dynamic Learning Online (see the inside front cover for more information).

The introductory chapter explains the terms anatomy and physiology and introduces you to some of the anatomical terminology that you will need to become familiar with.

Each chapter gives an overview of each system and why it is of significance to a therapist, has a list of learning objectives and is full of interesting facts and information to help stimulate your learning.

At the end of each chapter, to help to put the subject into context, there is a link to other body systems, to show how the body systems work as a whole to keep us in balance, along with a revision summary.

As you study each chapter you are directed to accompanying digital material where you will find a range of activities to help test your learning. These include labelling drag and drop activities, interactive multiple choice questions and answers and animations.

Anatomy and physiology is a fascinating subject and I sincerely hope that you will enjoy learning using the variety of interactive resources provided.

Helen McGuinness

introduction to anatomy & physiology

Before we begin the fascinating journey of learning how the body works, let's look at an overview of terms associated with the study of the human body.

Anatomy is the study of the *structure* and *location* of body parts and **Physiology** is the study of the *function* of those body parts.

The terms anatomy and physiology are interlinked and starting with the study of where parts of the body are located will in turn help you to build up a picture as to how they function. An example of this in practice is to think of the structure of the heart and all its chambers and valves (the anatomy); by visualising the individual structures it can help us to understand how the blood flows through the heart and how the heart beats (i.e. we can relate to its function or physiology).

The body may be likened to a map and the key to locating and understanding the parts of the body starts with directional terms and references.

Pathology is the study of disease in the body. Towards the back of each chapter there is a section of common pathologies associated with each system and their causes.

Anatomical terminology

When studying anatomy and physiology, it is necessary to have a key or directional terminology to give precise descriptions when referring to the exact location of a body part or structure. In anatomical terminology, all parts of the body are described in relation to other body parts using a standardised body position called the **anatomical position**.

An anatomical position is determined from a central imaginary line running down the centre or mid-line of the body. In this position the body is erect and facing forwards, arms to the side, palms are facing forwards with the thumbs to the side, and the feet are slightly apart with toes pointing forwards.

Learning anatomical terminology is like learning a new language. The common anatomical descriptive terms you will need to become familiar with are as follows:

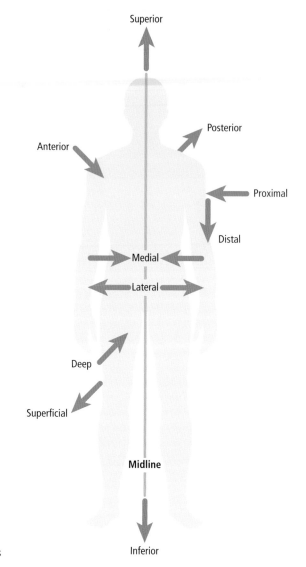

Fig 0.1 Anatomical terms

Anatomical term	Area of the body it relates to
Anterior	front surface of the body, or structure
Posterior	back surface of the body, or structure
Deep	further from the surface
Superficial	near the surface
Internal	nearer the inside
External	nearer the outside
Lateral	away from the mid-line
Medial	towards the mid-line
Superior	situated above or towards the upper part
Inferior	situated below or towards the lower part
Proximal	nearest to the point of reference
Distal	furthest away from the point of reference
Prone	lying face down in a horizontal position
Supine	lying face up in a horizontal position

Sagittal plane   **Frontal/coronal plane**   **Transverse plane**

Fig 0.2 Anatomical planes of the body

The anatomical planes of the body

In the study of anatomy there are three planes that separate the body into sections:

Frontal plane: divides the body into a front (anterior) portion and a rear (posterior) section.
Sagittal plane: this is a vertical plane that divides the body lengthwise into right and left sections.
Transverse plane: this is a horizontal plane that divides the body into top (superior) and bottom (inferior) sections.

The anatomical regions of the body

Just like a map, the anatomical regions of the body refer to a certain area of the body. The body is divided into:

- the head and neck
- the trunk
- the upper limbs (arms)
- the lower limbs (legs).

The table below will help you to learn the correct terminology for each region.

Anatomical regions of the head and neck

Anatomical term	Area of the body it relates to
cephalic	head
cervical	neck
cranial	skull
frontal	forehead
occipital	back of head
ophthalmic	eyes
oral	mouth
nasal	nose

Anatomical regions of the trunk (thorax and abdomen)

Anatomical term	Area of the body it relates to
axillary	armpit
costal	ribs
mammary	breast
pectoral	chest
vertebral	backbone
abdominal	abdomen
gluteal	buttocks
inguinal	groin
lumbar	lower back
pelvic	pelvis/lower part of abdomen
umbilical	navel
perineal	between anus and external genitalia
pubic	pubis

Anatomical regions of the upper limbs

Anatomical term	Area of the body it relates to
brachial	upper arm
carpal	wrist
cubital	elbow
forearm	lower arm
palmar	palm
digital	fingers (also relates to toes)

Anatomical regions of the lower limbs (legs)

Anatomical term	Area of the body it relates to
femoral	thigh
patellar	front of knee
pedal	foot
plantar	sole of foot
popliteal	hollow behind knee
digital	toes (also relates to fingers)

Body cavities

Body cavities are spaces within the body that contain the internal organs. There are two main cavities in the body:

- the **dorsal** cavity which is located in the posterior (back) region of the body
- the **ventral** body cavity which occupies the anterior (front) region of the trunk.

The dorsal cavity is subdivided into two cavities:

1 Cranial cavity	Encases the brain and is protected by the cranium (skull)
2 Vertebral/spinal cavity	Contains the spinal cord and is protected by the vertebrae

The **ventral cavity** is subdivided into:

1 The **thoracic cavity**	Surrounded by the ribs and chest muscles, the thoracic cavity contains the lungs, heart, trachea, oesophagus and thymus
	Separated from the abdominal cavity by the diaphragm muscle
2 The **abdominopelvic cavity**	
The abdominal cavity	Contains the stomach, spleen, liver, gallbladder, pancreas, small intestine and most of the large intestine
	The abdominal cavity is protected by the muscles of the abdominal wall and partly by the diaphragm and ribcage
The pelvic cavity	Contains the bladder, some of the reproductive organs and the rectum
	The pelvic cavity is protected by the pelvic bones.

Fig 0.3 Body cavities

cells and tissues

Introduction

The human body can be likened to a universe, as it is made up of very small structures which are organised to function as a whole.

It is incredible to think that the human body, a complicated and sophisticated machine, starts its journey of life with a single cell.

In order to understand how the body functions as a whole we need to first consider how the structure of the body is organised into its five basic levels: chemical, cellular, tissues, organs and systems.

Ultimately all the body systems, and the minute cells that are the basic components of all organs and tissues, are involved in maintaining health and keeping the body in a state of balance.

IN PRACTICE

It is important for therapists to have an understanding of cells and tissues as these are the foundation building blocks upon which the human body is formed.

Examining cells and tissues from the inside out is like looking at the body from the inside out. Understanding how the body functions from its cellular level will help therapists to understand how the body functions in both health and illness, and relate to the link between structure *and* function of the body's organs.

Objectives

By the end of this chapter, you will be able to recall and understand the following knowledge:

- the different levels of structural organisation in the body
- the importance of homeostasis and metabolism in correct body functioning
- parts of a cell's structure and their functional significance
- the structure and function of the main tissue types in the body
- the interrelationships between the cells and tissues and other body systems
- common pathologies associated with cells and tissues.

The different levels of structural organisation in the body

The human body as a whole is an organism that contains many parts to make up the whole. In order to appreciate the structure of the human body we need to study the five principal levels of structural organisation.

1 Chemical level

Every substance in the world is made up of basic particles such as atoms and molecules.

Atoms and molecules represent the lowest level of organisational complexity in the body and are essential for maintaining life. At the chemical level the smallest unit of matter is the atom.

An **atom** is the smallest particle of an element. An example is a hydrogen or oxygen atom.

A **molecule** is a particle composed of two or more atoms joined together. A common example is a water molecule (H_2O) made of one oxygen atom and two hydrogen atoms. Molecules combine to form cells.

2 Cellular level

Cells are the basic unit of all living organisms and are the basic structural and functional unit of the body. They are therefore the smallest units that show characteristics of life.

There are many different types of cells in the body, which vary in structure, size and shape according to their function. An example is white blood cells (leucocytes), which help fight infection in the body. Cells combine to form tissues.

3 Tissue level

A **tissue** is a group of similar cells that perform a particular function, for example epithelial, connective, muscular and nervous tissue. Two or more types of tissue combine to form organs.

4 Organ level

An **organ** is a specialised structure made up of different types of tissues that are grouped into structurally and functionally integrated units. Examples of organs in the body include the heart and the lungs. Organs combine to form systems.

5 System level

A **system** is a group of organs that works together to perform specific functions. The systems of the body include the circulatory, skeletal, skin, respiratory, reproductive, muscular, endocrine, nervous, urinary and digestive systems. Systems combine to form the living organism, i.e. the human body.

Homeostasis

Traditionally, the body is divided into different systems according to their specific functions. However, the ultimate purpose of each system is to maintain a constant internal environment for each cell to enable it to survive.

The human body is exposed to a constantly changing external environment. These changes are neutralised by the internal environment of blood, lymph and tissue fluids that bathe and protect the cells.

Fig 1.1 Levels of structural organisation in the body

Body parts function efficiently only when the concentrations of water, food substances, oxygen and the conditions of heat and pressure remain within certain narrow limits. The process by which the body maintains a stable internal environment for its cells and tissues is called **homeostasis**.

Homeostasis is like a fine-tuning mechanism that your body goes through automatically in order to restore balance among the body's systems.

When the body's systems are imbalanced through stress, pain, infection or depleted oxygen levels, the body's cells do not work at their optimal level and therefore signs of disorder and disease may be seen.

The body and its systems are constructed in such a way that all systems work synergistically with each other with one overall aim – to maintain homeostasis. Examples of homeostatic mechanisms in the body include the regulation of:

- body temperature
- blood pressure
- blood sugar levels
- pH levels.

Regulating the pH balance

The pH scale is a chemical table or rating scale used to measure the acid or alkaline (base) content of a substance. Acids have a pH from 0 to 7; alkalines (bases) have a pH of 7.0 to 14. The blood of the human body needs to be around 7.4. If the pH drops to below 7.0 to an acidic level, the condition is known as acidosis. If the pH goes above 7.8, the condition becomes alkalosis. Both acidosis and alkalosis can be life threatening.

In order to maintain the blood at a pH of 7.4 the body's systems work together by producing buffer substances which absorb excess hydrogen or hydrogen ions. The kidneys are also significant in maintaining homeostasis as they can detect if the pH of your body's fluids is too low (acidic).

Homeostasis is maintained by adjusting the metabolism of the body.

Metabolism

Metabolism is the term used to describe the physiological processes that take place in our bodies to convert the food we eat and the air we breathe into the energy we need to function. Metabolism is essentially the basic chemical working of the body cells and through metabolism food substances are transformed into energy or materials that the body can use or store.

Metabolism involves two processes:

- **Catabolism** – the chemical breakdown of complex substances by the body to form simpler ones, accompanied by the release of energy. The substances broken down include nutrients in food (carbohydrates and proteins) as well as the body's storage products (glycogen).
- **Anabolism** – the building up of complex molecules, such as proteins and fats, from simpler ones by living things. The rate at which a person consumes energy in activities and body processes is known as the **metabolic rate**. The minimum energy required to keep the body alive is known as the **basal metabolic rate**.

KEY FACT

The part of the brain called the hypothalamus is significant in maintaining homeostasis. Throughout the body, receptors in the blood vessels detect pressure, temperature, glucose levels and pH levels in the blood. These receptors send a signal through the nervous systems to the hypothalamus to initiate changes in the body to bring the body back to balance (an example of this is the secretion of insulin if the blood sugar levels get too high).

How elements contribute to the body's chemical make-up

When talking of the chemical make-up of the body, it is important to consider not only the common major elements and compounds that are involved in the body's make-up, but also how they relate to the physiological processes of the body.

Elements and compounds occur in one of three states: gas, liquid or solid. An example of this is water, which is usually a liquid (although it can become solid, as ice, or turn into gas if you think of steam). Salt and glucose are examples of solids, and carbon dioxide an example of a gas.

It takes energy to change the state of an element or a compound. The chemical bonds between the elements that make up the compounds are one of the ways that the body stores energy. This energy when released may be used in a variety of ways: to initiate chemical processes, to aid movement or for the body's growth, maintenance and repair.

The chemical make-up of a cell

Chemically, a cell is composed of the major elements carbon, oxygen, hydrogen and nitrogen and trace elements of several other elements such as sodium, calcium, chlorine, magnesium, iron, iodine, potassium, sulphur and phosphorus.

Cells are made up of approximately 80 per cent water, 15 per cent protein, 3 per cent lipids or fats, 1 per cent carbohydrates, 1 per cent nucleic acids.

Major compound	Elements present	Main significance in body
Water	Hydrogen and oxygen	Being like the body's reservoir, water provides a universal solvent for the facilitation of chemical reactions in the body's tissues Helps transport substances around the body
Carbohydrates	Carbon, hydrogen and oxygen	Main fuel for the body
Protein	Carbon, hydrogen, oxygen, nitrogen (may contain sulphur)	Main building blocks of the body's tissues
Fats/lipids	Carbon, hydrogen and oxygen	Energy source for the body's activities Energy store
Nucleic acids	Carbon, hydrogen, oxygen, nitrogen, phosphorus	Important molecules found inside cells (an example is deoxyribonucleic acid, which provides the genetic material inside the nucleus)

Cells

The cell is the fundamental unit of all living organisms and is the simplest form of life that can exist as a self-sustaining unit. Cells are therefore the building blocks of the human body.

Cells in the body take many forms, the size and shape being largely dependent on their specialised function. For example, some cells help fight

BODY FACT

BODY FACT

Each type of cell has a structure that is suited to its specific function. For example, a muscle cell is long and thin to enable it to contract and shorten, while skin cells are flat to aid the skin in providing a waterproof covering.

STUDY TIP

When examining the function of each organelle, it is helpful to think of the cell as the 'factory' and the organelles as a 'department' within the factory. Each cell organelle is responsible for the production of a certain product or substance that is used elsewhere in the cell or body.

KEY FACT

DNA is a long, twisted molecule found in the chromatin of the cell's nucleus. It is often called the body's blueprint, as it is a record of a person's height, bone structure, hair colour, body chemistry and other characteristics. When cells divide and multiply, DNA makes sure that the new cells are direct copies by passing on its hereditary information.

BODY FACT

If the spiral of DNA in the nucleus of just one human cell were stretched out in a single line, it would extend more than 6 feet.

disease, others transport oxygen or produce movement; some manufacture proteins and chemicals, and others store nutrients.

Parts of a cell's structure
Cell organelles

Molecules combine in very specific ways to form what is called cell organelles (little organs) which are the basic component parts of the cells. Each organelle has a particular functional significance within the cell that allows it to live.

Despite the great variety of cells in the body, they all have the same basic structure. When studying the cell's structure it is helpful to also think of it in three parts:

- the **outer part** called the **cell membrane**
- the **inner part** containing the **nucleus**
- the **middle layer** which contains a semi-fluid substance called the **cytoplasm**, which contains all the cell's organelles.

The outer part of the cell
Cell membrane

The cell membrane is a fine membrane that encloses the cell and protects its contents. This membrane is said to be semi-permeable in that it selectively controls the inward and outward movement of molecules into and out of the cell. Oxygen, nutrients, hormones and proteins are taken into the cell as needed, and cellular waste such as carbon dioxide passes out through the membrane. As well as governing the exchange of nutrients and waste materials, its function is to maintain the shape of the cell.

The inner part of the cell
Nucleus

The nucleus is the largest organelle in the cytoplasm and is the control centre of the cell, regulating the cell's functions and directing most metabolic activities. The nucleus governs the specialised work performed by the cell and the cell's own growth, repair and reproduction. All cells have at least one nucleus at some time in their existence. The nucleus is significant in that it contains all the information required for the cell to function and it controls all cellular operations.

The information required by the cell is stored in DNA (deoxyribonucleic acid), which carries the genetic materials for replication of identical molecules. The DNA strands are found in threadlike structures known as chromosomes.

A **chromosome** is one of the threadlike structures in the cell nucleus that carries the genetic information in the form of genes. The nucleus of a human cell contains 46 chromosomes, 23 of which are maternal and 23 of which are of paternal origin. Each chromosome can duplicate an exact copy of itself between each cell division so that each new cell formed receives a full set of chromosomes.

Chromatin

Chromatin is the substance inside the nucleus that contains the genetic material.

Nucleolus

Inside the nucleus is a dense spherical structure called a nucleolus which contains ribonucleic acid (RNA) structures that form ribosomes.

Nuclear membrane

The nucleus is surrounded by a perforated outer membrane called the nuclear membrane; materials move across it to and from the cytoplasm.

The middle part of the cell

Cytoplasm

The cytoplasm is the gel-like substance that is enclosed by the cell membrane. The cytoplasm contains the nucleus and the small cellular structures called organelles.

Most cellular metabolism occurs within the cytoplasm of the cell.

Centrosome

This is an area of clear cytoplasm found next to the nucleus and contains the centrioles.

Centrioles

Contained within the centrosomes are the small spherical structures called centrioles, which are associated with cell division, or mitosis. During cell division the centriole divides in two and migrates to opposite sides of the nucleus to form the spindle poles.

Chromatids

This is a pair of identical strands that are joined at the centromere and separate during cell division.

Centromere

The portion of a chromosome where the two chromatids are joined is the centromere.

Ribosomes

Ribosomes are tiny organelles made up of RNA and protein. They may be fixed to the walls of the endoplasmic reticulum (known as rough ER) or may float freely in the cytoplasm. Their function is to manufacture proteins for use within the cell and also to produce other proteins that are exported outside the cell.

Endoplasmic reticulum

This is a series of membranes continuous with the cell membrane. It can be thought of as an intracellular transport system, allowing movement of materials from one part of the cell to another. It links the cell membrane with the nuclear membrane and therefore assists movement and materials out of the cell.

It contains enzymes and participates in the synthesis of proteins, carbohydrates and lipids. The endoplasmic reticulum serves to store material, transport substances inside the cell, as well as detoxify harmful agents. Some endoplasmic reticulum appears smooth, while other appears rough due to the presence of ribosomes.

Mitochondria

Mitochondria are oval-shaped organelles that lie in varying numbers within the cytoplasm. The mitochondria are said to be the site of the cell's energy production. The mitochondria provide most of a cell's ATP (adenosine triphosphate), which is a compound that stores the energy needed by the cell.

The work of the mitochondria is assisted by enzymes which are proteins that speed up chemical changes. By means of cellular respiration, the mitochondria provide the energy which powers the cell's activities.

Lysosome

These are round sacs present in the cytoplasm. They contain powerful enzymes, which are capable of digesting proteins. Their function is to destroy any part of the cell that is worn out so that it can be eliminated – this is known as lysis.

Vacuole

These are empty spaces within the cytoplasm. They contain waste materials or secretions formed by the cytoplasm and are used for temporary storage, transportation or digestive purposes in different kinds of cells.

Golgi body/apparatus

This is a collection of flattened sacs within the cytoplasm. The golgi apparatus is typically located near the nucleus and attached to the

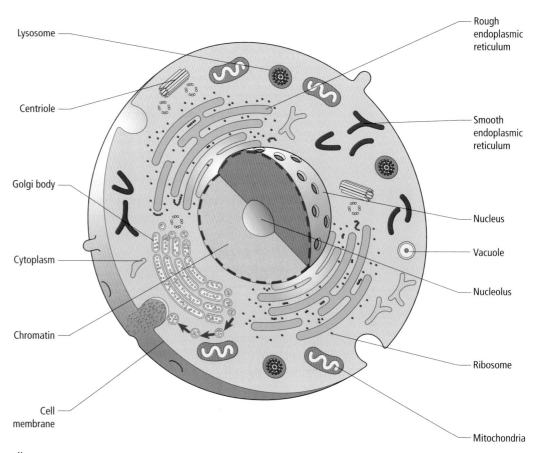

Fig 1.2 Structure of a cell

Student activity

Now complete Activity 1.1 in the resources for this book on Dynamic Learning Online.

endoplasmic reticulum. It is said to be the 'packaging department' of the cell as it stores the protein manufactured in the endoplasmic reticulum and later transports it out of the cell.

Functions of cells

In order for a cell to survive it must be able to carry out a variety of functions.

Respiration

Every cell requires oxygen for the process of metabolism. Oxygen is absorbed through the cell's semi-permeable membrane and is used to oxidise nutrient material to provide heat and energy. The waste products produced as a result of cell respiration include carbon dioxide and water. These are passed out from the cell through its semi-permeable membrane.

Growth

Cells have the ability to grow until they are mature and ready to produce. A cell can grow and repair itself by manufacturing protein.

Excretion

During metabolism various substances are produced which are of no further use to the cell. These waste products are removed through the cell's semi-permeable membrane.

Movement

Movement may occur in the whole or part of a cell. White blood cells, for instance, are able to move freely.

Irritability

A cell has the ability to respond to a stimulus, which may be physical, chemical or thermal. For example, a muscle fibre contracts when stimulated by a nerve cell.

Reproduction

When growth is complete in a cell, reproduction takes place. The cells of the human body reproduce or divide by the process of mitosis.

IN PRACTICE

Cell growth and reproduction rely on favourable conditions such as an adequate supply of food, oxygen, water, suitable temperatures and the ability to eliminate waste. Clients should be advised that if conditions become unfavourable for the skin, such as smoking, sun damage and air pollution, cell function will be impaired and skin cells may subsequently be destroyed, resulting in loss of elasticity, lines, wrinkles and dehydration.

As massage facilitates cell nutrition as well as increasing elimination of waste from the cells and tissues, clients should be encouraged to have treatments regularly to aid cell regeneration.

The cell's life cycle

It is vital for living cells to reproduce themselves in order to continue life, and cells undergo many divisions from the time of fertilisation to physical maturity. When a single cell undergoes division, it forms two daughter cells that are identical to the original cell. A cell may live from a few days to many years, depending on its type. Cells divide in two ways: **mitosis** and **meiosis**.

Mitosis

Mitosis is when a single cell produces two genetically identical daughter cells. It is the way in which new body cells are produced for both growth and repair. Division of the nucleus takes place in four phases (prophase, metaphase, anaphase and telophase) and is followed by the division of the cytoplasm to form the daughter cells.

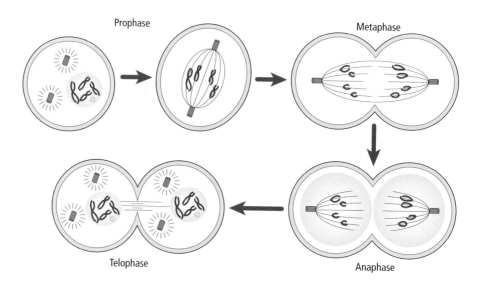

Fig 1.3 Stages of mitosis

Prophase
- Centrioles duplicate as chromatids in the nucleus change to become individual chromosomes.
- Centrioles separate and form spindles.

Metaphase
- Chromosomes align themselves in the centre of the cell, midway between the centrioles, as the nucleus and its protective membrane disappears.
- The centromere of each chromosome then replicates.

Anaphase
- Centromeres divide and identical sets of chromosomes move to opposite poles of the cell.

Telophase
- This is the final stage of mitosis.
- Nuclear membrane forms around each nucleus and spindle fibres disappear.
- Cytoplasm compresses and divides in half.

Meiosis

Meiosis is a type of cell division that produces four daughter cells, each having half the number of chromosomes of the original cell. Meiosis involves the production of a new organism, formed by the fusion of a sperm from the male and an egg from the female.

Before fertilisation there are only 23 chromosomes present in the sperm and the egg. After fertilisation has taken place the egg and the sperm fuse together to form a single cell called a zygote with 46 chromosomes (23 from each parent). The zygote is then able to reproduce itself by cell division or mitosis to form an embryo, foetus and eventually a fully formed individual.

Cellular respiration

All cellular functions depend on energy generation and transportation of substances within and among cells. In order to function properly a cell must maintain a stable internal environment and therefore the transport of materials has to be achieved without an excessive build-up of chemicals. The term cell respiration refers to the controlled exchange of nutrients (such as oxygen and glucose) and waste (such as carbon dioxide) by the cell to activate the energy needed for the cell to function.

In order for cells to carry out their work they need to produce enough energy or fuel. Fuel is provided by glucose from carbohydrate metabolism and in order for the glucose to be released or 'oxidised', oxygen is absorbed from the respiratory system into the bloodstream.

Cells are bathed in a fluid known as **tissue fluid** or interstitial fluid, which allows the interchange of substances between the cells and the blood, known as internal respiration.

The body's internal transport system, the blood, carries oxygen from the respiratory system and nutrients such as glucose from the digestive system to the cells and these are absorbed through the cell membrane in several different ways: **diffusion, osmosis, active transport** and **filtration**. When certain molecules are needed, such as glucose, the cell will take these in and discard other materials in order to preserve the equilibrium.

Diffusion

As chemicals become concentrated outside the cell, a flow of small molecules takes place through the cell membrane until a balance exists. This process in which small molecules move from areas of high concentration to those of lower concentration is called diffusion. Diffusion is the basis by which the cells lining the small intestines take in digestive products to be utilised by the body.

Diffusion

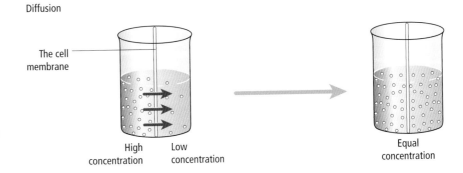

The cell membrane

High concentration   Low concentration

Equal concentration

Fig 1.4 Diffusion: the process in which small molecules move from an area of high concentration to lower concentration

Osmosis

This process refers to the movement of water through the cell membrane from areas of low chemical concentration to areas of high chemical concentration. This process allows for the dilution of chemicals, which are unable to cross the cell membrane by diffusion, in order to maintain equilibrium within the cell.

Fig 1.5 Osmosis: the movement of water through the cell membrane from low to high chemical concentration

Osmosis

The cell membrane

Area of low chemical concentration

Area of high chemical concentration

Equal concentration

Active transport

This is an energy-dependent process in which certain substances (including ions, some drugs and amino acids) are able to cross cell membranes against a concentration gradient. This is the process, using chemical energy, by which the cell takes in larger molecules that would be otherwise unable to enter in sufficient quantities. Carrier molecules within the cell membrane bind themselves to the incoming molecules, rotate around them and release them into the cell. This is the means by which the cell absorbs glucose.

Filtration

This is the movement of water and dissolved substances across the cell membrane due to differences in pressure. The force of the weight of the fluid pushes against the cell membrane, thereby moving it into the cell. One site of filtration in the body is in the kidneys. Blood pressure forces water and small molecules through plasma membranes of cells and the filtered liquid then enters the kidneys for filtration.

Tissues

Tissues are defined as a group of similar cells that act together to perform a specific function. The study of tissues is known as **histology**.

Due to the complexity of the human body it is not possible for every cell to carry out all the functions required by the body. Some cells, therefore, become specialised to form of a group of cells or tissues. There are four major types of tissues in the human body:

- **epithelial** tissue
- **connective** tissue
- **muscle** tissue
- **nervous** tissue.

BODY FACT

All four types of tissue have special purposes and therefore correspondingly have varying different rates of cellular regeneration. Epithelial tissue is renewed constantly by the process of cell division or mitosis. Bone tissue and adipose connective tissue are highly vascular and therefore heal quickly. Muscle tissue takes longer to regenerate. Nervous tissue regenerates very slowly. The less vascular forms of connective tissue such as ligaments and tendons are even slower to heal than muscle tissue, and cartilage is amongst the slowest to heal.

The following table gives an overview of the four major types of tissue in the body.

Type of tissue	Main function
Epithelial tissue	Provides a protective covering for surfaces inside and outside of the body
Connective tissue	Protects, binds and supports the body and its organs
Muscle tissue	Provides movement
Nervous tissue	Initiates and transmits nerve impulses

Epithelial tissue

Epithelial tissue consists of sheets of cells which cover and protect the external and internal surfaces of the body and line the inside of hollow structures. They specialise in moving substances in and out of the blood during secretion, absorption and excretion. As they are subject to a considerable amount of wear and tear, epithelial cells reproduce very actively.

Usually there is little matrix (a ground material or base) present in epithelial tissues. The matrix present tends to form continuous sheets of cells, with the cells held very close together. A thin permeable basement membrane attaches epithelial tissues to the underlying connective tissue. Epithelial tissue, which consists of cells closely packed together, comes in various shapes. There are two categories of epithelial tissue:

- **simple** (single layered)
- **compound** (multi-layered).

Simple epithelium

Simple epithelium tissue has only one layer of cells over a basement membrane. Being thin, it is fragile and is found only in areas inside the body which are relatively protected, such as the lining of the heart and blood vessels and the lining of body cavities. It is also found lining the digestive tract and in the exchange surfaces of the lungs where its thinness is an advantage for speedy absorption across it. There are four different types of simple epithelium, named according to their shape and the functions they perform.

The table on page 21 summarises the structure, location and function of the different types of simple epithelial tissue.

Compound epithelium

The main function of compound epithelium is to protect underlying structures. Compound epithelium contains two or more layers of cells. There are two main types:

- **stratified**
- **transitional**

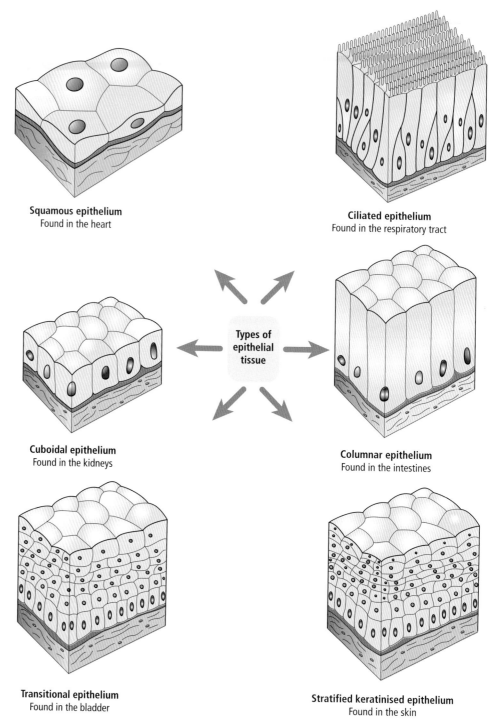

Squamous epithelium
Found in the heart

Ciliated epithelium
Found in the respiratory tract

Types of
epithelial
tissue

Cuboidal epithelium
Found in the kidneys

Columnar epithelium
Found in the intestines

Transitional epithelium
Found in the bladder

Stratified keratinised epithelium
Found in the skin

Fig 1.6 Types of epithelial tissue

Stratified epithelium is composed of a number of layers of cells of different shapes. In the deeper layers the cells are mainly columnar in shape and as they grow towards the surface they become flattened.

Type	Structure	Location	Function
Simple squamous	A single layer of flat, scale-like cells with a central nucleus. The cells fit closely together, rather like a pavement, producing a very smooth surface	Lines the alveoli of the lungs Lines blood and lymphatic vessels and the heart	Allows for exchange of nutrients, wastes and gases
Simple cuboidal	Single layer of cube-like cells	Ovaries, kidney tubules, thyroid gland, pancreas and salivary glands	Secretion and absorption
Simple columnar	Single layer of tall, cylindrical column cells with nucleus situated towards base of cell	Lines the small and large intestine, stomach and gall bladder	Secretion and absorption
Simple ciliated (columnar)	A form of columnar epithelium, single layer of rectangular cells that has hair-like projections (cilia) from its surface	Lines the upper part of respiratory system Also lines the uterine tubes	The beating of the cilia carries unwanted particles along with mucus out of the system Helps propel the ova towards the uterus

There are two types of stratified epithelium:

- **Non-keratinised stratified epithelium** – this is found on wet surfaces that may be subject to wear and tear such as the conjunctiva of the eyes, the lining of the mouth, the pharynx and the oesophagus.
- **Keratinised stratified epithelium** – this is found on dry surfaces such as the lining of the skin, hair and nails. The surface layers of keratinised cells are dead cells. They give protection and prevent drying out of the cells in the deeper layers from which they develop. The surface layer of cells is continually being rubbed off and is replaced from below.

Transitional epithelium is composed of several layers of pear-shaped cells which change shape when they are stretched. This type of tissue is found lining the uterus, bladder and pelvis of the kidney.

Connective tissue

Connective tissue is the most abundant type of tissue in the body. It connects tissues and organs by binding together the various parts of the body and helps to give protection and support. Connective tissue consists of a matrix or ground substance which contains cells called fibroblasts and fibres made of protein.

Connective tissue cells are often more widely separated from each other than those forming epithelial tissue, and the space between cells is larger and is filled with a large amount of non-living matrix. There may or may not be fibres in the matrix, which may be either a semi-solid jelly-like consistency or dense and rigid, depending on the position and function of the tissue.

There are several different types of connective tissue, which are summarised in the table on page 23.

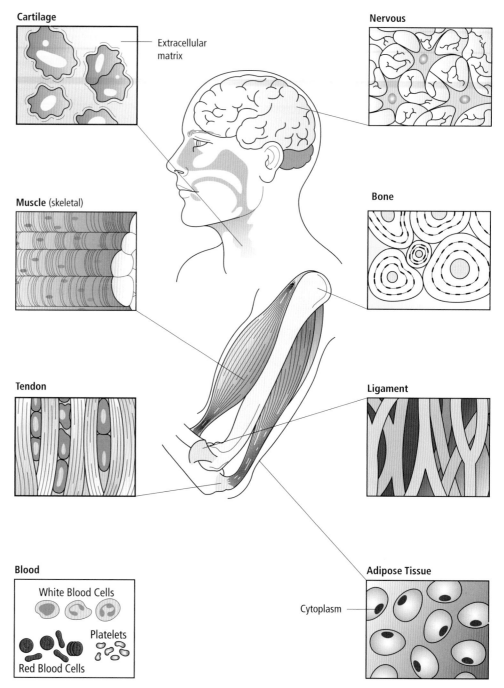

Fig 1.7 Types of connective tissue

Cartilage

For descriptive purposes, cartilage is divided into three types:

- **hyaline** cartilage
- **white fibrous** cartilage
- **yellow elastic** fibrocartilage.

Muscle tissue

Muscle tissue is very elastic and therefore has the unique ability to provide movement by shortening as a result of contraction. This tissue is made

Type	Structure	Location	Function
Areolar	Most widely distributed type of connective tissue in the body A loose, soft and pliable tissue containing collagen, elastin and reticular fibres	Under the skin, between muscles, supporting blood vessels and nerves and in the alimentary canal	Provides strength, elasticity, connects and supports organs
Adipose	A type of areolar tissue containing fat cells (adipocytes)	Surrounds organs such as kidneys and the heart Under the skin (subcutaneous layer) between bundles of muscle fibres In the yellow bone marrow of long bones and as a padding around joints	Provides insulation, support and protection; emergency energy reserve
White fibrous	Strong, connecting tissue made up of mainly closely packed bundles of white, collagenous fibres, with very little matrix Contains cells called fibrocytes between the bundles	Forms tendons which attach muscle to bone, ligaments which tie bones together and act as an outer protective covering for some organs such as the kidney and bladder	Provides strong attachment between different structures
Yellow elastic	Consists of branching yellow elastic fibres with fibrocytes in the spaces between the fibres	Arteries, trachea, bronchi and lungs	To allow the stretching of various organs, followed by a return to their original shape and size
Lymphoid	This tissue has a semi-solid matrix with fine branching fibres. The cells contained within this tissue are specialised and are called lymphocytes	In the lymph nodes, spleen, tonsils, adenoids, walls of the large intestine and glands in the small intestine	Forms part of the lymphatic system whose function is to protect the body from infection
Blood	Also known as liquid connective tissue. It contains the blood cells erythrocytes, leucocytes and thrombocytes which float within a fluid called plasma	Contained within blood vessels	Helps maintain homeostasis of the body by transporting substances throughout the body, by resisting infection and by maintaining heat
Bone	Hardest and most solid of all connective tissues Consists of tough, dense compact bones and slightly less dense cancellous bone	Bones	Protects and supports other organs and soft tissues
Cartilage	Much firmer tissue than any of the other connective tissues; matrix is quite solid	See table on page 24	See table on page 24

Type of cartilage	Description	Location	Function
Hyaline cartilage	Most abundant type of cartilage found in the body A smooth, bluish-white, glossy tissue Contains numerous cells called chondrocytes from which cartilage is produced	Found on the surfaces of the parts of bones which form joints Forms the costal cartilage which attaches the ribs to the sternum Forms part of the larynx, trachea and bronchi.	Provides a hard-wearing, low-friction surface within joints Provides flexibility in the nose and trachea
White fibrous cartilage	This type of cartilage is tough but slightly flexible It is composed of bundles of collagenous white fibres in a solid matrix with cells scattered among them	Found as pads between the bodies of the vertebrae called the intervertebral discs and in the symphysis pubis which joins the pubis bones together	Its function is one of support and to join together or fuse certain bones
Yellow elastic fibrocartilage	Consists of yellow elastic fibres running through a solid matrix, between which chondrocytes are situated	Found forming the pinna (lobe of the ear) and forming the epiglottis	To provide support and to maintain shape

up of contractile fibres, usually arranged in bundles and surrounded by connective tissue. There are three types of muscle tissue:

- **voluntary** (skeletal) tissue
- **involuntary** or smooth tissue
- **cardiac muscle** tissue.

The different types of muscle tissue are discussed in more detail in Chapter 4, 'The muscular system'.

Nervous tissue

Nervous tissue consists of cells called neurones which can pick up and transmit electrical signals by converting stimuli into nerve impulses. Nervous tissue has the characteristics of excitability and conductivity. Its functions are to coordinate and regulate body activity. Nervous tissue and neurones are discussed in more detail in Chapter 8, 'The nervous system'.

Membranes

Membranes are a thin, soft, sheet-like layer of tissue that covers a cell, organ or structure, that lines tubes or cavities or divides and separates one part of a cavity from another. There are three basic types of membranes in the body:

- **mucous** membrane
- **serous** membrane
- **synovial** membrane.

Types of membrane

Type of membrane	Description	Location	Function
Mucous membrane	Type of membrane that lines body cavities and outer layer of organs	Lines the respiratory, digestive, urinary and reproductive tracts	As well as lining the openings to the external environment, secretes a viscous slippery fluid called mucus that coats and protects underlying cells
Serous membrane	Type of membrane lining body cavities that are not open to the external environment and cover many of the organs Serous membranes consist of two layers: a parietal layer which lines the wall of body cavities and a visceral layer which provides an external covering to organs in body cavities	The pericardium of the heart Pleural membranes in the lungs The peritoneum lining the abdominal organs	As well as lining body cavities not open to the external environment, they secrete a thin, watery (serous) fluid that lubricates organs to reduce friction as they rub against one another and against the wall of the cavities
Synovial membrane	Type of membrane that lines the joint cavities of freely movable joints	Lines the spaces around certain joint cavities (shoulder, hip and knee)	Secretes synovial fluid that provides nutrition and lubrication to the joint so that it can move freely without undue friction.

Common pathologies of cells and tissues

Cancer/abnormal cell division

Cancerous diseases are characterised by the growth of abnormal cells that invade surrounding tissues and **metasasis** (the spread of cancerous cells to other parts of the body).

When cells in an area of the body divide without control, the excess tissue that develops is called a **tumour**, growth or **neoplasm**. The study of tumours is called **oncology** and a physician who specialises in this field is called an **oncologist**.

Tumours may be cancerous and sometimes fatal, or they may be quite harmless. A cancerous growth is called a **malignant** tumour and a non-cancerous growth is called a **benign** tumour. Benign tumours do not spread to other parts of the body but they may be removed if they interfere with a normal body function or are disfiguring. Cancers are classified according to their microscopic appearance and the body site from which they arise.

The name of the cancer is derived from the type of tissue in which it develops. Most human cancers are **carcinomas**, malignant tumours that arise from epithelial cells. **Melanomas**, for example, are cancerous growths of melanocytes, the skin cells that produce the pigment melanin.

Sarcoma is a general term for any cancer arising from muscle cells or connective tissues. For example, osteogenic sarcomas (bone cancer) is the most frequent type of childhood cancer, which destroys normal bone tissue and eventually spreads to other areas of the body.

Leukaemia is a cancer of blood-forming organs characterised by rapid growth and distorted development of leucoytes. **Lymphoma** is a malignant disease of lymphatic tissue such as the lymph nodes. An example is Hodgkin's disease.

Interrelationships with other systems

Cells and tissues link to the following body systems.

Skin
Keratinised stratified epithelium (a type of tissue containing layers of cells) is found on dry surfaces such as the skin, hair and nails.

Skeletal
Bone is the hardest and most solid type of connective tissue in the body which is needed for building the structures of the skeletal framework.

Muscular
There are three types of muscle tissue: skeletal muscle which controls voluntary movements, smooth muscle which controls involuntary movements and cardiac muscle which controls the heart.

Circulatory
Blood is a form of liquid connective tissue whose role is in transporting substances to and from the cells.

Respiratory
A type of tissue called ciliated columnar epithelium lines the respiratory tract, which carries unwanted particles out of the system.

Nervous
Neurones and neuroglia are the specialised cells that form nervous tissue which enables the body to receive and transmit nerve impulses in order to regulate and coordinate body activities.

Endocrine
The endocrine glands are made from epithelial tissue. They secrete hormones directly into the bloodstream to influence the activity of another organ or gland.

Digestive
The digestive system is lined with epithelial tissue with goblet cells that secrete mucus to aid the flow of the digestive processes.

Urinary
The bladder is lined with transitional epithelium which allows the bladder to expand when full and deflate when empty.

Key words associated with cells

atom	nucleus	centrioles
molecule	nucleolus	chromatid
cell	nuclear membrane	diffusion
tissue	lysosome	osmosis
organ	vacuole	active transport
system	ribosome	filtration
homeostasis	golgi body	cell respiration
metabolism	mitochondria	tissue fluid
cell membrane	centrosome	meiosis
cytoplasm	centromere	mitosis

Revision summary of cells

- The human body involves five levels of structural organisation – atoms and molecules, cells, tissues, organs and systems.
- **Atoms and molecules** are the lowest level of organisational complexity in the body.
- **Cells** are the smallest units that show characteristics of life.
- **Tissues** are a group of similar cells that perform a certain function.
- **Organs** are tissues grouped into structurally and functionally integrated units.
- **Systems** are a group of organs that work together to perform specific functions.
- The process by which the body maintains a stable internal environment for its cells and tissues is called **homeostasis**.
- Homeostatic mechanisms in the body include the regulation of body temperature, blood pressure, blood sugar levels and pH levels.
- **Metabolism** is the term used to describe the physiological processes that take place in our bodies to convert the food we eat and the air we breathe into the energy we need to function.
- The minimum energy required to keep the body alive is known as the **basal metabolic rate**.
- Major elements and compounds are involved in the body's make-up.
- Chemically, a cell is composed of the major elements carbon, oxygen, hydrogen and nitrogen.
- Cells are made up of approximately 80 per cent water, 15 per cent protein, 3 per cent lipids or fats, 1 per cent carbohydrates, 1 per cent nucleic acids.

- A **cell** is the basic, living, structural and functional unit of the body.
- The principal parts of the cell are the **cell membrane** and its **organelles** which play specific roles in cellular growth, maintenance, repair and control.
- The **cell membrane** encloses the cell and protects its contents. It is semi-permeable and governs the exchange of nutrients and waste materials.
- The **nucleus** controls the cell's activities and contains the genetic information.
- The **cytoplasm** is the substance inside the cell between the plasma membrane and the nucleus.
- The **ribosomes** are sites of protein synthesis.
- The **endoplasmic reticulum** links the cell membrane with the nuclear membrane and assists movement of materials out of the cell.
- The **Golgi body** processes, sorts and delivers proteins and lipids (fats) to the plasma membrane, lysosome and secretory vesicles.
- The **lysosome** is a round sac in the cytoplasm that contains powerful enzymes to help destroy waste and worn-out cell materials.
- The **mitochondria** are the 'powerhouses' of the cell.
- The **centrosome** is a dense area of cytoplasm, containing the centrioles.
- The **centrioles** are paired small spherical structures associated with cell division, or mitosis.
- The **chromatids** are a pair of identical strands that are joined at the centromere and separate during cell division.

- The **centromere** is the portion of a chromosome where the two chromatids are joined.
- Functions of cells include respiration, growth, excretion, movement, irritability and reproduction.
- Cell division is the process by which cells reproduce themselves.
- **Mitosis** is cell division that results in an increase in body cells and involves division of a nucleus.
- **Meiosis** is reproductive cell division and results in the fusion of an egg and a sperm into a zygote.
- Cells function through the exchange of fluids, nutrients, chemical and ions which are carried out by passive processes such as **diffusion, osmosis** and **filtration**, and active processes such as **active transport**.
- **Cell respiration** is the controlled exchange of nutrients such as oxygen and glucose and waste such as carbon dioxide by the cell to activate the energy needed for the cell to function.
- The fuel required by cells is provided by **glucose** from carbohydrate metabolism and **oxygen** absorbed from the respiratory system into the bloodstream.
- Cells are bathed in a fluid known as **tissue fluid** or interstitial fluid which allows the interchange of substances between the cells and the blood, known as internal respiration.

Key words associated with tissues

tissue	yellow elastic tissue	cuboidal epithelium
epithelial tissue	lymphoid tissue	columnar epithelium
simple epithelium	blood	ciliated epithelium
compound epithelium	bone	stratified epithelium
connective tissue	cartilage	transitional epithelium
areolar tissue	muscular tissue	mucous membrane
adipose tissue	nervous tissue	serous membrane
white fibrous tissue	squamous epithelium	synovial membrane

Revision summary of tissues

- A **tissue** is a group of similar cells that is specialised for a particular function.
- The tissues of the body are classified into four main types: **epithelial, connective, muscular** and **nervous**.
- **Epithelial tissue** provides coverings and linings of many organs and vessels.
- There are two categories of epithelial tissue: **simple** (single layer) and **compound** (multi layer).
- There are four different types of simple epithelium: **squamous, cuboidal, columnar** and **ciliated**.
- There are two different types of compound epithelium: **stratified and transitional**.
- **Connective tissue** is the most abundant type of body tissue. It connects tissues and organs to give protection and support.
- Connective tissue consists of the following different types: **areolar, adipose, white fibrous,** **yellow elastic, lymphoid, blood, bone** and **cartilage**.
- **Muscle tissue** is elastic and is therefore modified for contraction. It is found attached to bones (skeletal muscle), in the wall of the heart (cardiac muscle) and in the walls of the stomach, intestines, bladder, uterus and blood vessels.
- **Nervous tissue** is composed of nerve cells called neurones which pick up and transmit nerve signals.
- **Membranes** are thin, soft, sheet-like layers of tissue.
- **Mucous membrane** line cavities that open to the exterior such as the digestive tract.
- **Serous membranes** line body cavities that are not open to the external environment (the lungs and the heart).
- **Synovial membrane** lines joint cavities of freely moveable joints such as the shoulder, hip and knee.

Cells and tissues
Multiple-choice questions

1 The process by which the body maintains a stable internal environment of its cells and tissues is:
   a physiology
   b homeostasis
   c metabolism
   d anatomy

2 The pH scale of human blood needs to be:
   a 7.4
   b 7.0
   c 7.8
   d 0

3 The simplest form of life that can exist as independent self-sustaining units are:
   a tissues
   b atoms
   c organs
   d cells

4 Which of the following compounds are the building blocks of the body's tissues?
   a carbohydrates
   b water
   c fats
   d proteins

5 The process by which new body cells are produced for both growth and repair is:
   a meiosis
   b mitosis
   c metaphase
   d prophase

6 How many chromosomes does the nucleus of a human cell contains?
   a 43
   b 46
   c 23
   d 26

7 DNA is found within the:
   a nucleolus
   b cytoplasm
   c nuclear membrane
   d nucleus

8 The organelle that powers the cell activities is:
   a mitochondria
   b nucleus
   c lysosome
   d endoplasmic recticulum

9 The small spherical structures associated with cell division are:
   a centrosomes
   b centrioles
   c chromatids
   d centromeres

10 Tiny organelles concerned with the manufacture of protein within a cell are:
   a vacuoles
   b Golgi bodies
   c lysosomes
   d ribosomes

11 The process in which small molecules move from areas of high concentration to those of lower concentration is:
   a diffusion
   b osmosis
   c filtration
   d active transport

12 A collection of similar cells that group together to perform a certain function are:
   a organs
   b tissues
   c systems
   d atoms

13 Which of the following types of tissue takes the longest to heal?
   a bone
   b cartilage
   c muscle
   d epithelial tissue

14 The type of tissue that lines the internal and external organs of the body and lines vessels and body cavities is:
   a connective
   b serous
   c nervous
   d epithelial

15 Where would you find squamous epithelium?
   a brain
   b kidneys
   c lungs
   d ovaries

16 Where would you find ciliated epithelium?
   a kidney tubules
   b eyes
   c respiratory system
   d pancreas

17 Where would you find columnar epithelium?
   a stomach
   b small and large intestines
   c gall bladder
   d all of the above

18 The most widely distributed type of connective tissue in the body is:
   a adipose
   b epithelial
   c areolar
   d white fibrous

19 The most abundant type of cartilage found on the surface of parts of bones which form joints is:
   a elastic
   b hyaline
   c fibrocartilage
   d yellow elastic

20 Membranes that line openings to the outside of the body are called:
   a serous
   b synovial
   c mucous
   d epithelial

21 The excess tissue that develops when cells in an area of the body divide without control is known as a:
   a sarcoma
   b tumour
   c metastasis
   d lymphoma

2 the skin, hair and nails

Introduction

The skin

The skin is one of the largest organs in the body in terms of weight and surface area; it acts like a cell membrane, defining our parameters. Located within its layers are several types of tissues that carry out special functions such as protection, temperature regulation and excretion. The skin also forms natural openings for the mouth, nose and parts of the urino-genital systems. No other body system is more easily exposed to infections, disease, pollution or injury than the skin, yet no other body system is as strong and resilient.

The nail is an appendage of the skin and is a modification of the stratum corneum (horny) and stratum lucidum (clear) layers of the epidermis. Nails are non-living tissue. Their two main functions are protection for the fingers and toes and as tools for the manipulation of objects.

The hair is also an appendage of the skin and grows from a sac-like depression in the epidermis called a hair follicle. The primary function of hair is protection.

Objectives

By the end of this chapter you will be able to recall and understand the following knowledge:

- the structure and functions of the skin
- the characteristics of the different skin types
- the structure and functions of the nail
- the structure and functions of the hair
- the interrelationships between the skin and other body systems
- common pathologies associated with the skin, hair and nails.

The functions of the skin

The skin is so much more than an external covering. It is a highly sensitive boundary between our bodies and the environment. The skin has several important functions offering protection, temperature regulation, waste removal, as well as providing us with a sense of touch.

Sensitivity

The skin is considered as an extension of the nervous system. It is very sensitive to various stimuli due to its many sensory nerve endings which can detect changes in temperature, pressure and register pain.

Heat regulation

The skin helps to regulate body temperature in the following ways:

- When the body is losing too much heat, the blood capillaries near the skin surface contract, to keep warm blood away from the surface of the skin and closer to major organs.
- The erector pili muscles raise the hairs and trap air next to the skin when heat needs to be retained.
- The adipose tissue in the dermis and the subcutaneous layer helps to insulate the body against heat loss.
- When the body is too warm, the blood capillaries dilate to allow warm blood to flow near to the surface of the skin, in order to cool the body.
- The evaporation of sweat from the surface of the skin will also assist in cooling the body.

Absorption

The skin has limited absorption properties. Substances which can be absorbed by the epidermis include fat soluble substances such as oxygen, carbon dioxide, fat soluble vitamins and steroids, along with small amounts of water.

Protection

The skin acts as a protective organ in the following ways:

- The film of sebum and sweat on the surface of the skin, known as the acid mantle, acts as an antibacterial agent to help prevent the multiplication of micro-organisms on the skin.
- The fat cells in the subcutaneous layer of the skin help protect bones and major organs from injury.
- Melanin, which is produced in the basal cell layer of the skin, helps to protect the body from the harmful effects of ultraviolet radiation.
- The cells in the horny layer of the skin overlap like scales to prevent micro-organisms from penetrating the skin and to prevent excessive water loss from the body.

Excretion

The skin functions as a mini excretory system, eliminating waste through perspiration. The eccrine glands of the skin produce sweat, which helps to remove some waste materials from the skin such as urea, uric acid, ammonia and lactic acid.

Storage

The skin also acts as a storage depot for fat and water. About 15 per cent of the body's fluids are stored in the subcutaneous layer.

Vitamin D production

The skin synthesises vitamin D when exposed to ultraviolet light. Modified cholesterol molecules in the skin are converted by the ultraviolet rays in sunlight to vitamin D. It is then absorbed by the body for the maintenance of bones and the absorption of calcium and phosphorus in the diet.

The structure of the skin

Before looking at the structure of the skin, let's consider a few facts:

- The skin is a very large organ covering the whole body.
- It varies in thickness on different parts of the body. It is thinnest on the lips and eyelids, which must be light and flexible, and thickest on the soles of the feet and palms of the hands, where friction is needed for gripping.
- As the skin is the external covering of the body, it can be easily irritated and damaged and certain symptoms of disease and disorders may occur.
- Each client's skin varies in colour, texture and sensitivity and it is these individual characteristics that make each client unique.

Let's take a closer look at the structure of the skin. There are two main layers of the skin:

- the **epidermis**, which is the outer, thinner layer
- the **dermis**, which is the inner, thicker layer.

Below the dermis is the **subcutaneous layer**, which attaches to underlying organs and tissues.

Although the skin is technically a single organ, the two main layers do have different structures and functions.

The epidermis

The **epidermis** is the most superficial layer of the skin and consists of five layers of cells:

- the basal cell layer (stratum germinativum) – **innermost layer**
- the prickle cell layer (stratum spinosum)
- the granular layer (stratum granulosum)
- the clear layer (stratum lucidum)
- the horny layer (stratum corneum) – **outermost layer**.

In most areas of the body the epidermis is approximately 35–50 micrometres thick. It is thicker on the palms and soles of the feet (up to several millimetres) and thinner around the eye.

The epidermis holds a large amount of water, with the basal cell layer holding the highest percentage (approximately 80 per cent). Water is held in the spaces between the cells; each subsequent layer has less water, with the horny layer containing approximately 15 per cent.

BODY FACT

The skin accounts for approximately 15 per cent of your total body weight.

BODY FACT

The epidermis varies in thickness from 0.1 mm on the eyelids to more than 1 mm on the palms and soles of the feet.

IN PRACTICE

The appearance of the skin reflects a client's physiology. Observation of a client's skin will indicate their nutrition, circulation, age, immunity, genetics as well as environmental factors which all play a significant role in the skin's colour, condition and tone.

BODY FACT

The skin's capacity to retain water decreases with age, making the ageing skin more vulnerable to dehydration and wrinkles.

Hair
Pain receptor
Touch receptor
(Meissner's corpuscle)
Capillary network
Sebaceous gland
Erector pili muscle
Heat receptor
(Ruffini endings)
Hair follicle
Cold receptor
(Krause corpuscle)
Motor nerve
Hair bulb
Vein
Artery
Nerve endings
Subcutaneous fat

Epidermis
Dermis
Subcutaneous layer

Subdermal
muscle layer
Deep
fascia
Sweat (eccrine)
gland
Pacinian corpuscle
(pressure receptor)

Fig 2.1 Structure of the skin

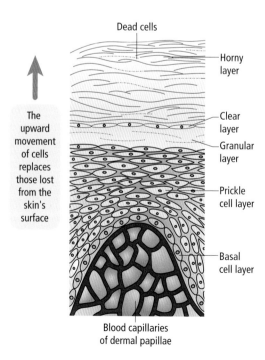

Dead cells
Horny layer
Clear layer
Granular layer
Prickle cell layer
Basal cell layer

The upward movement of cells replaces those lost from the skin's surface

Blood capillaries
of dermal papillae

Fig 2.2 Layers of the epidermis

Functions of the epidermis

The epidermis has three primary functions:

- protecting the body from the external environment, particularly the sun
- preventing excessive water loss from the body
- protecting the body from infection.

The basal cell layer (stratum germinativum)

This is the deepest of the five layers and therefore lies at the base of the epidermis. It consists of a single layer of column cells on a basement membrane, which separates the epidermis from the dermis. This layer of the epidermis is concerned with **cell regeneration**. The basal cells within this layer are constantly reproducing, producing new cells that constantly divide. As new cells are formed by division, they push adjacent cells towards the skin's surface.

Approximately 95 per cent of the cells within the epidermis are **keratinocytes**, which produce a protein substance called **keratin**. Keratin is what makes the epidermal cells more resilient and protective as they are pushed towards the skin's surface.

At intervals between the column cells, which divide to reproduce, are the large star-shaped cells called **melanocytes**, which form the pigment **melanin**, the skin's main colouring agent. This layer also contains tactile **(Merkel) discs** that are sensitive to touch.

Prickle cell layer (stratum spinosum)

This is the thickest layer of the epidermis. It is known as the prickle cell layer because each of the rounded cells contained within it has short projections which make contact with the neighbouring cells and give them a prickly appearance. The tiny hair-like structures on the prickle cells will eventually become **desmosomes**, which are small disc-shape attachments that provide strength and integrity by holding the upper level of epidermal cells together.

The cells of this layer are living and are therefore capable of dividing by the process mitosis.

The cells of this layer make special fats called **sphingolipids**, and when these cells reach the top layer (horny layer), these lipids play an important role in the retention of moisture in the skin.

It is in the prickle cell layer that the keratinocyte has a major role to play in skin barrier defence. Keratinisation refers to the process that skin cells undergo when they change from living cells with a nucleus to dead cells without a nucleus. The keratinisation process is well under way in the upper cells of this layer as the cells migrate upwards.

This layer also includes **Langerhan cells**, which set up an immune response to foreign bodies. These special defence cells are spread out among the keratinocytes and their role is to mop up invading foreign bodies that have found their way into the body and transport them to specialised white blood cells where they are neutralised.

Granular layer (stratum granulosum)

This layer consists of distinctly shaped cells that resemble granules, which are filled with keratin and produce **intercellular lipids** (the substances that

IN PRACTICE

The intercellular lipids in between the epidermal cells are responsible for hydration, epidermal firmness and smoothness. They protect against transepidermal water loss, which can result in dehydration. They also provide protection against any offending or injuring substances invading the skin.

One very important group of these lipids is **ceramides**, which are also contained within the ingredients of some skin-care products.

It is important to recognise that the cell renewal process is responsible for the production of these essential lipids, and if the cell cycle slows down, the production of lipids slows down and results in dryness and dehydration.

fill the spaces between the upper epidermal cells) from structures called **lamellar bodies**.

These lipids help form a strong cement-like structure to prevent the absorption of harmful substances by the skin and help to maintain hydration of the lower layers. The cells of this layer ultimately create an appearance of a wall of bricks (cells) and mortar (lipids).

As the cells move into the granular layer, a number of changes occur to the keratinocyte. The keratinocyte becomes less flexible, more granular in appearance, and the keratin within the cell has become completely hardened, thereby completing the keratinisation process.

As the cells move further up into the granular layer, further changes to the keratinocyte occur. The **desmosomes** begin to dissolve, preparing the **corneocyte** (dead skin cell) for **desquamation**, the process in which the outer layer of dead cells is continually being shed.

Clear layer (stratum lucidum)

This layer consists of transparent cells which permit light to pass through. The cells in the clear layer are filled with a substance called **eleidin**, which is produced from **keratohyalin** and is involved in the keratinisation process.

This layer is considered to be an important transitional stage in the development of the top layer of the epidermis (the horny layer). The keratinocyte has almost reached its final destination by the time it reaches this layer; during its upward movement it has gone through a process of change, which eventually will result in the formation of dead skin cells, known as **corneocytes**. Keratinisation is therefore complete by the time cells have reached the clear layer.

The clear layer is very shallow in facial skin, but thick on the soles of the feet and the palms of the hands, and is generally absent in hairy skin.

Horny layer (stratum corneum)

This is the most superficial outer layer, consisting of dead, flattened keratinocytes, now known as **corneocytes**. The horny layer is thought of as a permeability barrier, as the cells of this layer form a waterproof covering for the skin and help to prevent the penetration of bacteria.

The horny layer is the end result of the change that occurs when new live cells are produced in the basal layer, then pushed upwards by newer cells until they reach the surface where they dry out and are sloughed off. The outer layer of dead cells is continually being shed through desquamation.

Life span of the epidermal cells

In normal skin, it takes approximately 28–30 days for a cell produced by the basal layer to move through the epidermis to the surface. The rate of regeneration is partly determined by the rate at which the outer layer is being desquamated. With age this process is greatly reduced and by the age of 50, it is said to take about 37 days to complete the same process.

When the cells of the horny layer are lost quickly (for instance due to skin injury or sunburn), the process speeds up as the cells are replaced more

IN PRACTICE

The horny layer of the epidermis is an important layer in relation to understanding skin problems, as it is the part of the skin that is directly affected by the external environment. It also plays a key role in helping to contain moisture in the rest of the skin and in regulating the natural moisture flow out from the deeper layers to be lost eventually in evaporation from the skin surface. This natural moisture flow is known as **transepidermal water loss (TEWL)**.

Without adequate retained moisture, skin can become dry and unhealthy.

Under normal conditions, up to 15 per cent of the horny layer consists of water, which is vital to enable the stratum corneum to work. The natural functions of the skin do not work as efficiently when the horny layer contains less than 10 per cent of water and it becomes dry.

quickly from below. Removing the outer layers of the skin with a chemical peel will also speed up replacement.

Summary of the journey of cell regeneration through the epidermal layers

Epidermal layer	Significance
Horny layer	Keratinocytes become corneocytes (dead skin cells) and are subject to desquamation
Clear layer	Important transitional stage in the development of the horny layer Keratinisation is complete by the time cells have reached the clear layer
Granular layer	Keratinocytes becomes less flexible, more granular in appearance and hardened, thereby completing the keratinisation process
Prickle cell layer	The cells of this layer are living and are therefore capable of dividing by the process mitosis The keratinisation process is well under way in the upper cells of this layer as the keratinocytes migrate upwards
Basal cell layer	This layer is concerned with cell regeneration As new cells are formed by division, they push adjacent cells towards the skin's surface

The dermis

The **dermis** lies below the epidermis and is the deeper, thicker layer of the skin. It can be as much as 3 mm thick. The dermis contains several types of tissue that provide a supporting framework to the skin, as well as blood vessels, nerves, hair roots, sweat and sebaceous glands.

The functions of the dermis include:

- providing nourishment to the epidermis
- removing waste products from the epidermis
- giving a supporting framework to the tissues by providing shape and holding all its structures together
- contributing to skin colour.

The dermis has two layers: a superficial **papillary layer** and a deeper **reticular layer**.

The papillary layer

The superficial papillary layer is made up of fatty connective tissue and is connected to the underside of the epidermis by cone-shaped projections called **dermal papillae**, which contain nerve endings and a network of blood and lymphatic capillaries.

The fine network of capillaries in this layer bring oxygen and nutrients to the skin and carry the waste away. The many dermal papillae of the papillary layer form indentations in the overlying epidermis, giving it an irregular or ridged appearance. It is these ridges that leave fingerprints on objects that are handled.

The key function of the papillary layer of the dermis is to provide vital nourishment to the living layers of the epidermis above.

The reticular layer

The deeper reticular layer is formed of tough, fibrous connective tissue which helps to give the skin strength and elasticity and support and hold all structures in place.

The protein **collagen**, which accounts for about 75 per cent of the weight of the dermis and is organised in bundles running horizontally throughout the dermis, is buried in a jelly-like material called the **ground substance**. Collagen is responsible for giving the skin resilience and elasticity.

The collagen bundles are held together by elastic fibres running through the dermis. These are made of a protein called **elastin** that makes up less than 5 per cent of the weight of the skin.

The protein **elastin** contributes to the elasticity of the skin due to the fact that it helps holds the collagen fibres together. Both collagen and elastin fibres are made by cells called **fibroblasts**, which are found throughout the dermis.

An important substance that forms part of the tissue that surrounds the collagen and elastin fibres is **hyaluronic acid**. This special substance has the ability to attract and bind hundreds of times its weight in water. In this way it acts as a natural moisturising ingredient for maintaining moisture and for plumping the skin's tissues.

Special substances found in the ground substance of the dermis are the **glycoproteins**, which are capable of holding large amounts of water and are necessary for maintaining an accumulation of water in the dermis.

In addition to fibroblasts, other cells present in the dermis include:

- **mast** cells, which secrete histamine (involved in allergies), causing dilation of blood vessels to bring blood to the area
- **phagocytic** cells (**macrophages**), which are white blood cells that are able to travel around the dermis destroying foreign matter and bacteria.

Blood supply

Unlike the epidermis, the dermis has an abundant supply of blood vessels which run through the dermis and the subcutaneous layer. Arteries carry oxygenated blood to the skin via arterioles and these enter the dermis from

BODY FACT

Damage to collagen and elastin fibres as they break down is the primary cause of ageing and wrinkles. Also the amount of hyaluronic acid and glycoproteins produced in the skin decreases. Hence the skin becomes less resilient and loses elasticity.

below and branch into a network of capillaries around active or growing structures. These **capillary networks** form in the dermal papillae to provide the basal cell layer of the epidermis with food and oxygen. They also surround the sweat glands and erector pili muscles, two appendages of the skin.

The capillary networks drain into venules, small veins which carry the deoxygenated blood away from the skin and remove waste products. The dermis is therefore well supplied with capillary blood vessels to bring nutrients and oxygen to the germinating cells in the basal cell layer of the epidermis and to remove waste products from them.

Lymphatic vessels

There are numerous lymphatic vessels in the dermis. They form a network in the dermis, facilitating the removal of waste from the skin's tissue. The lymphatic vessels in the skin generally follow the course of veins and are found around the dermal papillae, glands and hair follicles.

Nerves

Nerves are widely distributed throughout the dermis. Most nerves in the skin are **sensory**, sending signals to the brain, and are sensitive to heat, cold, pain, pressure and touch. Branched nerve endings, which lie in the papillary layer and hair root, respond to touch and temperature changes. Nerve endings in the dermal papillae are sensitive to gentle pressure and those in the reticular layer are responsive to deep pressure.

Sensory nerves

There are at least five different types of sensory nerve endings in the skin:

- sensory
- pain
- touch
- temperature
- pressure.

The sensory nerve endings are also called receptors because they are part of the nervous system at which information is received.

Touch receptors

These receptors are located immediately below the epidermis. They are stimulated by light pressure on the skin, which enables a person to distinguish between different textures such as rough, smooth, hard and soft.

Pressure receptors

These receptors are situated beneath the dermis and are stimulated by heavy pressure.

Pain receptors

These receptors consist of branched nerve endings in the epidermis and dermis. They are quite evenly distributed throughout the skin and are important in that they provide a warning signal of damage or injury in the body.

Temperature receptors

There are separate hot and cold receptors in the skin that are stimulated by sudden changes in temperature. The dermis also has **motor nerve endings**, which relay impulses from the brain and are responsible for the dilation and constriction of blood vessels, the secretion of perspiration from the sweat glands and the contraction of the erector pili muscles attached to hair follicles.

The subcutaneous layer

This is a thick layer of connective tissue found below the dermis. The type of tissue found in this layer (fatty tissue) helps support delicate structures such as blood vessels and nerve endings. It also cushions the dermis from underlying tissues such as muscles and bones.

The subcutaneous layer contains the same collagen and elastin fibres as the dermis and contains the major arteries and veins which supply the skin and form a network throughout the dermis. The fat cells contained within this layer help to insulate the body by reducing heat loss.

Below the subcutaneous layer lies the subdermal muscle layer.

Appendages of the skin

The appendages are accessory structures that lie in the dermis of the skin and project onto the surface through the epidermis. These include the **hair**, **erector pili muscle**, **sweat** and **sebaceous glands** and the **nail**.

Hair is an important appendage of the skin which grows from a sac-like depression in the epidermis called a hair follicle. Hair grows all over the body, with the exception of the palms of the hands and the soles of the feet, and is a sexual characteristic.

One of the primary functions of hair is physical protection. The eyelashes act as a line of defence by preventing the entry of foreign particles into the eyes and helping shade the eyes from the sun's rays. Eyebrow hairs help to divert water and other chemical substances away from the eyes. Hairs lining the ears and the nose trap dust and help to prevent bacteria from entering the body. Body hair acts as a protective barrier against the sun and helps to protect us against the cold with the help of the erector pili muscle.

Another function is preventing friction. Underarm and pubic hair protects the skin and cushions against friction caused by movement.

The structure of a hair

The hair is composed mainly of the protein keratin and therefore is a dead structure. Longitudinally, the hair is divided into three parts:

- **hair shaft** – the part of the hair lying above the surface of the skin
- **hair root** – the part found below the surface of the skin
- **hair bulb** – the enlarged part at the base of the hair root.

Internally, the hair has three layers which all develop from the matrix (the active, growing part of the hair).

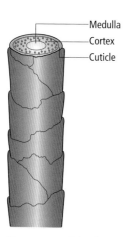

- Medulla
- Cortex
- Cuticle

Fig 2.3 Structure of the hair

> ### KEY FACT
>
> As we grow older, the amount of fat starts to decrease in the subcutaneous layer and eventually results in a bonier look to the facial contours.

Hair layer	Location	Description	Function
Cuticle	Outer layer	Made up of transparent protective scales which overlap one another	Protects the cortex and gives the hair its elasticity
Cortex	Middle layer	Made up of tightly packed keratinised cells containing the pigment melanin, which gives the hair its colour	Helps to give strength to the hair
Medulla	Inner layer	Made up of loosely connected keratinised cells and tiny air spaces	Determines the sheen and colour of hair due to the reflection of light through the air spaces

Hair colour is due to the presence of melanin in the cortex and medulla of the hair shaft. In addition to the standard black colour, the melanocytes in the hair bulb produce two colour variations of melanin: brown and yellow. Blond, light-coloured and red hair has a high proportion of the yellow variant. Brown and black hair possesses more of the brown and black melanin.

The structure of a hair in its follicle

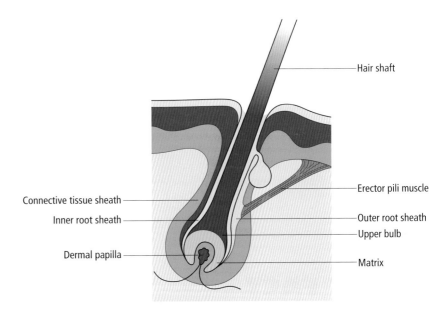

Fig 2.4 A hair in its follicle

The individual parts of a hair's structure are shown below.

Structure	Location	Function
Connective tissue sheath	Surrounds hair follicle and sebaceous gland	Supplies follicle with nerves and blood. Main source of sustenance for the follicle
Outer root sheath	Forms the follicle wall and is continuous with the basal cell layer of the epidermis	Provides a permanent source of growing cells (hair germ cells) to enable the follicle to grow and renew cells during its life cycle
Dermal papilla	Elevation at the base of the hair bulb, which contains a rich blood supply	Crucial source of nourishment for hair, providing the hair cells with food and oxygen

(Continued)

Structure	Location	Function
Inner root sheath	Originates from the dermal papilla at the base of the follicle and grows upwards with the hair (it ceases to grow when level with the sebaceous gland)	Shapes and contours the hair, helping to anchor it into the follicle
Hair bulb	Enlarged part at the base of the hair root	Area where the cells grow and divide by the process of mitosis
Matrix	Lower part of the hair bulb	Area of mitotic activity of the hair cells

Types of hair

There are three main types of hair in the body: **lanugo**, **vellus** and **terminal** hair.

Type of hair	Description	Where found in body
Lanugo	Fine, soft hair; often unpigmented	Found on a foetus; grows from around the third to the fifth month of pregnancy and is eventually shed to be replaced by secondary vellus hairs, around the seventh to eight month of the pregnancy
Vellus	Soft, downy hair; often unpigmented and does not have a medulla or a well-developed bulb Lies close to the surface of the skin and therefore has a shallow follicle	Found all over the face and body, except for the palms of the hands, soles of the feet, eyelids and lips
Terminal	Longer, coarser hairs, most are pigmented They vary greatly in shape, diameter, length, colour and texture They are deeply seated in the dermis and have well-defined bulbs	Found on the scalp, under the arms, eyebrows, pubic regions, arms and legs

BODY FACT

If stimulated by an increase in blood circulation resulting from hormonal changes in the body (such as puberty, pregnancy or menopause) or medication, the shallow follicle of a vellus hair can grow downwards to become a coarse, dark terminal hair.

Facts about hair growth

- Hair begins to form in the foetus from the third month of pregnancy.
- The growth of hair originates from the matrix, which is the active growing area where cells divide and reproduce by mitosis.
- Living cells, which are produced in the matrix, are pushed upwards away from their source of nutrition, die and are converted to keratin to produce a hair.
- Hair has a growth pattern which ranges from approximately 4–5 months for an eyelash hair to approximately 4–7 years for a scalp hair.
- Hair growth is affected by illness, diet and hormonal influences.

The growth cycle of a hair

Each hair has its own growth cycle and undergoes three distinct stages of development: **anagen, catagen** and **telogen**.

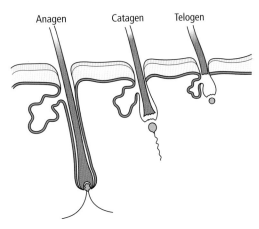

Fig 2.5 The hair growth cycle

Anagen
- Active growing stage.
- Lasts from a few months to several years.
- Hair germ cells reproduce at matrix.
- New follicle is produced which extends in depth and width.
- The hair cells pass upwards to form hair bulb.
- Hair cells continue rising up the follicle and as they pass through the bulb they differentiate to form individual structures of hair.
- Inner root sheath grows up with the hair, anchoring it into the follicle.
- When cells reach the upper part of bulb they become keratinised.
- Two-thirds of its way up the follicle, the hair leaves an inner root sheath and emerges onto surface of skin.

Catagen
- Lasts approximately 2–4 weeks.
- Transitional stage from active to resting.
- Hair separates from dermal papilla and moves slowly up the follicle.
- Follicle below retreating hair shrinks.
- Hair rises to just below level of sebaceous gland where the inner root sheath dissolves and the hair can be brushed out.

Telogen
- Short resting stage.
- Shortened follicle rests until stimulated once more.
- Hair is shed onto skin's surface.
- New replacement hair begins to grow.

Different types of hair growth

As there is a continuous cycle of hair growth, the amount of hair on the body remains fairly constant. However, hair growth will vary from client to client and from area to area. A new client coming to the salon for a hair removal treatment should be made aware of the fact that hair growth occurs in three stages which will result in the hair being at different lengths both above the skin and below it.

IN PRACTICE

While carrying out hair removal treatments, it is important to remember that the hair follicle is part of the skin's structure, therefore any treatment which affects the hair is also going to affect the skin. Once a hair has been removed, the maximum amount of blood will be sent straight to the area being treated to heal and protect the skin. This is a normal reaction of the skin and extra blood that has been sent to the treated area will soon be diverted again within a few hours of treatment. As the treated area of skin will have open follicles, it is vital that a client adheres strictly to after-care advice specified as open follicles offer bacteria an easy entry into the body.

Erector pili muscle

This is a small, smooth weak muscle made up of sensory fibres. It is attached at an angle to the base of a hair follicle which serves to make the hair stand erect in response to cold, or when experiencing emotions such as fright and anxiety.

Sweat glands

There are two types of sweat glands in the skin: **eccrine** and **apocrine**. The majority are **eccrine** glands which are simple coiled tubular glands that open directly onto the surface of the skin. There are several million of them distributed over the surface of the skin, although they are most numerous in the palms of the hands and the soles of the feet.

Their function is to regulate body temperature and help eliminate waste products. Their active secretion sweat is under the control of the sympathetic nervous system. Heat-induced sweating tends to begin on the forehead and then spreads to the rest of the body. Emotionally induced sweating, stimulated by fright, embarrassment or anxiety, begins on the palms of the hands and in the axilla and then spreads to the rest of the body.

Apocrine glands are connected with hair follicles and are found only in the genital and underarm regions. They produce a fatty secretion and breakdown of the secretion by bacteria leads to body odour.

Sebaceous glands

These glands are small sac-like pouches found all over the body, except for the soles of the feet and the palms of the hands. They are more numerous on the scalp, face, chest and back. Sebaceous glands commonly open into a hair follicle but some open onto the skin surface. They produce an oily substance called **sebum**, which contains fats, cholesterol and cellular debris.

Sebum is mildly antibacterial and antifungal and coats the surface of the skin and the hair shafts where it prevents excess water loss, lubricates and softens the horny layer of the epidermis, and softens the hair. The secretion of sebum is stimulated by the release of hormones, primarily androgens.

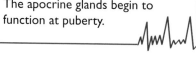

BODY FACT

The apocrine glands begin to function at puberty.

Student activity

Now complete Activity 2.1 in the resources for this book on Dynamic Learning Online.

The nail

The nail is an important appendage of the skin and is an extension of the stratum lucidum (clear layer) of the epidermis. It is composed of horny flattened cells which undergo a process of keratinisation, giving the nail a hard appearance. It is the protein keratin which helps to make the nail a strong but flexible structure. The part of the nail the eye can see is dead as it has no direct supply of blood, lymph and nerves. All nutrients are supplied to the nail via the dermis.

Functions of the nail

The nail has several important functions:

- It forms a protective covering at the ends of the phalangeal joints of the fingers and the toes, helping to support the delicate network of blood vessels and nerves at the end of the fingers.
- It is a useful tool enabling us to touch, manipulate small objects and scratch surfaces.

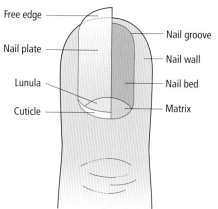

Free edge

Nail plate

Lunula

Cuticle

Nail groove

Nail wall

Nail bed

Matrix

Fig 2.6 Cross-section of a nail

The structure of the nail

The nail has several important anatomical regions.

Structure	Location	Function
Nail matrix	Situated immediately below the cuticle	The nail's most important feature. It is the area where the living cells are produced; receives a rich supply of blood which supplies oxygen to the nail and is vital to the production of new cells Area from which the health of the nail is determined
Nail bed	Immediately below the nail plate; is a continuation of the matrix part of the skin upon which the nail plate rests	Provides nourishment and protection for the nail Is richly supplied with blood vessels, lymph vessels and nerves from the underlying dermis
Cuticle	A fold of overlapping skin that surrounds the base of the nail	Protects the matrix and provides a protective seal against bacteria
Lunula	Light-coloured semicircular area of the nail, commonly called the half moon, that lies in between the matrix and the nail plate	Area of the nail where cells start to harden; the cells here are in a transitional stage (between hard and soft) Is a bridge between the living cells of the matrix and the dead cells of the nail plate
Nail plate	Main visible part of the nail which rests on the nail bed and ends at the free edge	Offers protection for the nail bed
Nail wall	The folds of skin overlapping the sides of the nails	Protects the edges of the nail plate from external damage
Nail groove	Deep ridges under the sides of the nail	Guides the growth of the nail up the fingers/toes, helping the nail to grow straight
Free edge	Part of the nail plate that extends beyond the nail bed	The part of the nail that is filed

The process of nail growth

BODY FACT

There are different names given to the different areas of the cuticle:
- The eponychium is the dead cuticle that adheres to the base of the nail, near the lanula.
- The peronychium is the cuticle that outlines the nail plate.
- The hyponychium is the cuticle skin found under the free edge of the nail.

Nail growth occurs from the nail matrix by cell division
As new cells are produced in the matrix, older cells are pushed forward and are hardened by the process of keratinisation, which forms the hardened nail plate
As the nail grows it moves along the nail grooves at the sides of the nail, which helps to direct the nail growth along the nail bed
It takes approximately six months for cells to travel from the lanula to the free edge of the nail
The growth of a nail does not follow a growth cycle and hence growth is continuous throughout life
The average growth rate of a nail is approximately 3 mm per month

Essential facts about nails

- Nails start growing on a foetus before the fourth month of pregnancy.
- The growth rate of nails will vary from person to person and from finger to finger, with the index finger generally being the fastest to grow.
- Toe nails have a slower rate of growth than fingernails.
- The rate of growth of a nail is faster in the summer due to an increase in cell division as a result of exposure to ultraviolet radiation.
- A good blood supply is essential to nail growth; oxygen and nutrients are fed to the living cells of the nail matrix and nail bed.
- Protein and calcium are good sources of nourishment for the nails.

Nail growth may be affected by the following factors:

- **Ill-health** – during illness the body receives a reduced blood supply to the nails as it attempts to restore the rest of the body to good health.
- **Diet** – a nutritional deficiency can result in a diminished blood supply to the nail.
- **Age** – during ageing the growth of a nail slows down due to the fact that the blood vessels supplying the matrix and the nail become less efficient.
- **Poor technique** – if a heavy pressure is used when using manicure implements such as a cuticle knife, damage may be caused to the matrix cells resulting in ridges to the nail. This may only be temporary as new cells produced in the matrix will replace the damaged ones, and depending on the extent of the damage the ridges may eventually grow out.
- **An accident** – such as shutting a finger in the door. This may result in bruising and bleeding of the nail or even the complete removal of a nail. It could result in permanent malformation of the nail if the nail bed has become damaged.

Nail diseases and nail disorders

Diseases of the nail are as a direct result of bacteria, fungi, parasites or viruses attacking the nail or surrounding tissues. Nail disorders may be caused by illness, physical and chemical damage, by general neglect or by poor manicuring techniques. Nail disorders do not contra-indicate manicure or pedicure treatments. However, nail diseases do as they may cause cross-infection.

A therapist must be able to recognise diseases and disorders so that the correct treatment or advice may be given.

Common nail diseases

Paronychia

Inflammation of the skin surrounding the nail. The tissues may be swollen and pus may be present which can develop into an abscess. It is a common condition on the fingers and is caused by bacterial or viral infection.

Initially, the cause may be due to prolonged immersion of the hands in water, poor manicure techniques, picking the cuticle or the nail wall separating from the nail. Infection with the herpes simplex virus can give rise to a whitlow, an abscess that forms around the nail.

Paronychia

Onychomycosis

This is a term given to fungal infections of the nail, commonly called Ringworm. It attacks the nail bed and nail plate, and presents as white or yellow scaly deposits at the free edge, which may spread down to invade the nail walls or bed. The nails become thickened, brittle, opaque or discoloured. The nail plate will appear spongy and furrowed.

In its advanced stages, the nail plate may separate from the nail bed (a condition known as onycholysis (see below). There may also be accompanying dryness and skin scaling at the base of the fingers and on the palms.

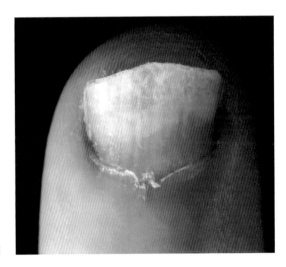

Ringworm of the nail

Onychia

This is a generic term used to describe any disease of the nail but more specifically refers to inflammation of the nail bed. In this condition the nail matrix appears red. There may be swelling, tenderness and pus formation. This could lead to the nail being shed. This condition may be caused by wearing false nails for too long or by harsh manicuring, chemical applications or by a variety of infections or physical damage.

Onycholysis

This is separation or loosening of part or all of a nail from its bed. It may be due to disease, physical damage or may occur spontaneously without any apparent cause. It can occur if sharp instruments are used under the free edge. Penetration of the flesh line allows bacteria or other infection to enter the nail bed.

Nail disorders

Leuconychia

This is a term given to white or colourless nails, or nails with white spots, streaks or bands. There may also be evidence of ridging. It may be caused as a result of injury to the matrix or the effects of disease. The white spots will usually disappear as the nail grows.

Leuconychia

Onychophagy

This is the technical term for nail biting in which the free edge, nail plate and cuticle are bitten to leave the hyponychium exposed and the cuticle and surrounding skin ragged, inflamed and sore. Nail biting is usually a nervous or stress-induced habit.

Nail ridges/corrugations

Ridges in the nail may occur due to irregular formation of the nail or to physical/chemical injury of the nail matrix. Ridges may be vertical which are common in healthy nails due to uneven development of the nail tissue, poor manicuring techniques or the effects of harsh chemicals. Ridges may also be horizontal and can be indicative of abnormal nail growth, a symptom of body malfunction or disease. Deep horizontal lines are often associated with illness.

Hang nail

A hang nail is a small strip of skin that hangs loosely at the side of the nail, or a small portion of the nail itself splitting away. A hang nail may develop due to dry, torn or split cuticles. Common causes are hands being immersed in water for long periods, cutting the nails too close, digging the cuticles, improper filing or the effects of detergents and other chemicals.

Onychogryphosis

This is a term given to an ingrown fingernail or toe nail. The first signs are inflammation, followed by tenderness, swelling and pain. Infection may aggravate the condition. It is caused by ill-fitting shoes, cutting or filing nails too short or too close to the skin. It may also be due to a malformation of the nail when it was beginning to grow.

Pterygium

This is a condition where the cuticle becomes over-grown and excessive and grows forward. The cuticle at the base of the nail becomes dry and split and grows forward sticking to the nail plate. Pterygium may be due to faulty nail care or lack of nail care.

Koilonychia

This is the term given to concave spoon-shaped nails. In this condition the nails are thin, soft and hollowed. Koilonychia may be congenital or it may be due to lack of iron or other minerals. The spoon shape results from abnormal growth at the nail matrix.

Eggshell nails

This is a term given to thin, white nails that are more flexible than normal. In this condition the nail separates from the nail bed and curves at the free edges. The condition may be associated with illness.

Onychorrhexis

This is the term given to dry, brittle nails. In this condition the nail loses its moisture, becomes dry and the free edge splits. The nails may peel into layers very easily. There may be transverse or longitudinal splitting of the nail plate and inflammation, tenderness, pain, swelling and infection may be present. Frequent immersion in water and contact with detergents and chemicals contribute to this condition. It may also indicate an iron deficiency, anaemia, or incorrect filing, which causes the nail plate to split.

Factors affecting the skin

There are many factors, both external and internal, which affect a client's skin.

Internal factors affecting the skin

Age

The natural process of ageing naturally affects the skin, as cell regeneration starts to decrease with age (see chart on page 55 for information on the effects of ageing).

Free radicals

These also contribute to skin ageing. Free radicals are parts of molecules (e.g. oxygen molecules) that are found in the body. As a result of external factors, like ultraviolet radiation, nicotine or unhealthy food, the free radicals become prone to react. This means that they are constantly looking for other chemical substances to bond with. Hence, they attack the collagen fibres, cellular membrane and lipid layer of the skin. Free radicals change the inherited properties stored in the cell nucleus, so that the quality of newly formed skin cells deteriorates.

Stress and lifestyle

When the body is subjected to regular stress and tension it can cause sensitivity and allergies in the skin as well as encourage the formation of lines around the eyes and the mouth.

Hormones

The natural glandular changes of the body have an effect on the condition of the skin throughout life. During puberty, the sex hormones stimulate the sebaceous glands, which may cause some imbalance in the skin.

BODY FACT

The body protects itself against these aggressors through **antioxidant enzyme systems** (antioxidants). But from the age of 20 onwards, these natural defence mechanisms gradually decline, so that the skin can no longer defend itself. Therefore, one of the basic ideas of modern anti-ageing therapy consists of making up for the deficiencies in hormones and antioxidants caused by advanced ageing, i.e. by supplying the body with the appropriate hormone and vitamin supplements.

At the onset of menstruation the skin may erupt due to the adjustment of hormone levels at that time. During pregnancy, pigmentation changes may occur, but usually disappear after birth. During the menopause the activity of the sebaceous glands is reduced and the skin becomes drier.

Smoking

The effects of smoking have been linked to premature ageing and wrinkling of the skin. Nicotine weakens the blood vessels which supply blood to the tissues; this deprives the tissues of essential oxygen and therefore the skin may appear dull and grey in colour.

Smoking affects the skin's cells and destroys vitamins B and C, which are important for healthy skin. Smoking dulls the skin by polluting the pores and increases the formation of lines around the eyes and the mouth.

Medication

Medication can affect the skin by causing dehydration, or sensitivity and/or allergies.

Diet

A healthy body is needed for a healthy skin. The skin can be thought of as a barometer of the body's general health.

- **Vitamin A:** helps repair the body's tissues and helps prevent dryness and ageing.
- **Vitamin B:** helps improve the circulation and the skin's colour and is essential to cellular oxidation.
- **Vitamin C:** is essential for healing and to maintain levels of collagen in the skin.
- **Vitamin E:** helps to heal damaged tissues and can help heal structural damage to the skin.

Water consumption

The skin is approximately 70 per cent water. Drinking an adequate amount of water (approximately 6–8 glasses per day) aids the digestive system and helps to prevent a build-up of toxicity in the skin's tissues.

Alcohol

Alcohol has a dehydrating effect on the skin by drawing essential water from the tissues. Excess consumption causes the blood vessels in the skin to dilate, resulting in a flushed appearance.

Exercise

Regular exercise promotes good circulation, increased oxygen intake and blood flow to the skin.

Sleep

Sleep is essential to physical and emotional well-being and is one of the most effective regenerators for the skin.

External factors affecting the skin

Photoageing

Photoageing is the process by which the skin undergoes accelerated ageing after ultraviolet exposure. The sun and its ultraviolet rays are therefore one of the most dominant factors in how the skin ages.

As we age naturally, the collagen and elastin fibres in the dermis weaken. This natural occurrence is accelerated upon frequent exposure to ultraviolet rays, as exposure to the rays weakens the skin's collagen and elastin fibres, which causes wrinkling and sagging of the tissues.

It is important to note that tanning machines/sunbeds can also cause accelerated ageing of the skin due to the fact that they produce large quantities of longwave ultraviolet light (UVA). Over-exposure may lead to the same risks as with over-exposure to natural sunlight, i.e. sagging and wrinkling, and to an increased risk of some skin cancers.

Environmental exposure

Exposure to adverse weather conditions, pollutants or poor air quality can affect the condition of the skin, often resulting in dryness and dehydration.

Occupation

The client's occupation could be a factor involved in their skin condition. For instance, they could be working in a hot or humid environment, or in dusty and dirty conditions.

Poor care

Lack of, or incorrect, skin care can be a major factor affecting the skin. The use of products that are too aggressive can strip the skin and effectively damage the barrier function of the skin. The correct use of sunscreens can provide the best protection against premature ageing.

Skin types and their characteristics

When talking of skin types, the classifications are predetermined by genetics and ethnicity. DNA is carried in chromosomes and is the factor that programs and influences skin characteristics such as follicle size, skin thickness, circulation and nerve endings.

The primary factors in determining skin types are:

- level of lipid (fat) secretions produced between the skin cells (this determines how well the skin retains moisture)
- the amount of secretion produced by the sebaceous glands.

Skin types are generally broadly classified and they are often streamlined in the skin care industry to allow clearer marketing of product lines. Skin is generally classified into five main types:

1 normal
2 dry
3 oily
4 combination
5 sensitive.

1 Normal skin

Few clients will have normal skin, as this skin type is very rare indeed. Normal skin is balanced in that it has a good oil and water balance. The best example of normal skin is in children from birth up until puberty.

Distinguishing features:

- The skin is neither too dry nor too oily and therefore has perfect hydration.
- To the touch the skin should be soft and supple.
- There should be a smooth texture which is neither too thick nor too thin.
- The skin should feel slightly warm as it has a good blood supply.
- The skin should be a creamy, pink colour with a clear, even surface free from blemishes (see discussion of ethnic skin types, page 56).
- The pores should be fine and virtually non-apparent.
- The skin should feel firm to the touch and generally have good elasticity.

When questioned, the client will usually report that they have very few problems with their skin.

IN PRACTICE

The aim in treating a normal skin type is to maintain the skin's balance and protect it from damage.

2 Dry skin

A dry skin is so called because it is either lacking in sebum or moisture, or both. It develops as a result of under-activity of the sebaceous glands.

The skin's natural oil, sebum, lubricates the corneum layer and in the absence of this oily coating the dead cells start to curl up and flake. The sebum coating also helps to prevent moisture loss by evaporation. Therefore, due to a lack of sebum, dry skin has difficulty retaining inner moisture.

Although dry skin is hereditary, it can also develop as a result of the ageing process.

Distinguishing features:

- The skin looks dry, often parched.
- To the touch the skin will feel papery and even a little coarse.
- The texture will appear thin and coarse and there may be patches of flaking skin.
- The skin often takes on the appearance of 'parchment' and is often sensitive and prone to the formation of dilated capillaries and milia around the eye and upper cheek area.
- Due to the dryness this type of skin tends to age prematurely, with fine lines becoming evident around the eyes even as soon as in the early to mid 20s.
- The pores are small and tight due to the lack of sebum production.
- The skin does not usually have good elasticity.

When questioned, the client will usually report that their skin feels tight and dry. They may also complain of sensitivity and premature ageing.

IN PRACTICE

The primary aim in treating dry skin is to help to balance the moisture and oil of the skin, soften the texture of the skin, hydrate and moisturise. Dry skin also needs a lot of sun protection.

3 Oily skin

Oily skin is hereditary and develops due to an over-production of sebum from the sebaceous glands.

IN PRACTICE

The aim in the treatment of an oily skin is to help balance it by bringing the oil secretions under control through thorough cleansing and exfoliation. It is still important to protect oily skin by moisturising the surface with a water-based hydrating product designed for oily skin.

There is always a tendency for clients to over-treat their skin if it is oily. However, this can compound the problem as excessive stimulation will result in stripping and irritating the skin, making it become dry and unbalanced. The skin's natural protection mechanism will then respond by producing more oil.

Distinguishing features:

- The pores are large and noticeable due to a build-up of sebum, causing them to stretch open.
- The skin appears oily; a characteristic shine is often apparent, especially down the T-zone.
- To the touch the skin feels thick and coarse.
- The texture is usually uneven.
- The skin is sallow in colour as a result of excess sebum production and dead corneum cells being permitted to build up on the outer surface.
- Blemishes are often very apparent, with blocked pores, comedones, papules and pustules all being present to a greater or lesser degree. Often some scarring is evident from previous blemish sites, which lead to a very uneven surface colour.
- The skin usually feels firm to the touch and an oily skin ages least prematurely. The elasticity is generally good.

When questioned, the client will usually report that their skin develops a 'shine' during the course of a day and make-up runs or 'slips', and maybe a foundation changes to a more orange colour. They will probably complain that their skin often feels thick and dirty, due to the accumulation of sebum and dead cells clogging the surface. They will also suffer with blemishes.

4 Combination skin

This is actually the most common skin type classification. As its name suggests, this skin is a bit of a mixture. Typically the T-zone (central area of the face corresponding to the forehead, nose and chin) is oily and the cheeks and neck are dry/normal. Combination skin can therefore be both dry and oily at the same time.

Distinguishing features:

- The skin is dry on the cheeks and neck and oily on the T-zone.
- To the touch the skin will probably vary, with the dry areas feeling rough and fine and the oily areas feeling thicker and coarse.
- The skin will have a patchy colour and the T-zone will probably suffer from blemishes, such as blocked pores, comedones, papules and pustules.
- Milia may be present around the dryer skin areas, also some sensitivity and dilated capillaries may be evident.
- The pores should be fine and small on the cheeks and neck but larger in the T-zone.
- The skin's tone and elasticity will vary, being poor in the dry areas but good in the oily areas.

When questioned, the client will usually report that they have all the problems of an oily skin in the T-zone but dryness and tightness on the cheeks, neck and around the eyes.

5 Sensitive skin

While sensitivity is a condition that may affect any skin type, sensitive skin is more commonly referred to in its own classification and therefore most product lines now recognise and market products specifically for this skin type.

Distinguishing features:

- Pink tone, with or without dilated capillaries.
- Thin and translucent appearance.
- Usually feels quite warm to the touch.
- Even after a gentle cleanse the skin may show quite high colouring.
- Prone to dry, flaky patches.
- Easily irritated by products and other external factors such as the elements.
- Reddens easily from any form of stimulation.

When questioned, the client will probably say their skin reacts easily to external stimuli by becoming red and blotchy, and may feel uncomfortable when touched.

NB. Although all skins may be sensitive at times, due to misuse of products, medication or the environment, clients with genetically determined sensitive skins will have an impaired barrier function and reduced lipid protection, making them more susceptible to allergens and irritants. Caution is therefore essential with this skin type when choosing products and suitable forms of treatment.

Male skin

Although there is not specifically a 'male' skin type, it is important to consider the differences in make-up between male and female skins. Firstly, there are hormonal differences between men and women. Testosterone, the male hormone, gives men a thicker epidermis (approximately 2 mm compared with 1.5 mm in women). Male skin does have a tendency to be tougher, more elastic and less sensitive than female skin, although daily shaving can increase the risk of skin rashes, infections and in-growing hairs. It is also more acidic and has a more efficient supply of blood and sebum. This means it tends to age better than women's skin, remaining softer, firmer and more supple.

Ageing of the skin

Like all organs, the skin is affected by the ageing process. In contrast to other organs, changes in the skin become visible over the years. The signs of ageing start to show as early as the end of the second or the beginning of the third decade of a person's life.

The skin's ability to continuously renew itself is affected by ageing. Old skin needs on average twice as long – as much as eight weeks – before it has renewed itself. The antural acidic protective coating changes because the sweat and sebaceous glands no longer exercise their function so efficiently and the skin becomes drier and thinner as it can no longer retain enough moisture and oil.

How ageing affects the skin

Age	Skin ageing characteristics
Childhood	Smooth, healthy and undamaged
Adolescence	Increased sebaceous gland activity, which may result in spots, comedones and pustules and for some may be the start of acne
The 20s	Collagen starts to diminish (approx I per cent per year), start of fine lines and loss of elasticity in skin of upper eyelid
The 30s	Sagging due to stretching of the skin and continued reduction in collagen, more fine lines and wrinkles, loss of hydration, moderate decrease in dermal repair
The 40s	Loss of elasticity more apparent, lines deepen in nasolabial folds, skin sagging at jaw line, forehead wrinkles deepen, noticeable drop in skin hydration levels
Menopause	Loss of of oestrogen accentuates wrinkles and loss of elasticity, slowing of ability to synthesise collagen, lipid production is affected, causing dehydration
The 50s	Wrinkles and loss of elasticity in the neck more apparent, reduction in supporting fat leads to bonier appearance of face, skin tends to be drier
The 60s and beyond	Loss of subcutaneous fat, skin becomes thinner, sagging worsens, dilated capillaries often present, uneven pigmentation, age spots, skin tags, low production of sebum and collagen, compromised dermal repair, many wrinkles and deep lines

Summary of main skin types

Skin type	Main recognition factors	Pore size	Elasticity
Normal	Soft, supple, smooth Free from blemishes	Fine	Good; firm
Dry	Papery, thin, flaky	Small and tight	Generally not good
Oily	Shiny, thick, coarse and uneven Sallow colouring Blocked pores, comedones, papules and pustules may be present	Enlarged	Good; firm
Combination	Dry on cheeks and neck, oily/blemished in T-zone	Variable; enlarged in T-zone and fine and small on cheeks	Poor in dry areas; good in oily areas
Sensitive	Warm to touch, thin, dry and flaky, high colouring, easily irritated	Variable; tend to be small and tight	May be poor in areas of sensitivity

White skin

Ethnic skin types

All ethnic skin types vary in the degree of melanin they produce. Although all ethnic skin types have the same number of melanocytes cells, black skins have melanocytes capable of making large amounts of melanin.

Ethnic skin type	Colouring	Characteristics
White skin (British, Scandinavian, East and West European, North American, South Australian, Canadian, New Zealand origin)	Generally a pale buff; some skins may appear pinkish while others have a sallowish tone	• Relatively small amounts of melanin present in white skins, as melanin is produced to varying degrees • Ages faster than black skins and it is important, therefore, to start protecting the skin from ultraviolet radiation as early as possible • Other types of white skins tan more easily and are far less sensitive, and whilst being pale in the winter, may establish a golden tan easily without burning
Oriental/light Asian skin (Chinese, Japanese or Middle East origin)	Creamy colour with a tendency to yellow and olive tones with more melanin present	• Rarely shows blemishes and defies normal signs of ageing • Scars are more likely to occur and hyper-pigment, causing unevenness, troughs, pits and hollows on the skin's surface

Ethnic skin type	Colouring	Characteristics
Dark Asian skin (Pakistani, Indian, Sri Lankan or Malaysian origin)	Very dark skin colour which is deeply pigmented with melanin	<ul><li>Smooth and supple with minimal signs of ageing</li><li>Sweat glands are larger and more numerous in this skin type, which gives a sheen to the skin that is often mistaken for oiliness</li><li>Deeply pigmented, it does not reveal the blood capillaries</li></ul>
Mediterranean skin (Italian, Spanish, Greek, Portuguese, Yugoslavian, South American or Central American origin)	Looks sallow with some reddish pigment	<ul><li>Good degree of melanin present which obscures the colour of the blood vessels</li><li>Tends to have a generous coating of sebum and is therefore oily</li><li>Tans easily and deeply without burning</li></ul>
Afro-Caribbean/black skin (West Indian/African origin)	Darker with a higher degree of melanin	<ul><li>Open pores</li><li>Oily with higher degree of sebaceous glands</li><li>Thick and tough</li><li>Desquamates easily</li><li>Forms keloid scars when damaged</li><li>More likely to be affected by several different types of disfiguring bumps (see pages 53 and 69, DPN)</li></ul>
Mixed skin	Clients with a mixed skin will usually have a combination of characteristics of all of the above skin types	The shades of colour and characteristics will vary greatly depending on the mix

Oriental/light Asian skin

As black skin is thicker than white skins it is prone to congestion and comedones. Black skin generally ages at a much slower rate than white skin, mainly due to the extra protection afforded by the melanin. A disadvantage to having more melanin is that it makes the skin more 'reactive'. This means that almost any stimulus such as a rash, scratch or inflammation may trigger the production of excess melanin, resulting in dark marks or patches on the skin. This is known as **post-inflammatory hyperpigmentation**.

Occasionally some black skins develop a decrease in melanin, or **post-inflammatory** hypopigmentation in response to skin trauma. In either

Dark Asian skin

Mediterranean skin

Afro Caribbean/black skin

IN PRACTICE

A common example of allergies is with nuts, and in the case of a client with a nut allergy, care would need to be taken to ensure nut-based ingredients (which are common in lots of skin care products) were avoided.

It is possible for a client to develop an allergy to a product after years of use, and although immediate reactions are more likely with skin care products, constant exposure to a particular ingredient or product can also cause the body to develop an allergy.

This can be confusing to a client who may not understand that the product they have been using for years is suddenly responsible for a reaction.

IN PRACTICE

Comedones are a form of skin blockage and may be released manually, and with the use of a comedone extractor.

case (hypo or hyperpigmentation) the light or dark areas may be disfiguring and may take months or years to fade. The increased thickness of the horny layer of the skin in black skins can cause dehydration which leads to increased skin shedding. This can create a grey 'ashen' effect as the loose cells build up on the skin.

General terms associated with the skin

Allergic reaction

This disorder occours when the body becomes hypersensitive to a particular allergen. When irritated by an allergen, the body produces histamine in the skin as part of the body's defence or immune system. The effects of different allergens are diverse and they affect different tissues and organs. For example, certain cosmetics and chemicals can cause rashes and irritation in the skin. Certain allergens such as pollen, fur, feathers, mould and dust can cause asthma and hay fever. If severe, allergies may be extremely serious and result in anaphylactic shock with symptoms in different parts of the body at the same time, including rashes, swelling of the lips and throat, difficulty breathing and a rapid fall in blood pressure and loss of consciousness.

In the case of a client experiencing a rash or severe redness or burning with the use of a product, the appropriate action is immediately to remove all traces of the product from the skin and apply cool, wet compresses to soothe the skin.

It is advisable for the client to discontinue all use of products, preferably including make-up, until the reaction has stopped and all symptoms of the allergy have gone. Then clients may be encouraged to use products on the skin, one by one, each day adding another product to see if the offending product or ingredient may be identified. In the event of a severe allergic reaction, advise the client to seek medical advice.

Comedone

This is a collection of sebum, keratinised cells and waste which accumulate in the entrance of a hair follicle. It may be open or closed. An open comedone is a 'blackhead' contained within the follicle, whereas a closed comedone is a whitehead, trapped underneath the skin's surface.

Open comedones (blackheads) and closed comedones (red raised areas)

Crows feet

These are fine lines around the eyes caused by habitual facial expressions and daily movement. They are associated with ageing of muscle tissue, but premature formation may be due to over-exposure to UV light or eye strain.

Cyst

This is an abnormal sac containing liquid or a semi-solid substance. Most cysts are harmless.

Erythema

This is reddening of the skin due to the dilation of blood capillaries just below the epidermis in the dermis.

Fissure

This is a crack in the epidermis exposing the dermis.

Keloid

A keloid is the over-growth of an existing scar which grows much larger than the original wound. The surface may be smooth, shiny or ridged. The onset is gradual and is due to an accumulation or increase in collagen in the immediate area. The colour varies from red, fading to pink and white.

Lesion

A zone of tissue with impaired function, as a result of damage by disease or wounding is called a lesion.

Macule

A macule is a small, flat patch of increased pigmentation or discolouration such as a freckle.

Milia

Milia is sebum trapped in a blind duct with no surface opening. Usually found around the eye area, they appear as pearly, white and hard nodules under the skin.

IN PRACTICE

Milia may be removed with a sterile microlance.

Milia

Mole

Moles are also known as a pigmented naevi. They appear as round, smooth lumps on the surface of the skin. They may be flat or raised and vary in size and colour from pink to brown or black. They may have hairs growing out of them.

Naevus

This is a mass of dilated capillaries and may be pigmented as in a birthmark.

Papule

Papule is a small raised elevation on the skin, less than 1 cm in diameter which may be a red colour. It often develops into a pustule.

Pustule

This is a small, raised elevation on the skin containing pus.

Skin tag

Small growths of fibrous tissue, which stand up from the skin and sometimes are pigmented (black or brown).

Scar

A scar is a mark left on the skin after a wound has healed. Scars are formed from replacement tissue during the healing of a wound. Depending on the type and extent of damage, the scar may be raised (hypertrophic), rough and pitted (ice pick) or fibrous and lumpy (keloid). Scar tissue may appear smooth and shiny or form a depression in the surface.

IN PRACTICE

Skin tags may be surgically removed or may be cauterised by a qualified electrologist with advanced training. They are not contra-indicated to skin care treatment, although care should be taken to avoid catching them and causing any discomfort.

Skin tag

Telangiecstasis

This is the term for dilated capillaries, where there is persistent vaso-dilation of capillaries in the skin. Usually caused by extremes of temperature and over-stimulation of the tissues, although sensitive and fair skins are more susceptible to this condition.

Tumour

A tumour is formed by an over-growth of cells. Almost every type of cell in the epidermis and dermis is capable of benign or malignant over-growth. Tumours are lumpy and even when they cannot be seen, they can be felt underneath the surface of the skin.

Ulcer

An ulcer is a break or open sore in the skin extending to every layer.

Urticaria

This condition is also known as 'hives'. Lesions appear rapidly and disappear within minutes or gradually over a number of hours. The clinical signs are the development of red weals which may later turn white. The area becomes itchy or may sting. There are a number of causes of urticaria, some of which are an allergic reaction to certain foods such as strawberries, shellfish, penicillin, house dust and pet fur. Other causes include stress and sensitivity to light, heat or cold.

Vesicles

These are small sac-like blisters. A bulla is a vesicle larger than 0.5 cm and is commonly called a blister.

Wart

A wart is a well-defined benign tumour varying in size and shape. See 'Viral infections of the skin'.

Weal

A weal is a raised area of skin, containing fluid which is white in the centre with a red edge. It is seen in the condition urticaria.

Common pathologies of the skin

Disorders of the sebaceous gland

Acne vulgaris

A chronic inflammatory disorder of the sebaceous glands which leads to the over-production of sebum. It involves the face, back and chest and is characterised by the presence of greasy, oily skin with enlarged pores, inflammation in and around the sebaceous glands, papules, pustules and, in more severe cases, cysts and scars.

Acne vulgaris is primarily androgen induced and appears most frequently at puberty and usually persists for a considerable period of time. Although it is commonly associated with teenage and adolescent skin, it can actually affect many age groups at different stages of life.

IN PRACTICE

The skin is a complex organ and when symptoms of disease and disorders occur, it can affect both a client's health and wellbeing.

It is essential that a facial therapist is able to recognise skin conditions that require medical treatment to ensure a client receives the correct form of treatment, and to avoid cross-infection in the salon if the condition presented is infectious. It is equally as important to be able to be knowledgeable about skin lesions and disorders to ensure the correct form of treatment, advice and/or referral to a dermatologist is made.

BODY FACT

The scientific name of the bacteria that cause acne vulgaris is *Proprionbacterium acnes*. These bacteria are anaerobic, which means that they do not need oxygen to survive and grow. Although these bacteria are constantly present in all follicles in small numbers, they are prevented from reproducing to large numbers by the oxygen that is provided by an open follicle. However, once the follicle becomes blocked from the circulation of oxygen, these bacteria multiply and feed off of the sebum produced by the over-active sebaceous glands.

The typical stages of acne development are as follows:

Acne starts to develop when an increase in hormone production (commonly puberty) stimulates the sebaceous glands
Excess sebum production causes additional cell build-up in the follicles, which become comedones (plugs of sebum and dead cells)
The blocked follicle opening results in inflammation and irritation and the formation of papules
The blockage of sebum and dead skin cells prevents oxygen reaching the bottom of the follicle and hence bacteria form. The infected papules become pustules
The bacteria excrete an inflammatory fatty acid by-product which eventually results in blocking the follicle completely
The skin forms hardened tissue to prevent the spread of bacteria, creating cysts
The damage to collagen and elastin in the dermis can lead to depressed and raised scars (the scars resulting from cysts are called ice-pick scars)

Different grades of acne vulgaris

There are four different grades of acne, the grade being dependent on the severity of the disorder

Grade I acne	Presence of a few papules and pustules, minor breakout. Mainly open comedones present, with some closed comedones Grade I acne is typical in a teenager just beginning puberty
Grade II acne	Greater incidence of papules and pustules, presence of many closed comedones and more open comedones
Grade III acne	Skin appears very red and inflamed, with many papules and pustules present
Grade IV acne	Cysts present with comedones, papules, pustules. Skin appears inflamed

Acne vulgaris

Rosacea

A chronic inflammatory disease of the face in which the skin appears abnormally red. The condition usually occurs in adults after the age of 40, but can begin as early as age 20.

The condition is gradual and begins with what first seems like a tendency to blush easily, a red complexion or an extreme sensitivity to cosmetic products.

The distinctive redness appears in a characteristic butterfly pattern across the nose and cheeks. As the condition progresses, there may be papules and pustules present. Although the condition may resemble acne, unlike acne, the condition rosacea is rarely if ever accompanied by comedones. The other distinguishing feature of rosacea, as compared with acne, other than the distinctive flushing and extreme skin sensitivity, are the dry, flaky patches that may accompany dry or oily skin. As many of the symptoms of rosacea can look like those of acne, it is a condition that is often misdiagnosed.

The redness often persists after cold exposure or after exposure to irritants like soap. With time, small blood vessels develop, making the redness more noticeable. Many patients will develop stinging or burning sensations and the skin will often feel tight. The skin feels like mild sunburn with smiling, frowning or squinting. Sometimes this progresses to the point that everything the patient puts on her face stings, burns and irritates.

A progressive stage of rosacea is characterised by swelling and growth of the nose and central facial areas. At times the ears may be involved as well. This condition is known as rhinophyma and can be very disfiguring.

Aggravating factors of Rosacea include hot, spicy foods, hot drinks, alcohol, menopause, the elements and stress.

Rosacea

Sebaceous cyst

A round, nodular lesion with a smooth shiny surface which develops from a sebaceous gland. They are usually found on the face, neck, scalp and back. They are situated in the dermis and vary in size from 5 to 50 mm. The cause is unknown.

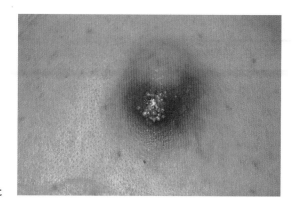

Sebaceous cyst

Seborrhoea

Defined as an excessive secretion of sebum by the sebaceous glands. In this condition the glands appear enlarged and the skin appears greasy, especially on the nose and the centre zone of the face. It can resemble acne in that there may be swellings and breakout. One of the main differences between acne and seborrhoea, however, is that in seborrhoea the increased oil production is often accompanied by scaly, greasy-looking thickened skin, especially on the scalp.

Seborrhoea is common where there is a high incidence of sebaceous glands (for instance the scalp and the sides of the nose). Seborrhoea can occur at any age, but is common in infancy (when it is called cradle cap) and at puberty due to glandular disturbances.

Seborrhoea

Disorders of the sweat glands

Hyperhidrosis

This is the excessive production of sweat affecting the hands, feet and underarms.

Bacterial infections

Boil

A boil begins as a small inflamed nodule which forms a pocket of bacteria around the base of a hair follicle or a break in the skin. Local injury or lowered constitutional resistance may encourage the development of boils.

Conjunctivitis

This is a bacterial infection following irritation of the conjunctiva of the eye. The inner eyelid and eyeball appear red and sore and there may be a pus-like discharge from the eye. The infection spreads by contact with the secretions from the eye of the infected person.

Folliculitis

This bacterial infection occurs in the hair follicles of the skin and appears as a small pustule at the base of a hair follicle. There is redness, swelling and pain around the hair follicle.

Conjunctivitis

Folliculitis

Impetigo

This is a superficial contagious inflammatory disease caused by streptococcal and staphylococcal bacteria. It is commonly seen on the face and around the ears and its features include weeping blisters which dry to form honey-coloured crusts. This bacteria is easily transmitted by dirty fingernails and towels.

Stye

This is an acute inflammation of a gland at the base of an eyelash, caused by a bacterial infection. The gland becomes hard and tender, and a pus-filled cyst develops at the centre.

Impetigo

Stye

Viral infections of the skin

Herpes simplex (cold sores)

Herpes simplex is normally found on the face and around the lips. It begins as an itching sensation, followed by erythema and a group of small blisters which then weep and form crusts. This condition will generally persist for approximately two or three weeks but will reappear at times of stress, ill health or exposure to sunlight.

Herpes simplex (cold sore)

Herpes zoster (shingles)

This is a painful infection along the sensory nerves due to the virus that causes chickenpox. Lesions resemble herpes simplex with erythema and blisters along the lines of the nerves. The areas affected are mostly on the back or upper chest wall. This condition is very painful due to acute inflammation of one or more of the peripheral nerves. Severe pain may persist at the site of shingles for months or even years after the apparent healing of the skin.

Herpes zoster (shingles)

Warts

A wart is a benign growth on the skin caused by infection with the human papilloma virus. Plane warts are smooth in texture with a flat top and are usually found on the face, forehead, back of the hands and the front of the knees. Plantar warts or verrucae occur on the soles of the feet and are usually the size of a pea.

Plane warts

Plantar wart

Fungal infections of the skin

Ringworm

This is a fungal infection of the skin which begins as small red papules that gradually increase in size to form a ring. The affected areas on the body vary in severity from mild scaling to inflamed itchy areas.

Ringworm

Tinea capitis

This is a type of ringworm and is a fungal infection of the scalp. It appears as painless, round, hairless patches on the scalp. Itching may be present and the lesion may appear red and scaly.

Tinea pedis (Athlete's foot)

This is a highly contagious fungal condition which is easily transmitted in damp, moist conditions such as swimming pools, saunas and showers. Athlete's foot appears as flaking skin between the toes which becomes soft and soggy. The skin may also split and the soles of the feet may occasionally be affected.

Tinea pedis

Infestation disorders of the skin

Pediculosis (lice)

This condition is commonly known as 'lice' and is a contagious parasitic infection, where the lice live off the blood sucked from the skin. Head lice are frequently seen in young children and if not dealt with quickly, may lead to a secondary infection of Impetigo as a result of scratching. With head lice, nits may be found in the hair. They are pearl-grey or brown, oval structures found on the hair shaft close to the scalp. The scalp may appear red and raw due to scratching.

Body lice are rarely seen. They will occur on an individual with poor personal hygiene and will live and reproduce in seams and fibres of clothing, feeding off the skin. Lesions may appear as papules, scabs and in severe cases as pigmented dry, scaly skin. Secondary bacterial infection is often present. A client affected by body lice will complain of itching, especially in the shoulder, back and buttock area.

Scabies

This is a contagious parasitic skin condition caused by the female mite burrowing into the horny layer of the skin where she lays her eggs. The first noticeable symptoms of this condition is severe itching which worsens at night. Papules, pustules and crusted lesions may also develop. Common sites for this infestation are the ulnar borders of the hand, palms of the hands and between the fingers and toes. Other sites include the axillary folds, buttocks, breasts in the female and external genitalia in the male.

Scabies

Pigmentation disorders

Albinism

This condition is caused by an inherited absence of pigmentation in the skin, hair and eyes, resulting in white hair, pink skin and eyes. The pink colour is produced by underlying blood vessels which are normally masked by pigment. Other clinical signs of this condition include poor eyesight and sensitivity to light.

Chloasma

This is a pigmentation disorder with irregular areas of increased pigmentation, usually on the face. It commonly occurs during pregnancy and sometimes when taking the contraceptive pill due to stimulation of melanin by the female hormone oestrogen.

Dermatosis papulosa nigra (DPN)

This is a unique benign skin condition that is common among black skins. It is characterised by multiple, small, hyperpigmented, asymptomatic papules.

It appears as small, dark bumps and most commonly affects the face, neck, chest and back. The cause of dermatosis papulosa nigra is uncertain. There is a strong genetic basis for the disorder and often the lesions can be seen in several members of the same family. Under the microscope, the lesions are a type of keratosis that is harmless.

Dermatosis papulosa nigra is not a skin cancer and it will not turn into a skin cancer. The condition is chronic, with new lesions appearing over time. No treatment is necessary other than for cosmetic concerns. In certain circumstances, if the lesions are symptomatic (painful, inflamed, itchy or catch on clothing), they can be treated via a minor surgical procedure.

Dermatosis papulosa nigra (DPN)

Ephelides

Another name for this is freckles. These are small, harmless pigmented areas of skin. They appear where there is excessive production of the pigment melanin (after exposure to sunlight).

Lentigo

These are also known as 'liver spots'. They are flat dark patches of pigmentation found mainly in the elderly on skin exposed to light.

Naevus

A naevus is a birthmark or clearly defined malformation of the skin. There are many different types of naevi:

- **Port wine stain** – also known as a 'deep capillary naevus'. Present at birth and may vary in colour from pale pink to deep purple. It has as an irregular shape but is not raised above the skin's surface. Usually found on the face but may also appear on other areas of the body.
- **Spider naevi** – a collection of dilated capillaries radiating from a central papule. Often appear during pregnancy or after 'picking a spot'.
- **Strawberry naevus** – usually develops before or shortly after a baby is born, but disappears spontaneously before the child reaches the age of ten. It is a red raised lump above the skin's surface.

Port wine stain

Vitiligo

Vitiligo

This condition is present on areas of the skin which lack pigmentation due to the basal cell layer of the epidermis no longer producing melanin. Its cause is unknown.

Hypertrophic disorders

Hypertrophic skin disorders refer to conditions which have resulted in an increase of size of a tissue or organ. This is caused by an enlargement of the cells.

Hyperkeratosis

Keratoses are generally defined as a build-up of cells. Hyperkeratosis is a rare skin disorder in which there is a gross thickening of the skin due to a mass of keratinocytes that builds up to a horny over-growth of skin cells.

Identifying skin cancers

It is important to be aware of the typical characteristics of skin cancer:

- An open sore, of any size, that bleeds, oozes or crusts and remains open for three or more weeks.
- A persistent, non-healing sore.

IN PRACTICE

Hyperkeratosis is a common problem for black skins and because of the increased cell turnover, black skins desquamate dead skin cells more readily. The accumulation of dead skin cells on the surface of the skin is what can give an ashen grey look to black skins.

Care needs to be taken in a treatment to avoid exfoliating too harshly to avoid irritation and sensitivity.

- A reddish patch or irritated area that does not go away and fails to responds to moisturisers or treatment creams.
- A smooth growth with a distinct rolled border and an indented centre.
- A shiny bump or nodule with a smooth surface that can be pink, red, white, back, brown or purple in colour.
- A white patch of skin that has a smooth, scarlike texture. The area of white stands out from the surrounding skin and can appear clear and taut.

There is a list of the A, B, C and D of identifying skin cancer:

- **Asymmetry** – one area of the suspected area is unlike the other.
- **Border** – there is an irregular, scalloped edge around the suspected lesion.
- **Colour** – colour varies from one area to another and may appear with shades of tan, brown, black, white, red or blue.
- **Diameter** – the area will generally be larger than 6 mm.

Basal cell carcinoma

This is a common form of skin cancer that originates in the basal cell layer of the epidermis. Often found on the face and other sun-exposed areas (especially in fair-skinned people). The most common type of basal cell carcinoma is a pearl-like bump, which may be pink or slightly flesh coloured, often with small capillaries running through it. Superficial basal cell carcinomas appear red, flat and scaly and may be misdiagnosed as other conditions, such as eczema.

Basal cell carcinomas rarely spread to other tissues or organs, and although not life threatening they can produce unpleasant scarring if not detected early.

Malignant melanoma

A malignant melanoma is a deeply pigmented mole which is life threatening if it is not recognised and treated promptly. Its main characteristic is a blue-black module which increases in size, shape and colour, and is most commonly found on the head, neck and trunk. Over-exposure to strong sunlight is a major cause and its incidence is increased in young people with fair skins.

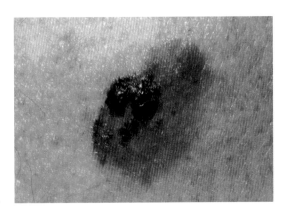

Malignant melanoma

Melanomas can occur in an existing mole or they may arise from normal skin. As they spread very quickly, early detection is essential.

Rodent ulcer

This is a malignant tumour which starts off as a slow-growing pearly nodule, often at the site of a previous skin injury. As the nodule enlarges, the centre ulcerates and refuses to heal. The centre becomes depressed, and the rolled edges become translucent, revealing many tiny blood vessels. Rodent ulcers do not disappear and if left untreated may invade the underlying bone. This is the most common form of skin cancer.

Rodent ulcer

Squamous cell carcinoma

This is a malignant tumour which arises from the prickle cell layer of the epidermis. It is hard and warty and eventually develops a 'heaped-up, cauliflower' appearance. It is most frequently seen in elderly people. Unlike basal cell carcinomas, squamous cell carcinomas can spread to other organs, or deeply within the skin. Fortunately, 90 per cent of squamous cell carcinomas are detected and removed before they spread or reappear.

Squamous cell carcinoma

IN PRACTICE

Care would need to be taken in the case of an inflammatory skin condition to avoid any form of stimulation (through product or treatment method) that may increase or worsen inflammation. If there is severe inflammation and the skin is broken, or there are any signs of infection, treatment would be avoided and the client would need to be referred to their medical practitioner.

Inflammatory skin conditions

Contact dermatitis

Dermatitis literally means inflammation of the skin. Contact dermatitis is caused by a primary irritant which causes the skin to become red, dry and inflamed. Substances which are likely to cause this reaction include acids, alkalis, solvents, perfumes, lanolin, detergent and nickels. There may be skin infection as well.

Eczema

This is a mild to chronic inflammatory skin condition characterised by itchiness, redness and the presence of small blisters that may be dry or weep if the surface is scratched. Eczema is non-contagious and the cause may be genetic or due to internal and external influences. It can cause scaly and thickened skin, mainly at flexures such as the cubital area of the elbows and the back of the knees.

Contact dermatitis

Eczema

Psoriasis

This is a chronic inflammatory skin condition. Psoriasis may be recognised as the development of well-defined red plaques, varying in size and shape, and covered by white or silvery scales. Any area of the body may be affected by psoriasis but the most commonly affected sites are the face, elbows, knees, nails, chest and abdomen. It can also affect the scalp, joints and nails. Psoriais is aggravated by stress and trauma but is improved by exposure to sunlight.

Psoriasis

Seborrhoeic dermatitis

This is a mild to chronic inflammatory disease of hairy areas well supplied with sebaceous glands. Common sites are the scalp, face, axilla and in the groin. The skin may appear to have a grey tinge or have a dirty yellow colour. Clinical signs include slight redness, scaling and dandruff in the eyebrows.

IN PRACTICE

A client with lupus should be referred to their medical practitioner. Lupus is not contagious, and with the appropriate medical advice on the client's condition, skin care treatments may be offered. In the event of a skin care service being offered, care would need to be taken to avoid stimulating products and/or treatments and any more aggressive forms of treatment. This condition has similar needs to a sensitive skin type and should be treated accordingly.

Auto-immune disorder of the skin

Systemic lupus erythematosus (SLE)

This is a chronic inflammatory disease of connective tissue affecting the skin and various internal organs. It is an auto-immune disease and can be diagnosed by the presence of abnormal antibodies in the bloodstream.

It is typically characterised by a red, scaly rash affecting the nose and cheeks. Other symptoms include joint pain, hair loss, swelling of the feet and fingers.

A form of lupus which primarily affects the skin is dicoid lupus erythematosus (DLE). This is where the skin forms round, firm lesions called discoids with red, raised bumps around the hair follicles. All forms of lupus are aggravated by sun exposure.

Systemic lupus erythematosus

Interrelationships with other systems

The skin links to the following body systems.

Skeletal

Vitamin D is produced by the skin upon exposure to ultraviolet light. This is needed in bone formation and bone maintenance.

Muscular

Muscles provide a supportive function to the skin. Muscles lie directly under the skin and therefore contribute to skin's tone and elasticity.

Circulatory

Blood clots at the site of an injury and forms a scab on the surface of the skin. This allows the skin to heal and protects underlying structures from any further damage.

Respiratory

Oxygen absorbed into the lungs upon inhalation is delivered to the cells of the skin, hair and nails to aid their renewal.

Nervous

There are numerous sensory nerve endings in the skin that respond to touch, tempertaure, pain and pressure.

Endocrine

The melanocyte-stimulating hormone (MSH) secreted by the central lobe of the pituitary stimulates the production of melanin in the basal cell layer of the skin. The sex hormones (gonadotrophice hormones) influence skin and hair growth during puberty, pregnancy and the menopause.

Digestive

Excess caloric consumption in the daily diet can result in adipose (fatty tissue) being stored in the subcutaneous layer of the skin.

Urinary

Water is lost from the skin as sweat. The kidneys regulate fluid balance in the body to prevent the skin from becoming dehydrated.

Key words associated with the skin, hair and nails

epidermis	reticular layer	medulla
dermis	adipose tissue	lanugo hair
subcutaneous layer	collagen	vellus hair
basal layer (stratum germinativum)	elastin	terminal hair
prickle-cell layer (stratum spinosum)	reticular fibres	anagen
granular layer (stratum granulosum)	hair	catagen
clear layer (stratum lucidum)	sebaceous gland	telogen
horny layer (stratum corneum)	eccrine gland	nail plate
cell regeneration	apocrine gland	nail bed
keratinisation	erector pili muscle	matrix
desquamation	hair shaft	nail wall
papillary layer	hair root	nail groove
	hair bulb	cuticle
	cuticle	lunula
	cortex	free edge

Revision summary of the skin, hair and nails

- The **skin** and the appendages derived from it (**hair, glands** and **nails**) make up the skin.
- The skin is one of the larger organs in the body.
- Functions of the skin include **protection, regulation of body temperature, sensation, excretion, storage, absorption** and **vitamin D production**.
- The principal parts of the skin are the outer **epidermis** and the inner **dermis**. Beneath the dermis lies the **subcutaneous layer**.
- The epidermis is the most superficial part and consists of five layers, from deepest to superficial: **basal cell layer** (stratum germinativum), **prickle cell layer** (stratum spinosum), **granular layer** (stratum granulosum), **clear layer** (stratum lucidum) and **horny layer** (stratum corneum).
- **Cell regeneration** occurs continuously in the **basal cell layer** and produces all other layers.
- It takes approximately a month for a new cell to complete its journey from the **basal cell layer**, where it is reproduced, to the **granular layer**, where it is keratinised to the **horny layer**, where it is **desquamated** or shed.
- The **dermis** is the deeper layer of the skin and provides support, strength and elasticity.
- It has a superficial **papillary** layer and a deeper **reticular** layer.
- The superficial **papillary** layer consists of **adipose connective tissue**, dermal papillae, nerve endings and a network of **blood** and **lymphatic capillaries**.
- The deeper **reticular** consists of tough **fibrous connective tissue** and contains **collagen, elastin** and **reticular** fibres.
- Appendages of the skin include the **hair**, glands (**sebaceous and sweat**) and **nails**.
- The **hair** is a dead keratinised structure and is divided into three parts: **hair shaft, root** and **bulb**.
- The role of a hair is protection.
- Internally the hair has three layers from the outer to inner layer: **cuticle, cortex** and **medulla**.
- The **matrix** and **hair bulb** is the area of mitotic activity for the hair cells.

- There are three main types of hair in the body: **lanugo, vellus** and **terminal**.
- Each hair has its own hair growth cycle.
- **Anagen** is the active growing stage, **catagen** is the transitional stage from active to resting and **telogen** is the short resting stage.
- Nails are made up of mainly **keratin** and are a modification of the horny and clear layers of the epidermis.
- The two main functions of the nail are protection for the fingers and toes, and for manipulation of objects.
- Parts of the nail's anatomical structure include the **nail plate, nail bed, matrix, nail wall, nail groove, cuticle, lunula** and **free edge**.
- Nail growth occurs from the nail **matrix** by cell division.
- As new cells are produced in the matrix, older cells are pushed forward and are hardened by **keratinisation** to form the hardened **nail plate**.
- Other related structures of the skin are the **erector pili muscle** and the glands.
- The **erector pili muscle** is the weak muscle associated with hair and will contract when you are cold or experiencing emotions such as fright or anxiety.
- **Sebaceous glands** are also known as oil glands. They have ducts and are attached to hair follicles.
- They secrete **sebum** which is mildly antibacterial and antifungal to lubricate the hair and the epidermis.
- **Sweat glands** are located in the **dermis** and secrete **sweat**.
- There are two types of sweat glands, **eccrine and apocrine**.
- **Eccrine glands** are the most numerous and are found in largest concentration in the palms of the hands, soles of the feet.
- **Apocrine glands** are attached to the hair follicles and are located in the axilla and groin.
- Factors affecting the skin include diet, water intake, sleep, stress and tension, exercise, alcohol, smoking, medication, chemicals, climate, environment, hormones and age.

The skin, hair and nails
Multiple-choice questions

1 In which of the following layers are epidermal cells constantly being reproduced?
   a horny layer
   b basal cell layer
   c clear layer
   d granular layer

2 Desquamation occurs in which layer of the epidermis?
   a horny layer
   b basal cell layer
   c prickle cell layer
   d clear layer

3 Which of the following is responsible for making the skin pigmentation darker?
   a keratin
   b sebum
   c carotene
   d melanin

4 The type of sweat glands that are widely distributed throughout the body are:
   a apocrine
   b eccrine
   c adipose
   d sebaceous

5 Which of the following is **not** a function of the skin?
   a protection
   b temperature regulation
   c transportation
   d excretion

6 The tough protein found in the epidermis, hair and nails is:
   a melanin
   b reticulin
   c keratin
   d collagen

7 In which layer of the skin would you find collagen fibres?
   a papillary layer
   b reticular layer
   c subcutaneous layer
   d basal cell layer

8 The function of the subcutaneous layer is to:
   a support blood vessels
   b insulate the body
   c support nerve endings
   d all of the above

9 Which of the following skin types is most likely to present with the best elasticity?
   a dry
   b sensitive
   c oily
   d mature

10 Which of the following is a fungal infection of the skin?
   a herpes simplex
   b ringworm
   c herpes zoster
   d impetigo

11 A chronic inflammatory skin disease in which the skin appears abnormally red is known as:
   a acne vulgaris
   b folliculitis
   c seborrhoea
   d rosacea

12 What is erythema?
   a small raised elevation in the skin
   b reddening of the skin due to the dilation of blood capillaries
   c mark left on the skin after a wound has healed
   d mass of dilated capillaries in the skin

13 Which of the following ethnic skin types is most likely to be affected by the condition Dermatosis papulosa nigra?
   a Afro-Caribbean/black
   b Oriental/light Asian
   c dark Asian
   d Mediterranean

14 A milia is:
   a a pearly hard white nodule under the skin
   b an abnormal sac containing fluid
   c a crack in the epidermis
   d a small, flat patch of increased pigmentation

15 Hair grows from a sac-like depression called the hair…
   a follicle
   b shaft
   c root
   d bulb

16 Which of the following provides a crucial source of nourishment for a hair?
   a connective tissue sheath
   b outer root sheath
   c dermal papilla
   d inner root sheath

17 The area of the nail where living cells are produced is the:
   a nail bed
   b lunula
   c cuticle
   d matrix

18 All nutrients are supplied to the nail via which layer of the skin?
   a subcutaneous layer
   b epidermis
   c subdermal layer
   d dermis

19 A common nail disease characterised by inflammation and bacterial infection of the skin surrounding the nail is:
   a onychomycosis
   b paronychia
   c pterygium
   d leuconychia

20 The most lethal type of skin cancer is:
   a squamous cell carcinoma
   b basal cell carcinoma
   c rodent ulcer
   d malignant melanoma

3

the skeletal system

Introduction

The skeleton is made up of no fewer than 206 individual bones, which collectively form a strong framework for the body.

The skeleton comprises bones that provide support and protection for our body. Bones must, however, be linked together in order to facilitate their supportive role and to allow movement. Joints provide the link between bones of the skeletal system. Joints, therefore, serve a dual purpose: they hold bones together via ligaments, offering stability for the joint, and give the skeletal system more flexibility by facilitating movement which is assisted by associated muscles and tendons.

IN PRACTICE

It is essential for therapists to have good working knowledge of the skeletal system, as bones are like landmarks in the body, and by tracing their outlines you can be accurate in describing the position of muscles, glands and organs. Learning the positions of the bones of the skeleton is, therefore, essential for learning the position of the muscles and for understanding joint movements, as bones must have muscle attachments to enable them to move.

◉ Objectives

By the end of this chapter you will be able to recall and understand the following knowledge:

- functions of the skeleton
- structure of bone
- growth and development of bone
- different types of bone in the body
- names and positions of the bones of the skeleton
- different types of joints and their range of movement
- the importance of good posture
- postural deformities
- the interrelationships between the skeletal and other body systems
- common pathologies of the skeletal system.

Functions of the skeleton

The skeletal system is made up of all types of bones which form the skeleton or bony framework of the body. Before learning the individual bones of the skeleton, it is important to understand the functions of the skeleton as a whole.

Support

The skeleton bears the weight of all other tissues. Without it we would be unable to stand up. Consider the bones of the vertebral column, pelvis, feet and legs which all support the weight of the body.

Shape

The bones of the skeleton give shape to structures such as the skull, thorax and limbs.

Protection of vital organs and delicate tissue

The skeleton surrounds vital organs and tissue with a tough and resilient covering, such as the rib cage protecting the heart and lungs and the vertebral column protecting the spinal cord.

Attachments for muscles and tendons

Bones are like anchors which allow the muscle to function efficiently.

Movement

This happens as a result of the coordinated action of muscles upon bones and joints. Bones are, therefore, levers for muscles.

Formation of blood cells

These develop in red bone marrow found in cancellous bone tissue.

Mineral reservoir

The skeleton acts as a storage depot for important minerals such as calcium which can be released when needed for essential metabolic processes like muscle contraction and the conduction of nerve impulses.

The structure of bone

Bone is one of the hardest types of connective tissue in the body and when fully developed is composed of water, calcium salts and organic matter. Bone tissue is a type of living tissue that is made from special cells called osteoblasts. There are two main types of bone tissue: **compact** and **cancellous**. All bones have both types of tissue, the amount being dependent on the type of bone.

Compact (dense) bone

This is the hard portion of the bone that makes up the main shaft of the long bones and the outer layer of other bones. It protects spongy bone and provides a firm framework for the bone and body. The bone cells in this type of bone (osteocytes) are located in concentric rings around a central haversian canal, through which nerves, blood and lymphatic vessels pass.

Cancellous (spongy) bone

In contrast, this is lighter in weight than compact bone. It has an open sponge-like appearance and is found at the ends of long bones or at the centre of other bones. It does not have a haversian system but consists of a web-like arrangement of spaces that are filled with red bone marrow and separated by the thin processes of bone. Blood vessels run through every layer of cancellous bone, conveying nutrients and oxygen.

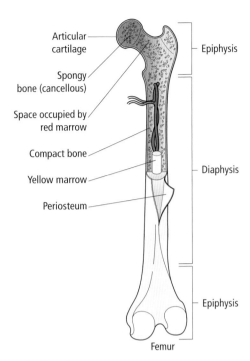

Articular cartilage
Spongy bone (cancellous)
Space occupied by red marrow
Compact bone
Yellow marrow
Periosteum
Epiphysis
Diaphysis
Epiphysis
Femur

Fig 3.1 Structure of a long bone

Bone marrow

Bones contain two types of marrow – red and yellow:

- Red marrow manufactures red blood cells. It is found at the end of long bones and at the centre of other bones of the thorax and pelvis.
- Yellow marrow is found chiefly in the central cavities of long bones.

Except for the ends that form joints, bones are covered with a thin membrane of connective tissue called the periosteum. The outer layer of the periosteum is extremely dense and contains a large number of blood vessels. The inner layer contains osteoblasts and fewer blood vessels. The periosteum provides attachment for muscles, tendons and ligaments.

The development of bone

The process of bone development is called **ossification**. The bones of a foetus are made of cartilage rods that are changed due to ossification into bone as the child develops and grows. This process begins in the embryo near the end of the second month and is not complete until about the 25th year of life.

Ossification takes place in three stages:

1 The cartilage-forming cells, called chondrocytes, enlarge and arrange themselves in rows similar to the bone they will eventually form.
2 Calcium salts are then laid down by special bone building cells called osteoblasts.
3 A second set of cells called osteoclasts, known as cartilage-destroying cells, brings about an antagonistic action, enabling the absorption of any unwanted bone.

A fine balance of osteoblast and osteoclast activity helps to maintain the formation of normal bone. Osteocytes are mature bone cells that maintain bone during our lifetime.

Cartilage

Cartilage is a dense connective tissue that consists of collagen and elastin fibres embedded in a strong gel-like substance. It is a flexible and durable type of tissue, cushioning and absorbing shock, thereby preventing direct transmission to bones.

There are three types of cartilage:

- **hyaline** – covers the articular bone surfaces
- **fibrous** – a strong and rigid type of cartilage between the discs of the spine
- **elastic** – a very flexible type of cartilage found in the auditory canal of the ear.

Cartilage has no blood supply and therefore does not repair or renew itself as easily as bone.

Ligaments

Ligaments are dense, strong flexible bands of white fibrous connective tissue that link bones together at a joint. They are inelastic but flexible, strengthening the joint and allowing the bones to move freely within a safe range of movement.

Tendons

Tendons are tough white fibrous cords of connective tissue that attach muscles to the periosteum (fibrous covering) of a bone. Tendons enable bones to move when skeletal muscles contract.

Types of bone

Bones are classified according to their shape. They are classified as **long bones, short bones, flat bones, irregular bones** and **sesamoid bones.**

Overview of the different types of bone

Bone type	Characteristics	Examples
Long	Weight-bearing bones designed to provide structural support	Arms and legs
Short	Look like blocks, allow a wider range of movement than larger bones	Wrist and ankle bones
Flat	Designed for protection	Skull, scapula, ribs, sternum, pelvic bones
Irregular	Have a variety of shapes; usually have projections that muscles, tendons and ligaments can attach to	Vertebral column, some facial bones
Sesamoid	Small rounded bone embedded in a tendon	Kneecap/patella

Long bones

Long bones have a long shaft (diaphysis) and one or more endings or swellings (epiphysis). Smooth hyaline cartilage covers the articular surfaces of the shaft endings. Between the diaphysis and epiphysis of growing bone is a flat plate of hyaline cartilage called the epiphyseal cartilage or growth plate. This is the site of bone growth and as fast as this cartilage grows it is turned into bone, allowing the bone to continue to grow in length.

A growth spurt is often seen during puberty through the influence of the sex hormones oestrogen and testosterone, both of which promote the growth of long bone. At around 25 years of age the entire plate becomes ossified.

All bones of the limbs are long bones (except the wrist and ankle bones).

Short bones

These bones are generally cube shaped with their lengths and widths being roughly equal. The bones of the wrist and the ankle are examples of short bones.

Flat bones

Flat bones are plate like structures with broad surfaces. Examples include the ribs and the scapulae.

Irregular bones

Irregular bones have a variety of shapes. Examples include the vertebrae and some of the facial bones.

Sesamoid bones

These are small rounded bones embedded in a tendon. The largest sesamoid bone is the patella which is embedded in the quadriceps femoris tendon.

The bones of the skeleton

The skeletal system is divided into two parts: the axial skeleton made up of 80 bones and the appendicular skeleton made up of 126 bones.

The axial skeleton forms the main axis or central core of the body and consists of the following parts:

- skull
- vertebral column
- sternum
- ribs.

The appendicular skeleton supports the appendages or limbs and gives them attachment to the rest of the body. It consists of the following parts:

- shoulder girdle
- bones of the upper limbs
- bones of the lower limbs
- bones of the pelvic girdle.

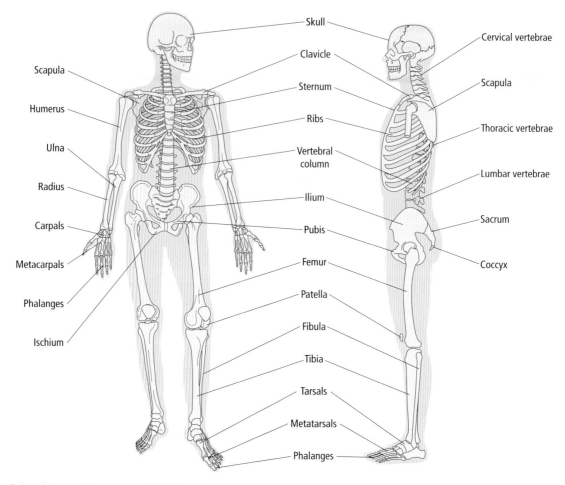

Fig 3.2 Bones of the skeleton (anterior and side)

The skull

The skull rests upon the upper end of the vertebral column, weighs around 11 pounds and consists of 22 bones. Eight bones make up the skull or cranium and 14 bones form the facial skeleton. The skull encloses and protects the brain and provides a surface attachment for various muscles of the skull.

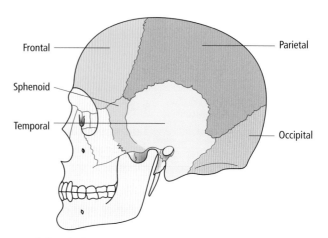

Fig 3.3 Bones of the skull

Student activity

Now complete Activity 3.1 in the resources for this book on Dynamic Learning Online.

The eight bones of the skull are as follows:

Name of bone/s	Position
Frontal × 1	Forms the anterior part of the roof of the skull, the forehead and the upper part of the orbits or eye sockets
Parietal × 2	Form the upper sides of the skull and the back of the roof of the skull
Temporal × 2	Form the sides of the skull below the parietal bones and above and around the ears
Sphenoid × 1	Located in front of the temporal bone and serves as a bridge between the cranium and the facial bones
Ethmoid × 1	Forms part of the wall of the orbit, the roof of the nasal cavity and part of the nasal septum
Occipital × 1	Forms the back of the skull

The bones of the face

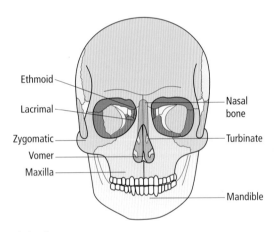

Fig 3.4 Bones of the face

There are 14 facial bones in total. These are mainly in pairs, one on either side of the face:

Name of bone/s	Position
Maxilla × 2	Largest bones of the face and they form the upper jaw and support the upper teeth
Mandible × 1	The only moveable bone of the skull and forms the lower jaw and supports the lower teeth. The mandible is the largest and heaviest bone in the skull
Zygomatic × 2	The most prominent of the facial bones and form the cheekbones
Nasal × 2	These small bones form the bridge of the nose
Lacrimal × 2	The smallest of the facial bones, located close to the medial part of the orbital cavity

(Continued)

BODY FACT

A cleft palate occurs when the palatine bones don't fuse during fetal development. Consequently, with the palatine unconnected, an opening exists between the roof of the mouth and the nasal cavity.

Name of bone/s	Position
Turbinate × 2	Layers of bone located either side of the outer walls of the nasal cavities
Vomer × 1	A single bone at the back of the nasal septum
Palatine × 2	L-shaped bones which form the anterior part of the roof of the mouth

The sinuses

There are four pairs of air-containing spaces in the skull and face called the sinuses. The function of the sinuses is to lighten the head, provide mucus and act as a resonance chamber for sound. The pairs of sinuses are named according to the facial bones by which they are located. They are the **frontal** sinuses, the **sphenoidal** sinuses, the **ethomoidal** sinuses and the **maxillary** sinuses which are the largest.

Student activity

Now complete Activity 3.2 in the resources for this book on Dynamic Learning Online.

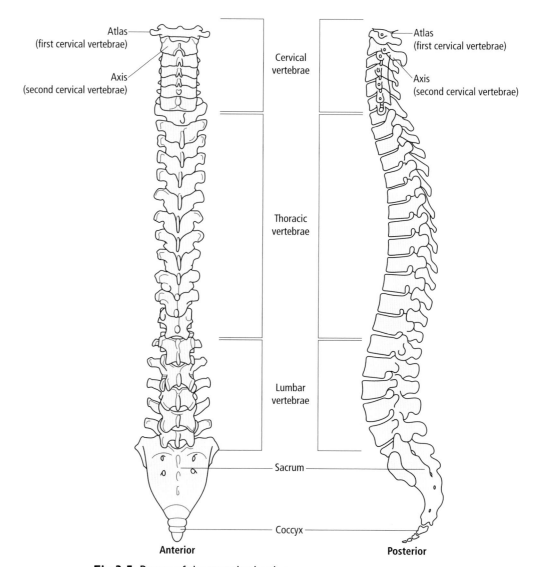

Fig 3.5 Bones of the vertebral column

The vertebral column

The vertebral column lies on the posterior of the skeleton, extending from the skull to the pelvis, providing a central axis to the body. It consists of 33 individual irregular bones called vertebrae. However, the bones of the base of the vertebral column, the sacrum and coccyx, are fused to give 24 movable bones in all.

The vertebral column is made up of the following:

Vertebrae	Number	Position	Description
Cervical	7	Vertebrae of the neck	Smallest vertebrae in the vertebral column The top two vertebrae, C1 the atlas and C2 the axis, allow the head and neck to move freely
Thoracic	12	Vertebrae of the mid spine; lie in the thorax where they articulate with the ribs	These vertebrae lie flatter and downwards to allow for muscular attachment of the large muscle groups of the back. They can be easily felt as you run your fingers down the spine
Lumbar	5	In the lower back	These are much larger in size than the vertebrae above them as they are designed to support more body weight These vertebrae can be easily felt on the lower back due to their large shape and width
Sacral	5	Lie in between the pelvic bones	This is a flat, triangular-shaped bone It is made up of five bones which are fused together A characteristic feature of the sacrum is the eight sacral holes. It is through these holes that nerves and blood vessels penetrate
Coccygeal	4	Base of spine below the sacrum	These are made up of four bones which are fused together and are sometimes referred to as the coccyx (tail bone)

BODY FACT

In between the vertebrae lies a padding of fibrocartilage called the intervertebral discs. These give the vertebrae a certain degree of flexibility and also act as shock absorbers in between the vertebrae, cushioning any mechanical stress that may be placed upon them.

Functions of the vertebral column

Now we have covered the individual structure of the vertebrae, let us consider the functions of the vertebral column as a whole:

- The vertebral column provides a strong and slightly flexible axis to the skeleton.
- By way of its different shaped vertebrae with their roughened surfaces, it is able to provide a surface for the attachment of muscle groups.
- The vertebral column also has a protective function as it protects the delicate nerve pathways of the spinal cord.

Therefore, the vertebral column mirrors the primary functions of the skeleton in its supportive and protective roles.

The thoracic cavity

This is the area of the body enclosed by the ribs, providing protection for the heart and lungs.

Essential parts contained within this cavity include:

- the sternum
- the ribs
- 12 thoracic vertebrae.

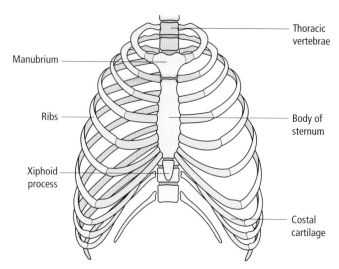

Fig 3.6 The thoracic cavity

The sternum

This is commonly referred to as the breast bone and is a flat bone lying just beneath the skin in the centre of the chest. The sternum is divided into three parts:

- **manubrium**, the top section
- **main body**, the middle section
- **xiphoid process**, the bottom section.

The top section of the sternum articulates with the clavicle and the first rib. The middle section articulates with the costal cartilages that link the ribs to the sternum. The bottom section provides a point of attachment for the muscles of the diaphragm and the abdominal wall.

The ribs

There are 12 pairs of ribs. They articulate posteriorly with the thoracic vertebrae. Anteriorly, the first ten pairs attach to the sternum via the costal cartilages, the first seven directly (known as the true ribs), the remaining three indirectly (known as the false ribs). The last two ribs have no anterior attachment and are called the floating ribs.

The appendicular skeleton

This consists of the shoulder girdle, the bones of the upper and lower limbs and the pelvic girdle.

The shoulder girdle

The shoulder girdle connects the upper limbs with the thorax and consists of four bones – two **scapula** and two **clavicle**.

The **scapula** is a large flat bone, triangular in outline which forms the posterior part of the shoulder girdle. It is located between the second and the seventh rib. The scapula articulates with the clavicle and the humerus and serves as a point of muscle attachment which connects the shoulder girdle with the trunk and upper limbs.

The **clavicle** is a long slender bone with a double curve. It forms the anterior portion of the shoulder girdle. At its medial end it articulates with

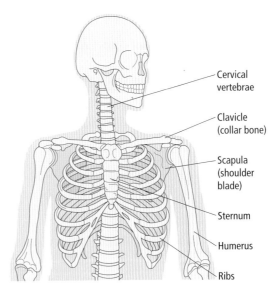

Fig 3.7 Bones of the neck, chest and shoulder girdle

the top part of the sternum and at its lateral end it articulates with the scapula. The clavicle acts as a brace to hold the arm away from the top of the thorax.

The clavicle provides the only bony link between the shoulder girdle and the axial skeleton. The arrangement of bones and the muscle attached to the scapula and the clavicle allow for a considerable amount of movement of the shoulder and the upper limbs.

The upper limb

The upper limb consists of the following bones:

humerus	Long bone forming the upper arm
radius	Long bone of the forearm (thumb side)
ulna	Long bone of the forearm (little finger side)
carpals	8 bones forming the wrist
metacarpals	5 long bones forming the palm of the hand
phalanges	14 bones forming the fingers and thumb

Humerus

The humerus is the long bone of the upper arm. The head of the humerus articulates with the scapula, forming the shoulder joint. The distal end of the bone articulates with the radius and ulna to form the elbow joint.

Radius and ulna

The ulna and radius are the long bones of the forearm. The two bones are bound together by a fibrous ring which allows a rotating movement in which the bones pass over each other. The ulna is the bone of the little finger side and is the longer of the two forearm bones. The radius is situated on the

Fig 3.8 Bones of the upper limb

thumb side of the forearm and is shorter than the ulna. The joint between the ulna and the radius permits a movement called pronation. This is when the radius moves obliquely across the ulna so that the thumb side of the hand is closest to the body. The movement called supination takes the thumb side of the hand to the lateral side. The radius and the ulna articulate with the humerus at the elbow and the carpal bones at the wrist.

Carpals

The wrist consists of eight small bones of irregular size which are collectively called carpals. They fit closely together and are held in place by ligaments. The carpals are arranged in two groups of four. Those of the upper row articulate with the ulna and the radius and the lower row articulates with the metacarpals. The upper row nearest the forearm is called scaphoid, lunate, triquetral and pisiform. The lower row is called the trapezium, trapezoid, capitate and hamate.

Metacarpals

There are five long metacarpal bones in the palm of the hand. Their proximal ends articulate with the wrist bones and the distal ends articulate with the finger bones.

Phalanges

There are 14 phalanges. These are the finger bones, two are in the thumb or pollex and three are in each of the other digits.

The lower limb

The lower limb consists of the following bones:

femur	Long bone forming the thigh
patella	Bone forming the kneecap
tibia	Long bone of the lower leg (anterior, medial side)
fibula	Long bones of the lower leg (lateral side)
tarsals	7 bones forming the ankle
metatarsals	5 bones forming the dorsal (top) surface of the foot
phalanges	14 bones forming the toes

Femur

The femur is the bone of the thigh. It is the longest bone in the body and has a shaft and two swellings at each end. The proximal swelling has a rounded head like a ball which fits into the socket of the pelvis to form the hip joint. Below the neck are swellings called trochanters, which are sites for muscle attachment. The distal ends of the femur articulate with the patella or kneecap.

Patella

The patella or kneecap is located anterior to the knee joint. Its main function is to provide stabilisation, cushion the hinge joint at the knee and protect the knee by shielding it from impact.

Fig 3.9 Bones of the lower limb

Tibia and fibula

The tibia and fibula are long bones of the lower leg. The tibia is situated on the anterior and medial side of the lower leg. It has a large head where it joins the knee joint and the shaft leads down where it forms part of the ankle. The tibia is the larger of the two bones of the lower leg and thus carries the weight of the body. The fibula is situated on the lateral side of the tibia in the lower leg and is the shorter and thinner of the two bones. The end of the fibula forms part of the ankle on the lateral side.

The foot

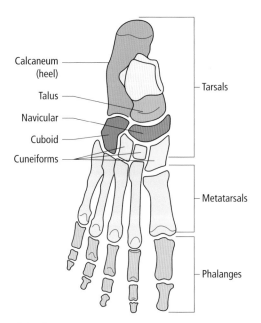

Fig 3.10 Bones of the foot

Tarsals

There are seven bones in the foot, which collectively are called the tarsals. Each tarsal is an irregular bone that slides minutely over the next bone to collectively provide motion. The individual tarsals are as follows:

- **Talus** – the talus bone is the main tarsal. It articulates with the tibia and fibula to form the ankle joint. The talus is significant in that it bears the weight of the entire body when standing or walking.
- **Calcaneum** – the calcaneum is also known as the heel bone. It is the largest and most posterior tarsal bone. The calcaneum is an important site for attachment of muscles of the calf.
- **Cuboid** – the cuboid is situated between the fourth and fifth metatarsals and the calcanuem on the lateral (outer) border of the foot.
- **Cuneiform** – there are three cuneiform bones which are located between the navicular bone and the first three metatarsal bones. They are numbered medially to laterally from I through to III (the most medial being I, the middle being II and the most lateral being III).
- **Navicular** – the navicular bone is situated between the talus bone and the three cuneiforms.

- **Metatarsals** – there are five metatarsals forming the dorsal surface of the foot.
- **Phalanges** – 14 phalanges form the toes, two of which are in the hallux or big toe and three to each of the other digits.

Arches of the foot

The bones of the feet form arches which are designed to support body weight and to provide leverage when walking. The arches of the foot are maintained by ligaments and muscles. They give the foot resilience in bearing the body's weight when running or walking. The arches of the foot are the:

- **medial longitudinal arch** – this runs along the medial side of the foot from the calcaneum bone to the end of the metatarsals
- **lateral longitudinal arch** – this runs along the lateral side of the foot from the calcaneum bone to the end of the metatarsals
- **transverse arch** – this runs between the medial and lateral aspect of the foot and is formed by the navicular, three cuneiforms and the bases of the five metatarsals.

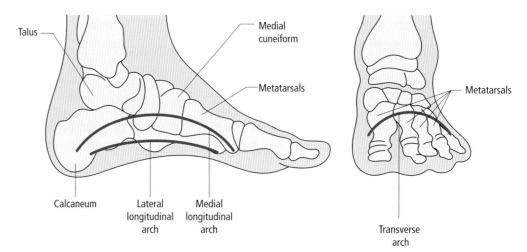

Fig 3.11 Arches of the feet

The pelvic girdle

The pelvic girdle consists of two hip bones which are joined together at the back by the sacrum and at the front by the symphysis pubis.

Fig 3.12 Bones of the pelvic girdle

Each hip bone consists of three separate bones which are fused together. They are the:

- ilium
- ischium
- pubis.

Pelvic bone	Position	Description
Ilium	Forms superior (upper part) of the pelvic girdle	The largest and most superior pelvic bone in the pelvic girdle Upper border is iliac crest; an important site of attachment for muscles of the anterior and posterior abdominal walls
Ischium	Forms the inferior (lower) and posterior (back) part of pelvic girdle	The ischial tuberosity is a bony protrusion which is the part of the ischium that you sit on It receives the weight of the body when sitting and provides muscle attachments for the muscles such as the hamstrings and the adductors
Pubis	Collective name for the two pubic bones in the most anterior (front) portion of the pelvis	Two pubic bones resemble a wishbone and are linked via a piece of cartilage called the symphysis pubis The pubic bones provide attachment sites for some of the abdominal muscles and fascia

Student activity

Now complete Activity 3.3 in the resources for this book on Dynamic Learning Online.

Functions of the pelvic girdle

Like the vertebral column, the pelvic girdle mirrors the primary functions of the skeleton – it has a role in supporting the vertebral column and the body's weight and offers protection by encasing delicate organs such as the uterus and bladder.

Joints

A joint is formed where two or more bones or cartilage meet and is otherwise known as an articulation. Where a bone is a lever in a movement, the joint is the fulcrum or the support which steadies the movement and allows the bone to move in certain directions.

Types of joint

Joints are classified according to the degree of movement possible at each one. There are three main joint classifications:

- **fibrous** – no movement is possible (also known as fixed joints)
- **cartilaginous** – slight movement is possible
- **synovial** – freely moveable joints.

Fibrous joints

These are immovable joints with tough fibrous tissue between the bones. Often the edges of the bones are dovetailed together into one another, as in the sutures of the skull. Some examples of fibrous joints include the joints between the teeth and between the maxilla and mandible of the jaw.

Cartilaginous joints

These are slightly movable joints which have a pad of fibrocartilage between the end of the bones making the joint. The pad acts as a shock absorber.

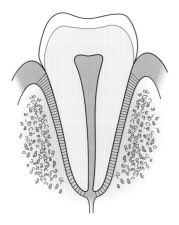

Fig 3.13 A fibrous joint

Some examples of cartilaginous joints are those between the vertebrae of the spine and at the symphysis pubis, in between the pubis bones.

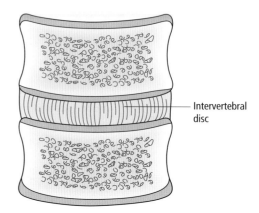

Intervertebral disc

Fig 3.14 A cartilaginous joint

Synovial joints

These are freely movable joints which have a more complex structure than the fibrous or cartilaginous joints. Before looking at the different types of synovial joints it is important to have an understanding of the general structure of a synovial joint.

The general structure of a synovial joint

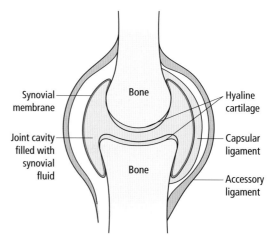

Synovial membrane

Joint cavity filled with synovial fluid

Bone

Bone

Hyaline cartilage

Capsular ligament

Accessory ligament

Fig 3.15 A synovial joint

- A synovial joint has a space between the articulating bones which is known as the synovial cavity.
- The surface of the articulating bones is covered by hyaline cartilage which is supportive to the joint by providing a hard-wearing surface for the bones to move against one another with the minimum of friction.
- The synovial cavity and the cartilage are encased within a fibrous capsule which helps to hold the bones together to enclose the joint. This joint

capsule is reinforced by tough sheets of connective tissue called ligaments which bind together the articular ends of bones.

- The joint capsule is reinforced enough to allow strength to resist dislocation but is flexible enough to allow movement at the joint.
- The inner layer of the joint capsule is formed by the synovial membrane which secretes a sticky oily fluid called synovial fluid which lubricates the joint and nourishes the hyaline cartilage.
- As the hyaline cartilage does not have a direct blood supply, it relies on the synovial fluid to deliver its oxygen and nutrients and to remove waste from the joint which is achieved via the synovial membrane.

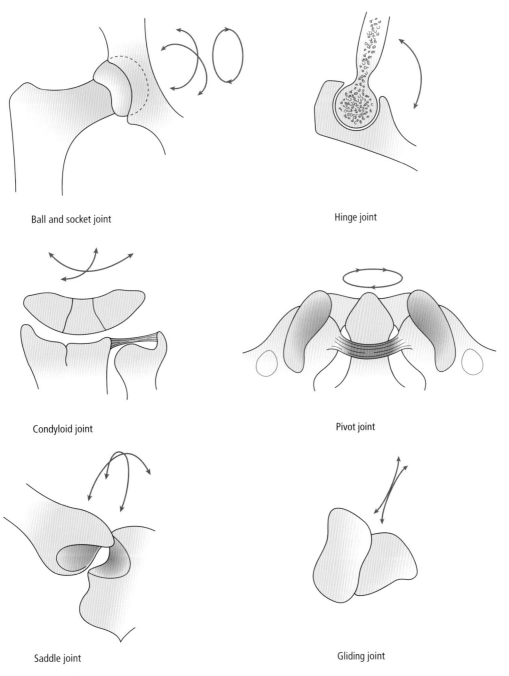

Ball and socket joint

Hinge joint

Condyloid joint

Pivot joint

Saddle joint

Gliding joint

Fig 3.16 Types of synovial joint

Types of synovial joints

Synovial joints are classified into six different types according to their shape and the movements possible at each one. The degree of movement possible at each synovial joint is dependent on the type of synovial joint and its articulations.

Type of synovial joint	Description	Movement	Example
Ball and socket	Formed when the rounded head of one bone fits into a cup-shaped cavity of another bone	Allows movement in many directions around a central point; flexion, extension, adduction, abduction, rotation and circumduction	Hip and shoulder joints
Hinge	Where the rounded surface of one bone fits the hollow surface of another bone	Movement is possible in only one plane; allows flexion and extension	Knee and elbow joints, joints in between the phalanges
Condyloid	The joint surfaces are shaped so that the concave surface of one bone can slide over the convex surface of another bone in two directions	Although a condyloid joint allows movement in two directions, one movement dominates. Movements possible include flexion, extension, adduction and abduction	Wrist joint and joint between the metacarpals and phalanges (metacarpophlangeal joints)
Gliding	Often referred to as synovial plane joints as they occur where two flat surfaces of bone slide against one another	Allow only a gliding motion in various planes (side to side/back and forth)	Joints between vertebrae and sacroiliac joint
Pivot	Occurs where a process of bone rotates in a socket; one component is shaped like a ring and the other component is shaped so that it can rotate within the ring	Only permits rotation	Joint between the first and second cervical vertebrae (atlas and axis) and joint at the proximal ends of the radius and the ulna
Saddle	Shaped like a saddle; articulating surfaces of bone have both rounded and hollow surfaces so that the surface of one bone fits the complementary surface of the other	Movements possible at this joint include flexion, extension, adduction, abduction and a small degree of axial rotation	Thumb joint

Glossary of angular movements possible at joints

Anatomical term	Description	Illustration
Flexion	Bending of a body part at a joint so that the angle between the bones is decreased	
Extension	Straightening of a body part at a joint so that the angle between the bones is increased	
Dorsiflexion	Upward movement of the foot so that feet point upwards	
Plantar flexion	Downward movement of the foot so that feet face downwards towards the ground	

(Continued)

Anatomical term	Description	Illustration
Adduction	Movement of a limb towards the midline	
Abduction	Movement of a limb away from the midline	
Rotation	Movement of a bone around an axis (180 degrees)	
Circumduction	A circular movement of a joint (360 degrees)	
Supination	Turning the hand so that the palm is facing upwards	

Anatomical term	Description	Illustration
Pronation	Turning the hand so that the palm is facing downwards	
Eversion	Soles of the feet face outwards	
Inversion	Soles of the feet face inwards	

Posture

Posture is a measure of balance and body alignment and is the maintenance of strength and tone of the body's muscles against gravity. Good posture is said to be when the maximum efficiency of the body is maintained with the minimum effort. When evaluating posture, an imaginary line is drawn vertically through the body. This is called the centre of gravity line. From the front or back this line should divide the body into two symmetrical halves. Good posture is as follows:

- with feet together the ankles and knees should touch
- hips should be the same height
- shoulders should be level

Fig 3.17 Good posture

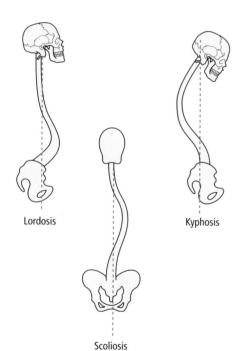

Fig 3.18 Postural defects

- sternum and vertebral column should run down the centre of the body in line with the centre of gravity line
- head should be erect and not tilted to one side.

Posture varies considerably in individuals and is influenced by factors such as body frame size, heredity, occupation, habits and personality. Additional factors which may also affect posture include clothing, shoes and furniture.

Good posture is important as it:

- allows a full range of movement
- improves physical appearance
- keeps muscle action to a minimum, thereby conserving energy and reducing fatigue
- reduces the susceptibility of injuries
- aids the body's systems to function efficiently.

Poor posture may have the following effects on the body:

- produce alterations in body function and movement
- waste energy
- increase fatigue
- increase the risk of backache and headaches
- impair breathing
- increase the risk of muscular, ligament or joint injury
- affect circulation
- affect digestion
- give a poor physical appearance.

Postural defects

Kyphosis
This is an abnormally increased outward curvature of the thoracic spine. In this condition the back appears round as the shoulders point forward and the head moves forward. A tightening of the pectoral muscles is common in this condition.

Lordosis
This is an abnormally increased inward curvature of the lumbar spine. In this condition the pelvis tilts forward and as the back is hollow, the abdomen and buttocks protrude and the knees may be hyperextended. Typical problems associated with this condition are tightening of the back muscles followed by a weakening of the abdominal muscles. Hamstring problems are common because of the anterior tilt of the pelvis. Increased weight gain or pregnancy may cause or exacerbate this condition.

Scoliosis
This is a lateral curvature of the vertebral column, either to the left or right side. Evident signs of this condition include unequal leg length, distortion of the rib cage, unequal position of the hips or shoulders and curvature of the spine (usually in the thoracic region).

Common pathologies of the skeletal system

Ankylosing spondylitis

This is a systemic joint disease characterised by inflammation of the intervertebral disc spaces, costo-vertebral and sacroiliac joints. Fibrosis, calcification, ossification and stiffening of joints are common and the spine becomes rigid. Typically, a client will complain of persistent or intermittent lower back pain. Kyphosis is present when the thoracic or cervical regions of the spine are affected and the weight of the head compresses the vertebrae and bends the spine forward. This condition can cause muscular atrophy and loss of balance and falls. Typically this disease affects young male adults.

Arthritis – gout

This is a joint disorder due to deposition of excessive uric acid crystals accumulating in the joint cavity. It commonly affects the peripheral joints, commonly the metatarsophalangeal joint of the big toe. Kidneys can be affected. Other cartilage may be involved including the ear pinna.

Arthritis – osteoarthritis

This is a joint disease characterised by the breakdown of articular cartilage, growth of bony spikes, swelling of the surrounding synovial membrane and stiffness and tenderness of the joint. It is also known as degenerative arthritis. It is common in the elderly and takes a progressive course. This condition involves varying degrees of joint pain, stiffness, limitation of movement, joint instability and deformity. It commonly affects the weight bearing joints – the hips, knees, lumbar and cervical vertebrae.

Arthritis – rheumatoid

This is a chronic inflammation of peripheral joints resulting in pain, stiffness and potential damage to joints. It can cause severe disability. Joint swellings and rheumatoid nodules are tender.

Bunion

This is a swelling of the joint between the big toe and the first metatarsal. Bunions are usually caused by ill-fitting shoes and are made worse by excessive pressure.

Bursitis

This condition is the inflammation of a bursa (small sac of fibrous tissue that is lined with synovial membrane and filled with synovial fluid). It usually results from injury or infection and produces pain, stiffness and tenderness of joint adjacent to the bursa.

Dupuytren's contracture

This is the forward curvature of the fingers (usually the ring and little fingers) caused by contracture of the fibrous tissue in the palm and fingers.

IN PRACTICE

In the case of a client with a joint disorder, position the client according to individual comfort. Remember that extra cushioning and support may be required.

IN PRACTICE

Avoid forcibly mobilising ankylosed joints and in the case of cervical spondylitis avoid hyperextending the neck.

IN PRACTICE

In the case of a client with arthritis, passive and gentle friction movements around the joint may be beneficial where there is minimal pain, but excessive movement may cause joint pain and damage. Always ask the client to demonstrate the range of movement possible at each joint and this will guide you as to the limitations of treatment.

IN PRACTICE

Although therapeutic treatments such as massage cannot cure arthritis, they can help to prevent its progress through relaxation and reduction of discomfort. Always ensure there is no pain and that care is taken when gently mobilising a joint.

Treatment is generally of shorter duration as clients may be taking pain killers and be unable to give adequate feedback.

Fracture

A fracture is a breakage of a bone, either complete or incomplete. There are six different types:

- A **simple fracture** involves a clean break with little damage to surrounding tissues and no break in the overlying skin (also known as a closed fracture).
- A **compound fracture** is an open fracture where the broken ends of the bone protrude through the skin.
- A **comminuted fracture** is where the bone has splintered at the site of impact and smaller fragments of bone lie between the two main fragments.
- A **greenstick fracture** only occurs in children and is a partial fracture in which one side of the bone is broken and the other side bends.
- An **impacted fracture** is where one fragment of bone is driven into the other.
- A **complicated fracture** occurs when a broken bone damages tissues and/or organs around it.

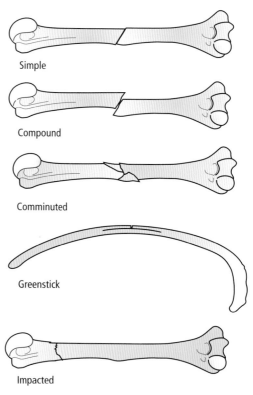

Simple

Compound

Comminuted

Greenstick

Impacted

Fig 3.19 Drawings of the six types of fracture

Frozen shoulder (adhesive capsulitis)

This chronic condition causes pain and stiffness and reduced mobility (or locking) of the shoulder joint. This may follow an injury, stroke or myocardial infarction or may develop due to incorrect lifting or a sudden movement.

Osteoporosis

This condition is caused by brittle bones due to ageing and the lack of the hormone oestrogen which affects the ability to deposit calcium in the matrix of bone. This can also result from prolonged use of steroids. Vulnerability to osteoporosis can be inherited. Bones can break easily and vertebrae can collapse.

Spina bifida

This is a congenital defect of the vertebral column in which the halves of the neural arch of a vertebra fail to fuse in the midline.

Sprain

A sprain is the injury to a ligament caused by overstretching or tearing. A sprain occurs when the attachments to a joint are stressed beyond their normal capacity, resulting in pain and swelling. The ankle joint and lower back are often sprained.

Stress

Stress can be defined as any factor which affects physical or emotional health. Examples of excessive stress on the skeletal system include poor posture, stiff joints and repetitive strain injuries.

Synovitis

This is the inflammation of a synovial membrane in a joint.

Temporo-mandibular joint tension (TMJ syndrome)

This is a collection of symptoms and signs produced by disorders of the temporo-mandibular joint. It is characterised by bilateral or unilateral muscle tenderness and reduced motion. It presents with a dull aching pain around the joint often radiating to the ear, face, neck or shoulder. The condition may start off as clicking sounds in the joint. There may be protrusion of the jaw or hypermobility and pain on opening the jaw. It slowly progresses to decreased mobility of the jaw and locking of the jaw may occur. Causes include chewing gum, biting nails, biting off large chunks of food, habitual protrusion of the jaw, tension in the muscles of the neck and back and clenching of the jaw. It may also be caused by injury and trauma to the joint or through a whiplash injury.

Whiplash

This condition is caused by damage to the muscles, ligaments, intervertebral discs or nerve tissues of the cervical region by sudden hyperextension and/or flexion of the neck. The most common cause is a road traffic accident when acceleration/deceleration causes sudden stretch of the tissue around the cervical spine. It may also occur as a result of hard impact sports. It can present with pain, limitation of neck movements with muscle tenderness which can start hours to days after the accident and may take months to recover.

IN PRACTICE

The condition whiplash may last for a few months or years. In the acute stages, avoid manipulating the neck and moving it vigorously.

Interrelationships with other systems

The skeletal system links to the following body systems:

Skin

The role of vitamin D production in the skin helps bones absorb calcium in order to keep them strong and healthy.

Muscular

Mucles pull on bones at joints in order to effect movement.

Circulatory

Erythrocyres are produced in the bone marrow of long bones.

Digestive

Food ingested in the digestive system is broken down and vital nutrients, such as calcium and phopsorus, are carried in the blood to the bones.

Nervous

Muscles require stimulation from a nerve impulse in order to contract and produce movement.

Endocrine

Growth hormones produced by the pituitary gland are responsible for the growth rate of bones in childhood.

Key words associated with the skeletal system

bone	thoracic vertebrae	tarsals
compact	lumbar vertebrae	metatarsals
cancellous	sacral vertebrae (sacrum)	medial longitudinal arch
ossification	coccygeal vertebrae (coccyx)	lateral longitudinal arch
cartilage	thoracic cavity	transverse arch
ligament	sternum	ilium
tendon	ribs	ischium
axial skeleton	appendicular skeleton	pubis
frontal	shoulder girdle	joint
parietal	upper limb	fibrous
temporal	lower limb	cartilaginous
sphenoid	pelvic girdle	synovial
ethmoid	scapula	ball-and-socket joint
occipital	clavicle	hinge
maxilla	humerus	condyloid
mandible	radius	gliding joint
zygomatic	ulna	pivot joint
nasal	carpals	saddle joint
lacrimal	metacarpals	synovial cavity
turbinate	phalanges	fibrous joint capsule
vomer	femur	synovial membrane
palatine	tibia	synovial fluid
cervical vertebrae	fibula	

Revision summary of the skeletal system

- The functions of the skeleton are support, shape, protection, movement, attachment for muscle and tendons, formation of blood cells and mineral storage.
- **Bone** is the hardest type of connective tissue in the body.
- There are two types of bone tissue: **compact** (hard) and **cancellous** (spongey).
- The process of bone development is called **ossification** and is not complete until around the 25th year of life.
- **Cartilage** is a strong and rigid type of connective tissue that cushions and supports bone.
- A **ligament** binds bones to other bones.
- A **tendon** attaches a muscle to bone.
- Bones are classified according to shape: **long, short, flat, irregular** and **sesamoid**.
- The **axial skeleton** forms the main core of the body and consists of the skull, vertebral column, sternum and ribs.
- There are eight bones of the skull: one **frontal**, two **parietal**, two **temporal**, one **sphenoid**, one **ethmoid** and one **occipital**.
- There are 14 bones of the face: two **maxillae**, one **mandible**, two **zygomatic**, two **nasal**, two **lacrimal**, two **turbinate**, one **vomer** and two **palatine**.
- There are 33 bones in the vertebral column: seven **cervical vertebrae** in the neck, 12 **thoracic vertebrae** in the mid spine, five **lumbar vertebrae** in the lower back, five **sacral vertebrae** (forming the sacrum) and four **coccygeal vertebrae** (forming the coccyx at the base of the spine).
- The **thoracic cavity** protects vital organs in the chest and includes the **sternum**, 12 pairs of **ribs** and the 12 **thoracic vertebrae**.
- The **appendicular skeleton** supports the appendages or limbs and consists of the **shoulder girdle, bones of the upper and lower limbs** and **bones of the pelvic girdle**.
- The shoulder girdle consists of two **scapulae** (posteriorly) and two **clavicle** bones (anteriorally).
- The upper limb consists of the **humerus** in the upper arm, **radius** and **ulna** in the forearm, eight **carpals** in the wrist, five **metacarapals** in the palm and 14 **phalanges** in the fingers.
- The lower limb consists of the **femur**, bone of the upper leg, **tibia** and **fibula** in the lower leg, seven **tarsals** in the ankle, five **metatarsals** in the dorsum of the foot and 14 **phalanges** in the toes.
- There are three arches in the foot designed to support body weight and to provide leverage when walking: **medial longitudinal arch, lateral longtudinal arch** and the **transverse arch**.
- The pelvic girdle consists of the **ilium, ischium** and the **pubis**.
- A **joint** is a point of contact between two or more bones.
- Joints hold bones together via **ligaments** and provide flexibility by facilitating movement.
- Structurally joints are classified as **fibrous, cartilaginous** or **synovial**.
- **Fibrous** joints are immovable such as the sutures of the skull bones.
- **Cartilaginous** joints are slightly movable such as between the vertebrae of the spine.
- **Synovial** joints are freely movable joints and there are several different types: **ball and socket** (hip), **hinge** (knee and elbow), **condyloid** (wrist), **gliding** (between the vertebrae), **pivot** (between the first and second cervical vertebrae), **saddle** (between the trapezium and metacarpal of the thumb).
- Features of a synovial joint include a **joint (synovial) cavity**, a **fibrous joint capsule**, a **synovial membrane** containing **synovial fluid**.

1 How many bones is the skeleton made up of?
   a 208
   b 106
   c 80
   d 206

2 Mature bone cells are called:
   a osteoblasts
   b osteoclasts
   c osteocytes
   d chondrocytes

3 How many bones are there, in total, in the skull?
   a 24
   b 22
   c 14
   d 11

4 The bone of the skull which forms the upper sides and back of the roof of the skull is the:
   a occipital
   b sphenoid
   c temporal
   d parietal

5 The largest bone in the face is the:
   a mandible
   b zygomatic
   c nasal
   d maxilla

6 The vertebral column consists of how many movable bones?
   a 24
   b 33
   c 12
   d 9

7 Which type of bone are the vertebrae classified as?
   a short
   b long
   c irregular
   d sesamoid

8 The portion that makes up the main shaft of long bone is:
   a cancellous bone
   b compact bone
   c red bone marrow
   d yellow bone marrow

9 The bone forming the posterior part of the shoulder girdle is the:
   a scapula
   b sternum
   c manubrium
   d clavicle

10 The long bone of the upper arm is the:
   a radius
   b ulna
   c humerus
   d hamate

11 The type of joint that permits free movement is:
   a synovial
   b fibrous
   c cartilaginous
   d hyaline

12 The largest and most superior pelvic bone is the:
   a ilium
   b pubis
   c ischium
   d sacrum

13 The largest tarsal bone, that forms the heel, is the:
   a cuneiform
   b calcaneum
   c cuboid
   d talus

14 How many tarsal bones are found in the foot?
   a 7
   b 8
   c 9
   d 10

15 A hinge joint permits:
   a rotation
   b circumduction
   c adduction
   d flexion and extension

16 The hip is classified as a:
   a pivot joint
   b ball and socket joint
   c gliding joint
   d hinge joint

17 The type of fracture where the broken ends of the bone protrude through the skin is known as:
   a comminuted
   b compound
   c compact
   d complicated

18 An example of where a gliding joint may be found in the body is:
   a the elbow
   b the ankle
   c the wrist
   d between the vertebrae

19 An abnormal inward curvature of the lumbar spine is known as:
   a lordosis
   b kyphosis
   c scoliosis
   d spina bifida

20 The joint disease characterised by the breakdown of articular cartilage, swelling and stiffness of the joints is:
   a rheumatoid arthritis
   b osteoarthritis
   c gout
   d ankylosing spondylitis

4 the muscular system

Introduction

The muscular system comprises over 600 individual muscles which are primarily concerned with movement and body coordination. The muscular system is closely related to the skeletal system; there is an intimate relationship between muscle and bone as both contribute to creating a movement in the body.

You will have learned from the skeletal system that bones and joints provide the leverage in a movement, but it is in fact a muscle which provides the pull upon the bone to effect the movement. The key to learning the anatomical position and action of muscles is to first learn the individual position of the bones. It is then a logical step to learn the muscle attachments in relation to bone and what movements those muscles create.

IN PRACTICE

It is essential for therapists to have a good working knowledge of the muscular system as they are primarily working on the muscles and associated connective tissues that make up about half of the body's soft tissue mass.

Having knowledge of the position and action of muscles allows therapists to be more accurate in their treatment applications to ensure effective results, and to recognise the varying degrees of muscle tone. Understanding how muscles contribute to movement in the body will help therapists appreciate how pathological disorders often result in muscle dysfunction.

◎ Objectives

By the end of this chapter, you will be able to recall and understand the following knowledge:

● functions of the muscular system
● structure and functions of the different types of muscle tissue
● structure and function of the different types of attachments of muscles
● how muscles contract
● definition of the terms 'muscle tone' and 'muscle fatigue'
● the effects of temperature and increased circulation on muscle contraction
● position and action of the main superficial muscles of the face and body
● the interrelationships between the muscular and other body systems
● common pathologies of the muscular system.

The functions of the muscular system

The muscular system consists largely of skeletal muscle tissue which covers the bones on the outside and connective tissue which attaches muscles to the bones of the skeleton. Muscles, along with connective tissue, help to give the body its contoured shape.

The muscular system has three main functions.

Movement

Consider the action of picking up a pen that has dropped onto the floor. This seemingly simple action of retrieving the pen involves the coordinated action of several muscles pulling on bones at joints to create movement. Muscles are also involved in the movement of body fluids such as blood, lymph and urine. Consider also the beating of the heart which is continuous throughout life.

Maintaining posture

Some fibres in a muscle resist movement and create slight tension in order to enable us to stand upright. This is essential since without body posture we would be unable to maintain normal body positions such as sitting down or standing up.

The production of heat

As muscles create movement in the body they generate heat as a by-product which helps to maintain our normal body temperature.

Muscle tissue

Muscle tissue makes up about 50 per cent of your total body weight and is composed of:

- 20 per cent protein
- 75 per cent water
- 5 per cent mineral salts, glycogen and fat.

There are three types of muscle tissue in the body:

- **skeletal** or **voluntary** muscle tissue which is primarily attached to bone
- **cardiac** muscle tissue which is found in the walls of the heart
- **smooth** or **involuntary** muscle tissue which is found inside the digestive and urinary tracts, as well as in the walls of blood vessels.

All three types of muscle tissue differ in their structure and functions and the degree of control the nervous system has upon them.

Overview of the three types of muscle tissue

Muscle type	Description	Location	Function
Voluntary/skeletal	Striped appearance Have many nuclei Held together by connective tissue	Attached to bones, skin or other muscles	Facilitates movement of bones Moves blood and lymph Heat production Maintenance of posture
Cardiac	Striped appearance Branched structure Has a single nucleus Has intercalated discs in between each cardiac muscle cell	Heart	Provides a consistent flow of blood throughout the body
Smooth/involuntary	Non-striated Shaped like spindles Has a single nucleus	In walls of stomach, intestines, bladder, uterus and in blood vessels	Moves substances through the various tracts (digestive, genito-urinary)

Voluntary muscle tissue

Voluntary muscle tissue is made up of bands of elastic or contractile tissue bound together in bundles and enclosed by a connective tissue sheath which protects the muscle and helps to give it a contoured shape.

Voluntary or skeletal muscle tissue has very little intercellular tissue. It consists almost entirely of muscle fibres held together by fibrous connective tissue and penetrated by numerous tiny blood vessels and nerves. The long slender fibres that make up muscle cells vary in size. Some are around 30 cm in length, whereas others are microscopic.

Each muscle fibre is enclosed in an individual wrapping of fine connective tissue called the endomysium. These are further wrapped together in bundles, known as fasciculi and are covered by the perimysium (fibrous sheath) which is then gathered to the muscle belly (main part of the muscle) with its own sheath – the fascia epimysium.

The relatively inelastic parts of each of the muscles are tendons and these are usually made up of the continuation of the endomysium and perimysium.

Each muscle fibre is made up of even thinner fibres called myofibrils, which are the contractile elements of a skeletal muscle fibre. These consist of long strands of microfilaments, made up of two different types of protein strands called actin and myosin. It is the arrangement of actin and myosin filaments which gives the skeletal muscle its striated or striped appearance when viewed under a microscope. Muscle fibre contraction results from a sliding movement within the myofibrils in which actin and myosin filaments merge.

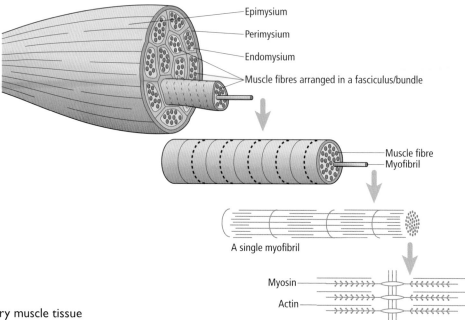

Fig 4.1 The structure of voluntary muscle tissue

Most skeletal muscles are made up of a combination of the following types of fibres.

Fast twitch fibres (white)

These have fast, strong reactions but tire quickly. They are well adapted for rapid movements and short bursts of activity. They have a rich blood supply and mainly use the energy stores of glucose in the muscles which can be transferred into mechanical energy without oxygen.

Slow twitch fibres (red)

These fibres have greater endurance but do not produce as much strength as fast twitch fibres. They are therefore suited to slower and more sustained movements and are relatively resistant to fatigue. Their energy comes from the breaking down of glucose by oxygen and they depend on a continuous supply of glucose for endurance. Slow twitch fibres have a good circulation (the red colour comes from both the circulation and from the presence of a red pigmented protein that stores the oxygen).

During low-intensity work, such as walking, the body is working well below its maximal capacity and only slow twitch fibres are working. As muscle intensity increases and the exercise becomes more anaerobic, fast twitch fibres are activated. Whatever the intensity of movement, only a small number of fibres are used at any one time to prevent damage and injury to the tissues.

The way in which the bundles of fibres lie next to one another in muscle will determine its shape. The contractile force of a muscle is partly attributable to the architecture of its fibres. Common muscle fibre arrangements include the following:

BODY FACT

Each person is born with a set number of muscle fibres which cannot be increased. An increase in the size of a muscle is due to exercise which will cause an increase in the individual fibres. However, with disuse these will shrink again as the muscle atrophies. It is interesting to note that men are more able to enlarge their muscles through exercise than women due to the effects of male hormones.

- **Parallel fibres** – muscles with parallel fibres can vary from short, flat muscles to spindle-shaped (fusiform) muscles to long straps.
- **Convergent** – this is where the muscles fibres converge towards a single point for maximum concentration of the contraction. The direction of movement is determined by which sections of the muscle are activated. The muscle may be a triangular sheet (the pectoralis major muscle or the latissimus dorsi). These muscles often cross joints that have a large range of possible movements. They provide a strong but steady pull, fine-tuning the angle of movement and thus balancing movement with continuing stability in the joint.
- **Pennate** – this is where the fibres lie at an angle to the tendon and, therefore, also to the direction of pull. They have lots of short fibres so the muscle pull is short but strong. They may be further classified as follows:

  - **Uni-pennate** – diagonal fibres attach to one side of the tendon only such as the soleus.
  - **Bi-pennate** – the fibres converge onto a central tendon from both sides such as the rectus femoris.
  - **Multipennate** – the muscle has several tendons of origin such as the deltoid.

BODY FACT

Every time a muscle is used, the muscle fibres shorten along their length, therefore tension often accumulates in lines in the longer muscles (particularly those with parallel fibres such as the paravertebral muscles). In muscles with shorter fibre pennates and convergent fibres tension is often in knots rather than in lines.

a Parallel   b Fusiform   c Unipennate   d Multipennate   e Bipennate

Fig 4.2 The six muscle shapes

Voluntary muscle works intimately with the nervous system and will, therefore, only contract if a stimulus is applied to it via a motor nerve. Each muscle fibre receives its own nerve impulse so that fine and varied motions are possible. Voluntary muscles also have their own small stored supply of glycogen which is used as fuel for energy. Voluntary muscle tissue differs from other types of muscle tissue in that the muscles tire easily and need regular exercise.

Cardiac muscle

Cardiac muscle is a specialised type of involuntary muscle tissue found only in the walls of the heart. Forming the bulk of the wall of each heart

Fig 4.3 Cardiac muscle tissue

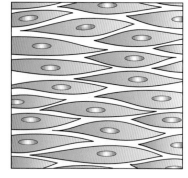

Fig 4.4 Smooth/involuntary muscle tissue

chamber, cardiac muscle contracts rhythmically and continuously to provide the pumping action necessary to maintain a relatively consistent flow of blood throughout the body. Cardiac muscle resembles voluntary muscle tissue in that it is striated due to the actin and myosin filaments. However, it differs in two ways:

● It is branched in structure.
● It has intercalated discs in between each cardiac muscle cell which form strong junctions to assist in the rapid transmission of impulses throughout an entire section of the heart, rather than in bundles.

The contraction of the heart is automatic. The stimulus to contract is stimulated from a specialised area of muscle in the heart called the sinoatrial (SA) node which controls the heart rate.

As the heart has to alter its force of contraction due to regional requirements, its contraction is regulated not only by nerves but also by hormones such as adrenaline in the blood which can speed up contractions.

Smooth muscle

Smooth muscle is also known as involuntary muscle, as it is not under the control of the conscious part of the brain. It is found in the walls of hollow organs such as the stomach, intestines, bladder, uterus and in blood vessels.

The main characteristics of smooth muscle are:

● The muscle cells are spindle-shaped and tapered at both ends.
● Each muscle cell contains one centrally located oval-shaped nucleus.

Smooth muscle has no striations due to the different arrangement of the protein filaments actin and myosin which are attached at their ends to the cell's plasma membrane.

The muscle fibres of smooth muscle are adapted for long, sustained contraction and, therefore, consume very little energy. One of the special features of smooth muscle is that it can stretch and shorten to a greater extent and still maintain its contractile function. Smooth muscle will contract or relax in response to nerve impulses, stretching or hormones but it is not under voluntary control.

Smooth muscle, like voluntary muscle, has muscle tone and this is important in areas such as the intestines where the walls have to maintain a steady pressure on the contents.

Muscle contraction

Muscle tissue has several characteristics which help contribute to the functioning of a muscle:

● **Contractibility** – the capacity of the muscle to shorten and thicken
● **Extensibility** – the ability to stretch when the muscle fibres relax
● **Elasticity** – the ability to return to its original shape after contraction
● **Irritability** – the response to stimuli provided by nerve impulses.

Muscles vary in the speed at which they contract. The muscle in your eyes will be moving very fast as you are reading this page, whilst the muscles in your limbs assisting you in turning the pages will be contracting at a moderate speed. The speed of a muscle contraction is, therefore, modified to meet the demands of the action concerned and the degree of nervous stimulus it has received.

Stimulus to contract

Skeletal or voluntary muscles are moved as a result of nervous stimulus which they receive from the brain via a motor nerve. Each skeletal fibre is connected to the fibre of a nerve cell. Each nerve fibre ends in a motor point which is the end portion of the nerve and is the part through which the stimulus to contract is given to the muscle fibre. A single motor nerve may transmit stimuli to one muscle fibre or as many as 150, depending on the effect of the action required.

The site where the nerve fibre and muscle fibre meet is called a neuromuscular junction. In response to a nerve impulse, the end of the motor nerve fibre secretes a neurotransmitter substance called acetylcholine which diffuses across the junction and stimulates the muscle fibre to contract.

Cardiac and smooth muscle are innervated by the autonomic nervous system.

The contraction of voluntary muscle tissue

The functional characteristic of muscle is its ability to transform chemical energy into mechanical energy in order to exert force. Muscles exert force by contracting or making themselves shorter.

The role of actin and myosin

A voluntary or skeletal muscle consists of many long cylindrical fibres. Each of these fibres is in turn filled with long bundles of even smaller fibres called myofibrils. A myofibril resembles stacked blocks. In each block (or sarcomere) thick filaments containing the protein myosin overlap thin filaments containing the protein actin. Sarcomeres are divided into dark Z lines with their centres known as H zones. As the muscle contracts, its sarcomeres shorten, reducing the distance between the Z lines and the width of the H zone. Muscle fibre contraction results from a sliding movement within the myofibrils in which the actin and myosin filaments merge. Actin and myosin affect contraction in the following way:

- During contraction a sliding movement occurs within the contractile fibres (myofibrils) of the muscle in which the actin protein filaments move inwards towards the myosin and the two filaments merge.
- Cross-bridges of myosin filaments form linkages with actin filaments.
- This action causes the muscle fibres to shorten and thicken and then pull upon their attachments (bones and joints) to effect the movement required.
- The attachment of myosin cross-bridges to actin requires the mineral calcium.
- The nerve impulses leading to contraction cause an increase in calcium ions within the muscle cell.
- During relaxation the muscle fibres elongate and return to their original shape.
- The force of muscle contraction depends upon the number of fibres in a muscle which contract simultaneously. The more fibres involved, the stronger and more powerful the contraction will be.

KEY FACTS

The basic contractile process is the same in cardiac, smooth and voluntary muscles, with movement being achieved through the action of the protein filaments actin and myosin. However, since the requirements are different in terms of speed and force of contraction, the structure of cardiac and smooth muscles are slightly different to voluntary muscle tissue.

The energy needed for muscle contraction

A certain amount of energy is needed to effect the mechanical action of the muscle fibres. This is obtained principally from carbohydrate foods such as glucose in the arterial blood supply. Glucose, which is not required immediately by the body, is converted into glycogen and is stored in the liver and the muscles. Muscle glycogen, therefore, provides the fuel for muscle contraction. The process is as follows:

- During muscle contraction glycogen is broken down by a process called oxidation, where glucose combines with oxygen and releases energy. Oxygen is stored in the form of haemoglobin in the red blood cells and as myoglobin in the muscle cells.
- During oxidation, a chemical compound called ATP (adenosine triphosphate) is formed. Molecules of ATP are contained within voluntary muscle tissue and their function is to temporarily store energy produced from food.
- When the muscle is stimulated to contract, ATP is converted to another chemical compound, ADP (adenosine diphosphate), which releases the energy needed to be used during the phase of muscle contraction.
- During the oxidation of glycogen, a substance called pyruvic acid is formed.
- If plenty of oxygen is available to the body, as in rest or undertaking moderate exercise, then the pyruvic acid is broken down into waste products, carbon dioxide and water, which are excreted into the venous system. This is known as aerobic respiration.
- If insufficient oxygen is available to the body, as may be in the case of vigorous exercise, then the pyruvic acid is converted into lactic acid. This is known as anaerobic respiration.

The effects of increased circulation on muscle contraction

During exercise muscles require more oxygen to cope with the increased demands made on the body. The body is then active in initiating certain circulatory and respiratory changes to the body to meet the increased oxygen requirements of the muscles.

Circulatory changes that occur in the body during muscle contraction

During exercise there is an increased return of venous blood to the heart, owing to the more extensive movements of the diaphragm and the general contractions of the muscles compressing the veins. With the rate and output of each heart beat being increased, a greater volume of blood is circulated around the body which leads to an increase in the amount of oxygen in the blood.

More blood is distributed to the muscle and less to the intestine and skin to meet the needs of the exercising muscles. During exercise a muscle may receive as much as 15 times its normal flow of blood.

Respiratory changes

The presence of lactic acid in the blood stimulates the respiratory centre in the brain increasing the rate and depth of breath, producing panting. The

KEY FACT

The waste product lactic acid, which diffuses into the bloodstream after vigorous exercise, causes the muscles to ache. This condition is known as muscle fatigue which is defined as the loss of the ability of a muscle to contract efficiently due to insufficient oxygen, exhaustion of energy supply and the accumulation of lactic acid.

rate and depth of breath remains above normal for a while after strenuous exercise has ceased. Large amounts of oxygen are taken in to allow the cells of the muscles and the liver to dispose of the accumulated lactic acid by oxidising it and converting it to glucose or glycogen. Lactic acid is formed in the tissues in amounts far greater than can be immediately disposed of by available oxygen. The extra oxygen needed to remove the accumulated lactic acid is what is called the oxygen debt which must be repaid after the exercise is over.

The effects of temperature on muscle contraction

Exercising muscles produces heat, which is carried away from the muscle by the bloodstream and is distributed to the rest of the body. Exercise is, therefore, an effective way to increase body temperature. When muscle tissue is warm, the process of contraction will occur faster due to the acceleration of the chemical reactions and the increase in circulation. However, it is possible for heat cramps to occur in muscles which are exercised at high temperatures, as increased sweating causes loss of sodium in the body, leading to a reduction in the concentration of sodium ions in the blood supplying the muscle.

Cramp occurs when muscles become over-contracted and hence go into spasm. This is usually caused by an irritated nerve or an imbalance of mineral salts such as sodium in the body. Cramp most commonly affects the calf muscles or the soles of the feet. Cramp can be very painful as it is a sudden involuntary contraction of the muscle.

Treatment to relieve the pain of cramp includes stretching the affected muscle group and using soothing effluerage movements to help to relax the muscles. Conversely, as muscle tissue is cooled, the chemical reactions and circulation slow, causing the contraction to be slower. This causes an involuntary increase in muscle tone known as shivering that increases body temperature in response to cold.

Muscle tone

Even in a relaxed muscle, a few muscle fibres remain contracted to give the muscle a certain degree of firmness. At any given time a small number of motor units in a muscle are stimulated to contract and cause tension in the muscle rather than full contraction and movement, whilst the others remain relaxed. The group of motor units functioning in this way change periodically so that muscle tone is maintained without fatigue. This state of partial contraction of a muscle is known as muscle tone and is important for maintaining body posture.

Good muscle tone may be recognised by the muscles appearing firm and rounded, wherseas poor muscle tone may be recognised by the muscles appearing loose and flattened.

Muscles with less than the normal degree of tone are said to be flaccid and when the muscle tone is greater than normal the muscles become spastic and rigid.

Muscle attachments

In order to understand how skeletal muscles produce movement, it is helpful to first understand how muscles are attached to the rest of the body.

Tendons

Tendons are tightly woven, white, glistening tough fibrous bands or cords that link muscle to bone. They do not stretch or contract the way muscles do and, therefore, are not at all elastic.

A tendon's blood supply is limited so it usually does not heal quickly or easily. Tendons are mechanically strong, as their primary role is to transmit the contractile force of the muscle to the bone. For this reason, tendons are relatively inflexible structures, designed to be strongest in the direction of tensile stress.

Despite their great strength, tendons are most susceptible to excessive tensile stress injuries. Luckily complete tendon tears or ruptures are infrequent (the most common ruptured tendon is the Achilles tendon).

Ligaments

Ligaments are strong, fibrous, elastic tissues that are usually cord-like in nature. They are placed parallel with or closely interlaced with one another which creates a white, shining silvery effect. A ligament is pliant and flexible so as to allow good freedom of movement but is also strong, tough and inextensible (does not stretch).

Their attachments to various skeletal components help to maintain the bones in correct relationship to one another, stabilising the joints. When torn, ligaments heal slowly due to the fact that they have a relatively poor blood supply compared with muscles and tendons.

The orientation of a ligament's fibres (parallel arrangements complemented by transverse fibres) gives the ligament an ability to resist stress in several different planes. Ligaments also contain a greater concentration of elastin than a tendon. This will allow the ligament a small degree of 'give' before it pulls taut at a particular joint. This small amount of 'give' is important because if ligaments were as rigid and 'ungiving' to tensile stress as a tendon, the frequency of ligament injuries would be much greater. The most common injury to a ligament is a sprain. Ligamentous tearing is generally referred to as a sprain.

Fascia

Fascia consists of fibrous connective tissue that envelops certain muscles which then forms partitions for others. Fascia is all encompassing. It packages, supports and envelops all the body's muscles and organs. It separates different muscles yet allows them to glide smoothly beside each other. The fascial planes provide pathways for nerves, blood vessels and lymphatic vessels.

Fascia, therefore, plays a key role in maintaining the 'health' of a muscle. When these cellophane-like sheets become adhered to neighbouring muscle tissue, efficiency and function can be significantly diminished. If the fascia becomes torn or over-stressed, its subsequent loss of elasticity will cause and maintain chronic tissue congestion.

Origins and insertions

Muscle attachments are known by the terms origin and insertion. Generally, the end of the muscle closest to the centre of the body is referred to as the origin, and the insertion is the furthest attachment.

BODY FACT

One of the most problematic features of fascia is its response to prolonged immobilisation. If the body is held in one position for long periods of time, the fascia has a tendency to adapt to that position. This is especially problematic when the fascia is held in a shortened position. When it is kept in this shortened position, it will structurally adapt to that position and resist an attempt to return to its normal length.

Origins are often shorter and broader and attach over a larger area, while insertions are commonly longer and the fibres are more densely concentrated, attaching to a smaller bone area. The insertion is generally the most movable point and, therefore, the point at which the muscle work is done.

Muscle movement

In the coordination of movement muscles work in pairs of groups. Muscles are classified by functions as agonists (prime movers), antagonists, synergists and fixators (stabilisers).

Although muscles are usually described as performing a particular action, they do not act alone. Any movement is the result of cooperation between a large number of muscles which is coordinated in the cerebellum in the brain for smooth efficient actions.

Antagonists
This is when two muscles or sets of muscles pull in opposite directions to each other. They don't actually work against one another but work in a reciprocal complementary way with one relaxing to allow the other to contract.

Agonists/prime movers
This is known as the main activating muscle. It is important to note that these terms are used in relation to a specific action. The roles are, therefore, relative to one another and are interchangeable. An example is the action of the biceps and triceps of the upper arm. Biceps are the agonist in flexion of the elbow joint, and triceps are the antagonist. In relation to extending or straightening the elbow the roles are reversed.

Synergysts
This term refers to muscles on the same side of a joint that work together to perform the same movement. An example of this is the flexing of the elbow. The biceps actually work synergistically with the brachialis muscle that lies underneath it.

Fixators
These are muscles that stabilise a bone to give a steady base from which the agonist works. For the biceps and triceps to flex and extend the elbow joint, muscles around the shoulder and upper back control the position of the arm.

Biomechanically, muscles do one of two things – stretch or contract. Muscular contractions can be isometric or isotonic. Isotonic contractions may be further classified as either concentric or eccentric. The opposite of contracting is stretching which extends the muscles.

Isometric contraction
This is when the muscle works without actual movements (*iso* means same and *metric* means length). Postural muscles work by isometric contraction.

STUDY TIP

Learning muscles can be daunting. It is first helpful to break down the information into manageable chunks and learn a few muscles at a time.

The following may help you when studying muscles:

a Is there a clue in the name of the muscle as to where it is located in the body (for example, the tibialis anterior muscle is located alongside the tibia bone in the front of the lower leg)?

b Try to visualise where the muscle is on your or a client's body.

c Look for information that will help you remember its action (see key facts in the last column of the table below).

d If you know where the muscle is located and attached you can work out its action by moving that body part and feeling the muscle contracting.

Isotonic contraction

This term refers to when the muscle force is considered to be constant (tonic meaning the same tone or tension) but the muscle length changes. There are two types of isotonic contraction:

- **Concentric contractions** (towards the centre) – this type of contraction occurs when the muscle shortens to move the attachments closer such as when the biceps bends up the forearm.
- **Eccentric contractions** (away from the centre) – this type of contraction occurs when a muscle is stretched as it tries to resist a force pulling the bones of attachment away from one another, such as when tensing the biceps and someone pulls your forearm straight.

During many everyday actions, both isometric and isotonic contractions occur simultaneously. As an example, in a standing position the quadriceps muscle straightens the knee when standing to keep you upright, thereby preventing your knee from bending (isometric contraction). If you sit down slowly, the muscle is stretched and an eccentric contraction controls the rate at which the knee bends to lower the body. If you then stand up, the muscle works concentrically to straighten the knee again.

The muscles of the head and neck

Name of muscle	Position	Attachments	Action/s	Key facts
Frontalis (front-**ta**-lis)	Extends over the forehead	Attaches to the skin of the eyebrows and the frontal bone at the hairline	Wrinkles the forehead and raises the eyebrows	Used when expressing surprise
Occipitalis (ok-sip-it-**ta**-lis)	Base/back of skull	Attached to the occipital bone and the skin of the scalp	Moves the scalp backwards	Is united to the frontalis muscle by a broad tendon called the epicranial aponeurosis which covers the skull like a cap
Temporalis (tem-po-ra-lis)	Fan-shaped muscle situated on the side of the skull above and in front of the ear	Attaches to the temporal bone and to the upper part of the mandible	Raises the lower jaw when chewing	Muscle becomes tightened with a tension headache
Orbicularis oculi (or-bik-**you**-la-**ris** ock-you-**ly**)	Circular muscle surrounding the eye	Attached to the bones at the outer edge and the skin of the upper and lower eyelids at the inner edge	Closes the eye	Used when blinking or winking It also compresses the lacrimal gland, aiding the flow of tears

Name of muscle	Position	Attachments	Action/s	Key facts
Orbicularis oris (or-bik-**you**-la-**ris** or-ris)	Circular muscle that surrounds the mouth	Its fibres attach to the maxilla, mandible, the lips and the buccinator muscle	Closes the mouth	Used when shaping the lips for speech and when kissing It also contracts the lips when tense
Corrugator (**kor**-u-gay-**tor**)	Located in between the eyebrows	Attached to the frontalis muscle and the inner edge of the eyebrow	Brings the eyebrows together	Used when frowning
Procerus (pro-**ser**-rus)	Located in between the eyebrows	Attached to the nasal bones and the frontalis muscle	Draws the eyebrows inwards	Creates a puzzled expression
Nasalis (nay-sa-**lis**)	Located at sides of the nose	Attached to the maxillae bones and the nostrils	Dilates and compresses the nostrils	Used when blowing the nose
Zygomatic major and minor/ zygomaticus (zi-go-**mat**-ik-**us**)	Lies in the cheek	Extends from the zygomatic bone to the angle of the mouth	Draws the angle of the mouth upward and laterally	Used when laughing or smiling
Levator labii superioris (le-vay-**tor** lay-be-eye soo-pee-**ri**-o-ris)	Above the lip, located towards the inner cheek beside the nose	Extends from the upper jaw to the skin of the corners of the mouth and the upper lip	Raises the upper lip and the corner of the mouth	Used to create a snarling expression
Levator anguli oris (le-vay-**tor** ang-you-**lie o**-ris)	Above the lip, located at an angle above the side of the mouth	Extends from the maxilla (upper jaw) to the angle of the mouth	Raises the corner of the mouth	Used when smiling, is also known as the caninus (kay-ni-nus) as its contraction can result in the teeth, especially the canine tooth, becoming visible
Depressor anguli oris (dee-**pres**-or ang-you-**lie o**-ris)	Side of chin extending down at an angle from the side of mouth	Extends from the mandible (lower jaw) to the angle of the mouth	Draws the corners of the mouth downwards	Used when expressing sadness or uncertainty
Depressor labii inferioris (dee-**pres**-or **lay**-be-eye in-fee-**ri**-o-**ris**)	Side of chin, extending down from lower lip	Extends from the mandible to the angle of the mouth	Pulls the lower lip downwards	Used when expressing sorrow, doubt or irony
Risorius (ri-sor-**ri**-us)	Triangular-shaped muscle lying horizontally on the cheek, joining at the corners of the mouth (lies above the buccinator)	Attached to the zygomatic bone at one end and the skin of the corner of the mouth at the other	Pulls the corner of the mouth sideways and outwards	Used when grinning

(Continued)

Name of muscle	Position	Attachments	Action/s	Key facts
Buccinator (buk-sin-**a**-tor)	Main muscle of the cheek	Attached to the maxilla and mandible and the muscles of the lips	Compresses the cheeks when sucking or blowing	Used when blowing a balloon or blowing a trumpet Helps hold food in contact with the teeth when chewing
Mentalis (men-**ta**-lis)	Radiates from the lower lip over the centre of the chin	Attached to the mandible and the skin of the lower lip	Elevates the lower lip and wrinkles the skin of the chin	Used when expressing displeasure and when pouting
Masseter (ma-**sa**-ter)	Thick, flattened muscle at sides of cheek/jaw	Extends from maxilla and zygomatic bone to the mandible	Raises the jaw and exerts pressure on the teeth when chewing	Main muscle of mastication Can be felt just in front of the ear when the teeth are clenched
Lateral pterygoids (lat-er-al ter-i-goyds)	Outer part of cheeks	Extends from the sphenoid bone to the mandible and temporomandibular joint	Opens the jaw and moves mandible when chewing	Tension in these muscles may be associated with dysfunction of the temporomandibular joint (TMJ syndrome)
Medial pterygoids (mee-dee-al ter-i-goyd)	Outer part of cheeks	Extends from the sphenoid bone to the internal surface of the mandible	Closes the jaw and moves the mandible when chewing	Tension in these muscles may be associated with dysfunction of the temporomandibular joint (TMJ syndrome)
Sternocleido-mastoid (ster-no-**kli**-do-**mas**-toyd)	Long muscle that lies obliquely across each side of the neck	Extends upwards from the sternum and clavicle at one end to the mastoid process (back of the ear)	When working together they flex the neck (pull the chin down towards the chest) and when working individually, they rotate the head to the opposite side	Spasm of the sternomastoid muscle results in a condition known as torticollis or wryneck Sternomastoid is the only muscle that moves the head but is not attached to any vertebrae
Platysma (pla-tiz-ma)	Superficial muscle that covers the front of the neck	Extends from the chest (fascia covering the upper part of pectoralis major and deltoid) up either side of the neck to the chin	Depresses the lower jaw and lower lips	Used in yawning and when creating a pouting expression

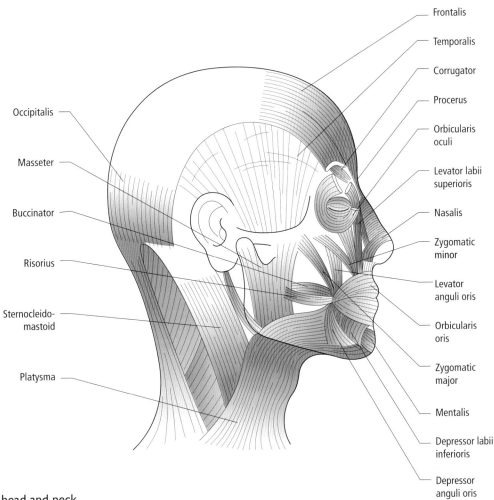

Occipitalis
Masseter
Buccinator
Risorius
Sternocleido-mastoid
Platysma

Frontalis
Temporalis
Corrugator
Procerus
Orbicularis oculi
Levator labii superioris
Nasalis
Zygomatic minor
Levator anguli oris
Orbicularis oris
Zygomatic major
Mentalis
Depressor labii inferioris
Depressor anguli oris

Fig 4.5 The muscles of the head and neck

Student activity

Now complete Activity 4.1 in the resources for this book on Dynamic Learning Online.

The muscles of the posterior of the neck

Name of muscle	Position	Attachments	Action/s	Key facts
Splenius capitis (**splee**-knee-**us** kap-**i**-tis)	Long muscle in posterior of neck	Extends from the spinous processes of C7–T3 (7th cervical to 3rd thoracic vertebrae) to the mastoid process of the temporal bone and the occipital bone	Extension of the head and neck, lateral flexion of the head and neck	Shaped like a bandage and attaches onto the head The right and left splenius captitis muscles form a 'V' shape
Splenius cervicus (**splee**-knee-**us** ser-**vi**-sis)	Long muscle in posterior of neck (fibres slightly thinner and longer than splenius capitis)	Extends from the spinous processes of T3–T6 (3rd thoracic to 6th thoracic vertebrae) to the transverse processes of C1–C3 (1st cervical to 3rd cervical vertebrae)	Extension of the neck, lateral flexion of the neck	Shaped like a bandage and attaches onto the cervical spine. The right and left splenius cervicus muscles form a 'V' shape

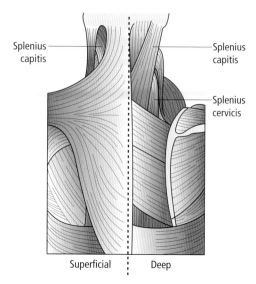

Splenius capitis

Splenius capitis

Splenius cervicis

Superficial | Deep

Fig 4.6 The muscles of the posterior of the neck

The muscles of the shoulder

Name of muscle	Position	Attachments	Action/s	Key facts
Trapezius (**tra**-pee-**zee**-us)	Large triangular-shaped muscle in upper back Its fibres are arranged in three groups – upper, middle and lower	Extends horizontally from the base of the skull (occipital bone) and cervical/thoracic vertebrae to scapula Its fibres are arranged in three groups – upper, middle and lower	The upper fibres raise the shoulder girdle, the middle fibres pull the scapula towards the vertebral column and the lower fibres draw the scapula and shoulder downwards	One of the most commonly found muscles to hold upper body tension, causing discomfort and restrictions in the neck and shoulder
Levator scapula (**le**-vay-**tor** skap-**you**-lee)	Strap-like muscle that runs almost vertically through the neck	Cervical vertebrae to the scapula	Elevates and adducts the scapula	Due to its attachments, tension in the levator scapula can affect mobility of both the neck and the shoulder
Rhomboids (**rom**-boyds)	Fibres of these muscles lie between the scapulae	They attach to the upper thoracic vertebrae at one end and the medial border of the scapula at the other end	Adduct the scapula	Also known as the 'Christmas tree' muscles, due to arrangement of fibres Tension in these muscles often results in aching and soreness in between the scapulae

Name of muscle	Position	Attachments	Action/s	Key facts
Supraspinatus (soo-pra-**spy**-nay-**tus**)	Located in the depression above the spine of the scapula	Attached to the spine of the scapula at one end and the humerus at the other	Abducts humerus, assisting the deltoid	Is the only muscle of the rotator cuff that does not rotate the humerus
Infraspinatus (in-fra-**spy**-nay-**tus**)	Deep muscle covering the lower part of the scapula	Attaches to the middle two-thirds of the scapula below the spine of the scapula at one end and the top of the humerus at the other	Rotates humerus laterally (outwards)	One of the four rotator cuff muscles Tension in this muscle can affect the range of mobility in the arm and the shoulder
Teres major (te-reez **may**-jor)	Deep, small muscle located between lower border of scapula and humerus	Attaches to the bottom lateral edge of the scapula at one end and the back of the humerus at the other	Adducts and medially (inwardly) rotates humerus	Sometimes referred to as the 'little helper' of the latissimus dorsi muscle because they run together between the scapula and the humerus
Teres minor (te-reez **my**-nor)	Deep, small muscle located above teres major	Attaches to the lateral edge of the scapula at one end and into the top of the posterior of the humerus at the other	Rotates humerus laterally (outwards)	One of the four rotator cuff muscles Although the teres major and minor may appear similar by name, they wrap around the humerus in opposite directions and therefore have opposite rotary actions
Subscapularis (sub-skap-u-la-**ris**)	Large muscle located beneath the scapula	Attaches to the inside surface of the scapula to the anterior of the top of the humerus	Rotates the humerus medially, draws the humerus forwards and down when the arm is raised	One of the four rotator cuff muscles Often implicated in the case of a frozen shoulder
Deltoid (del-toid)	Thick triangular muscle that caps the top of the humerus and shoulder	Attaches to the clavicle and the spine of the scapula at one end and to the side of the humerus at the other	Abducts arm, draws the arm backwards and forwards	The deltoid has anterior, lateral and posterior fibres and these give the shoulder its characteristic shape

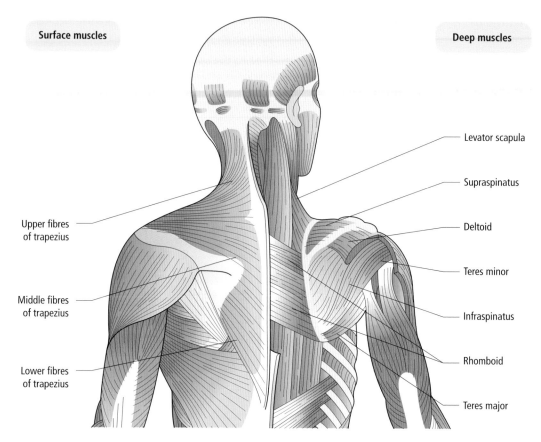

Surface muscles

Deep muscles

Levator scapula

Supraspinatus

Upper fibres of trapezius

Deltoid

Teres minor

Middle fibres of trapezius

Infraspinatus

Lower fibres of trapezius

Rhomboid

Teres major

Fig 4.7 The muscles of the shoulder

The muscles of the upper limb

Name of muscle	Position	Attachments	Action/s	Key facts
Coraco-brachialis (**kor**-a-**ko**-bra-**key**-al-**is**)	Medial surface of the upper arm	Extends from the scapula to the middle of the humerus	Flexes and adducts the humerus	Name of this muscle is related to the coracoid process (in the scapula) and the brachium (the arm)
Biceps (**by**-seps)	Anterior surface of upper arm (humerus)	Attaches to the scapula at one end and the radius and flexor muscles of the forearm at the other	Flexes the forearm at the elbow and supinates the forearm	Actions of the biceps muscle are likened to the action of removing a corkscrew from a wine bottle
Triceps (**try**-seps)	Posterior surface of the upper arm	Attaches to the posterior of the humerus and outer edge of the scapula at one end and to the ulna below the elbow at the other	Extension (straightening) of the forearm	Also referred to as the 'boxer's muscle' as it is used when delivering a 'knock-out' punch

Name of muscle	Position	Attachments	Action/s	Key facts
Brachialis (**bray**-key-**al**-is)	Lies beneath biceps	Attaches to the distal half of the anterior surface of the humerus at one end and the ulna at the other	Flexes the forearm at the elbow	Strong and fairly large muscle, which accounts for much of the contour of the biceps muscle
Pronator teres (pro-**nay**-tor **te**-reez)	Crosses the anterior aspect of the elbow	Attaches to the distal end of the humerus and the upper aspect of the ulna at one end and the lateral surface of the radius at the other	Pronates and flexes forearm	Due to the fact that the fibres of the pronator teres cross the elbow joint, irritation and inflammation of this muscle may contribute to the condition 'tennis elbow'
Supinator (**sue**-pin-**a**-tor)	Runs diagonally across forearm crossing the elbow joint to outer edge of radius	Attaches to the lateral aspect of the humerus and the radius	Supinates the forearm	Due to the fact that the fibres of the supinator cross the elbow joint, irritation and inflammation of this muscle may contribute to the condition 'tennis elbow' (as above)
Brachioradialis (**bray**-key-o-**ray**-dee-**al**-is)	Anterior of forearm; connects the humerus to the radius	Attaches to the distal end of the humerus at one end and the radius at the other end	Flexes forearm at the elbow	Can be felt as the bulge on the radial side of the forearm. Sometimes nicknamed the 'hitchhiker muscle' for its characteristic action of flexing the forearm in a position halfway between full pronation and full supination
Flexor carpi radialis (**fleks**-or **kar**-pie **ray**-dee-**a**-lis)	Along radial side of anterior of forearm	Extends from medial end of the humerus to radial side of forearm and the base of the second and third metacarpal	Flexion of the wrist	Any of the flexor muscles in the forearm can become easily inflamed due to excess pressure and overwork, a common example being working on a keyboard for extended periods of time
Flexor carpi ulnaris (**fleks**-or **kar**-pie ul-**na**-ris)	Along ulnar side of anterior of forearm	Extends from the medial end of the humerus to the pisiform and hamate carpal bones and the base of the fifth metacarpal	Flexion of the wrist	See above

(Continued)

Name of muscle	Position	Attachments	Action/s	Key facts
Flexor carpi digitorum (**fleks**-or **kar**-pie)	Largest flexor on anterior of forearm (lies beneath other flexors)	Extends from the medial end of the humerus, the anterior of the ulna and radius to the anterior surfaces of second to fifth fingers	Flexion of the fingers	See above
Extensor carpi radialis (eks-**ten**-sor **kar**-pie ray-dee-a-lis)	Extends along the radial side of the posterior of the forearm	From above the lateral end of the humerus to the posterior of the base of the second metacarpal	Extension of the wrist	Any of the extensor muscles in the foream can become easily inflamed due to excess pressure and overwork, a common example being working on a keyboard for extended periods of time
Extensor carpi ulnaris (eks-**ten**-sor **kar**-pie ul-**na**-ris)	Extends along the ulnar side of the posterior of the forearm	From above the lateral end of the humerus to the ulna and the posterior side of the base of the fifth metacarpal	Extension of the wrist	See above
Extensor digitorum (eks-**ten**-sor dij-i-**toe**-rum)	Along lateral side of posterior of forearm	Extends from the lateral end of the humerus to the second and fifth phalanges	Extension of the fingers	See above

The muscles of the hand

Thenar muscles

This is an eminence of soft tissue located on the radial side of the palm of the hand. There are three muscles of the thenar eminence:

- abductor pollicis brevis
- flexor pollicis brevis
- opponens pollicis.

Action – all three muscles move the thumb.

Hypothenar muscles

This is an eminence of soft tissue located on the ulnar side of the palm of the hand. There are three muscles of the hypothenar eminence:

- abductor digiti minimi manus
- flexor digiti minimi manus
- opponens digiti minimi.

Action – all three muscles move the little finger.

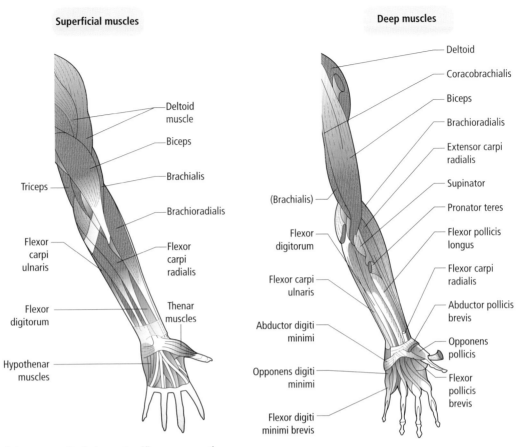

Fig 4.8 The muscles of the upper limb (anterior/flexor aspect)

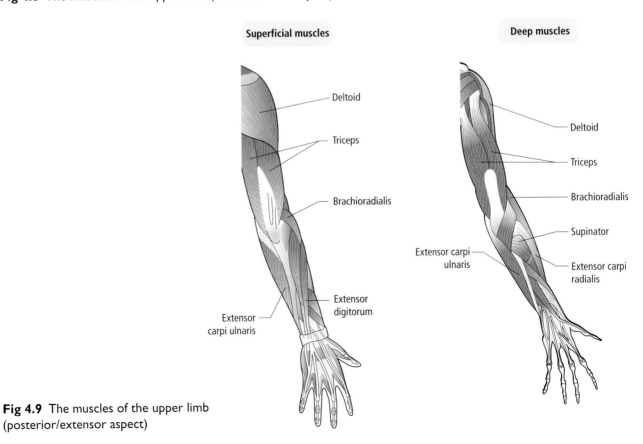

Fig 4.9 The muscles of the upper limb
(posterior/extensor aspect)

The muscles of the lower limb

Name of muscle	Position	Attachments	Action/s	Key facts
Quadriceps extensor (**quad**-ri-seps eks-**ten**-sor) The quadriceps is made up of four muscles: **rectus femoris**, **vastus lateralis**, **vastus intermedius**, **vastus medialis**	Anterior aspect of the thigh	Attached to the pelvic girdle (rectus femoris) and femur (vastus group) at one end and to the patella and tibia at the other end	As a group they extend the knee and flex the hip	The quadriceps is a group of strong muscles used for walking, kicking and raising the body from a sitting or squatting position
Sartorius (sar-**tor**-ee-us)	Crosses the anterior of the thigh	Attached to the ilium of the pelvis and the medial aspect of the tibia	Flexes the hip and knee and rotates the thigh laterally (turns it outwards)	Due to its unusual position, the sartorius can flex both the hip and the knee. Over contraction of the sartorius can lead to knee problems because turning the leg outwards puts pressure on the knee Sartorius is also the longest muscle in the human body
Adductors (ad-**duk**-tors This is a group of four muscles: **adductor brevis**, **adductor longus**, **adductor magnus** and **pectineus**	Situated on the medial aspect of the thigh	Attached to the lower part of the pelvic girdle at one end (pubic bones and the ischium) and the inside of the femur at the other end	As a group they adduct and laterally rotate the thigh They also flex the hip	The adductors are important muscles in the maintenance of posture Groin strains are common problems associated with these muscles
Gracilis (gra-**sil**-is)	Long strap-like muscle	Attached to the lower edge of the pubic bone at one end and the upper part of the medial aspect of the tibia at the other end	Adducts thigh, flexes knee and hip, medially (inwardly) rotates the thigh and tibia	Gracilis muscle is the second longest muscle in the human body
Hamstrings	Consist of three muscles – two situated on the inside of the thigh (**semitendinosus** and **semi-membranosus**) and one on the outside of the thigh (**biceps femoris**)	Posterior aspect of the thigh attaches to the lower part of the pelvis (ischium) and the lower part of the posterior of the femur to either side of the posterior of the tibia	Flex the knee and extend the hip	The hamstrings contract powerfully when raising the body from a stooped position and when climbing stairs

Name of muscle	Position	Attachments	Action/s	Key facts
Tensor fascia latae (**ten**-sor **fash**-ee-a **la**-tee)	Runs laterally down the side of the thigh	Attached to the outer edge of the ilium of the pelvis and runs via the long fascia lata tendon to the lateral aspect of the top of the tibia	Flexes, abducts and medially rotates thigh	Attached to a broad sheet of connective tissue (fascia lata tendon), which helps to strengthen the knee joint when walking and running
Gastrocnemius (**gas**-trok-**nee**-me-us)	Large superficial calf muscle with two bellies (central portion of the muscle) on the posterior of the lower leg	Attached to the lower aspect of the posterior of the femur across the back of the knee and runs via the Achilles tendon to the calcaneum at the back of the heel	Plantar flexes the foot and assists in knee flexion	Provides the push during fast walking and running
Soleus (**so**-lee-us)	Deep in the gastrocnemius in the calf	Attached to the tibia and fibula just below the back of the knee at one end and runs via the Achilles tendon to the calcaneum at the other end	Plantar flexes the foot	A thicker and flatter muscle than the gastrocnemius and accounts for the contours of the gastrocnemius being so visible
Tibialis anterior (tib-ee-a-lis an-**tee**-ri-or)	Anterior aspect of the lower leg	Attached to the outer side of the tibia at one end and the medial cuneiform	Dorsiflexes and inverts the foot	If the tibialis anterior muscle becomes weak, it can lead to the lower leg rolling inwards due to the collapse of the medial longitudinal arch of the foot
Tibialis posterior (tib-ee-**a**-lis pos-**tee**-ri-or)	Posterior aspect of the lower leg, very deeply situated in the calf	Attached to the back of the tibia and fibula at one end and to the navicular, third cuneiform and second, third and fourth metatarsals at the other end	Assists in plantar flexion and inverts the foot	Weakness in this muscle can cause the feet to turn out from the ankles rather than the knees. This causes the muscle to stretch and the medial longitudinal arch of the foot to drop
Peroneus longus/brevis (pero-knee-us long-us)	Situated on the lateral aspect of the lower leg	Attach to the fibula to the underneath of the first (longus) and fifth metatarsal (brevis)	Plantar flexes and everts the foot	Going over on to the outside of the ankle, as in a trip or a fall, can sprain the peroneal muscles in the lower leg. If the injury is not treated properly it can affect future stability of the ankle joint
Flexor digitorum longus (**fleks**-or dij-i-**toe**-rum **long**-us)	Medial to the tibialis anterior muscle	Extends from the middle third of the posterior of the tibia to the plantar surface of the second to fifth toes	Flexion of the toes, plantar flexion and inversion of the foot	Flexor and extensor muscles of the lower leg can become weak due to excess pressure and overuse in walking and running
Flexor hallicus longus (**fleks**-or hal-**oo**-sis **long**-us)	On the outer side of the lower leg, towards the back of the lower leg	Extends from the distal two-thirds of the posterior fibula to the plantar surface of the big toe	Flexion of big toe, plantar flexion and inversion of foot	See above

(Continued)

Name of muscle	Position	Attachments	Action/s	Key facts
Extensor digitorum longus (eks-**ten**-sor **long**-us)	Lateral to the tibialis anterior muscle	Extends from the proximal two-thirds of the anterior of the fibula to the dorsal surface of the second to fifth toes	Extension of second to fifth toes, dorsiflexion and eversion of foot	See above
Extensor hallicus longus (eks-**ten**-sor hal-**oo**-sis **long**-us)	Runs down the anterior of the lower leg	Extends from the middle third of the anterior of the fibula to the dorsal surface of the big toe	Extension of big toe, dorsiflexion and inversion of foot	See above

Fig 4.10 The muscles of the anterior of the lower limb

The muscles of the pelvic floor

The **levator ani** and the **coccygeus** are the muscles that form the pelvic floor. These muscles support and elevate the organs of the pelvic cavity such as the uterus and the bladder. They provide a counterbalance to increased intra-abdominal pressure which would expel the contents of the bladder, rectum and the uterus.

During childbirth these muscles can become weakened and need to be strengthened by pelvic floor exercises as soon as possible after the birth.

Superficial muscles

Gluteus medius

Gluteus maximus

Biceps femoris

Semitendinosus

Lateral head of gastrocnemius

Semimembranosus

Medial head of gastrocnemius

Deep muscles

Piriformis

Tendon of semitendinosus (cut)

Gracilis

Semimembranosus

Tendon of semi-tendinosus (cut)

Tibialis posterior

Flexor digitorum longus

Achilles tendon

Gluteus minimus

Tendon of long head of biceps femoris (cut)

Adductor magnus

Short head of biceps femoris

Tendon of long head of biceps femoris (cut)

Soleus

Peroneus longus

Flexor hallucis longus

Fig 4.11 The muscles of the posterior of the lower limb

The muscles of the anterior aspect of the trunk

Name of muscle	Position	Attachments	Action/s	Key facts
Pectoralis major (pek-to-ra-lis **may**-jor)	Thick, fan-shaped muscle covering the anterior surface of the upper chest	Attaches to the clavicle and the sternum at one end and to the humerus at the other end	Adducts arm, medially (inwardly) rotates arm	Tightness in this muscle can cause restrictions of the chest and postural disortions (rounded shoulders)
Pectoralis minor (pek-to-ra-lis **my**-nor)	Thin muscle that lies beneath the pectoralis major	Fibres attach laterally and upwards from the ribs at one end to the scapula at the other end	Draws the shoulder downwards and forwards	Used during forced expiration, as in coughing Accessory respiratory muscle
Serratus anterior (ser-**at**-tus an-**tee**-ri-or)	Broad, curved muscle located on the side of the chest/rib cage below the axilla	Attaches to the outer surface of the upper eighth or ninth rib at one end and to the inner surface of the scapula, along the medial edge nearest the spine	Pulls the scapula downwards and forwards	Has a serrated appearance which comes from attaching onto separate ribs
External obliques (**eks**-turn-al o-**bleek**)	Laterally at the sides of the waist	Fibres slant downwards from the lower ribs to the pelvic girdle and the linea alba (tendon running from the bottom of the sternum to the pubic symphysis)	Flexes, rotates and sidebends the trunk It compresses the contents of the abdomen	Often referred to as the pocket muscles as their fibres run in the direction in which you put your hands in your pocket
Internal obliques (in-turn-al o-**bleek**)	Broad, thin sheet of muscle located beneath the external obliques	Fibres run up and forward from the pelvic girdle to the lower ribs	Flexes, rotates and sidebends the trunk Compresses the contents of the abdomen	Fibres of the internal obliques are deeper and run at right angles to the external obliques
Rectus abdominis (**rek**-tus ab-**dom**-i-nis)	Long, strap-like muscle extending medially along the length of the abdomen	Attaches to the pubic bones at one end and the ribs and the sternum at the other	Flexes the vertebral column, flexes the trunk (as in a sit-up), compresses the abdominal cavity	Has three fibrous bands that give the muscle a segmented appearance and divides it into the so-called 'six pack'
Transversus abdominus (trans-**ver**-sus ab-**dom**-i-nis)	Large, deep muscle with fibres extending across anterior of abdominal cavity	Attaches to the inner surfaces of the ribs (last six) and iliac crest at one end and extends down to the pubis via the linea alba (a long tendon that extends from the bottom of the sternum to the pubic symphysis)	Compression of the abdominal contents and supports the organs of the abdominal cavity	Often called the corset muscle because it wraps around the abdomen like a corset

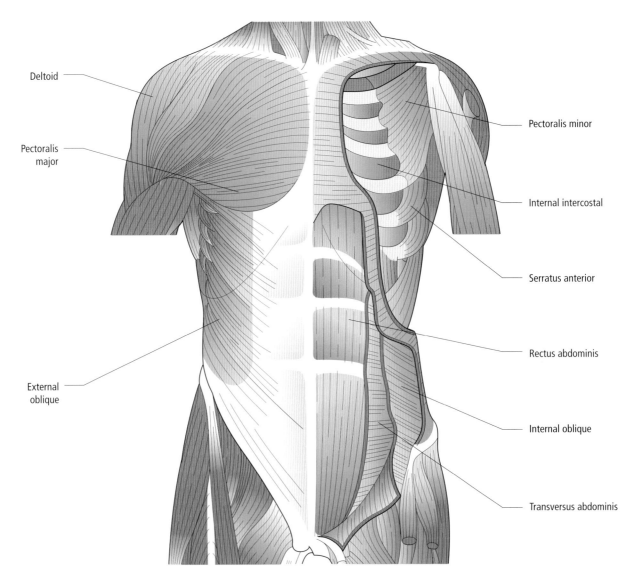

Deltoid

Pectoralis major

External oblique

Pectoralis minor

Internal intercostal

Serratus anterior

Rectus abdominis

Internal oblique

Transversus abdominis

Fig 4.12 The muscles of the anterior of the trunk

The muscles of respiration

Name of muscle	Position	Attachments	Action/s	Key facts
Diaphragm (**di**-a-fram)	Large, dome-shaped muscle that separates the thorax from the abdomen	Attaches to the lower part of the sternum, lower six ribs and upper three lumbar vertebrae and its fibres converge to meet on a central tendon in the abdominal cavity	On contraction the diaphragm flattens to expand the volume of the thoracic cavity to assist inspiration. Upon relaxation and expiration it returns to its dome shape	An unusual muscle in that it is under both unconscious control, as in the regulation of breathing from the brain, and conscious control (in that we can choose to override the brainstem control to hold our breath, sigh, sing or talk)

Name of muscle	Position	Attachments	Action/s	Key facts
External intercostals (**eks**-turn-al in-ter-**kos**-tals)	Superficial muscles that occupy the space between the ribs (positioned on the outside)	Attach to the spaces between the ribs	Help to elevate the rib cage during inhalation	Help to increase the depth of the thoracic cavity
Internal intercostals (**in**-turn-al in-ter-**kos**-tals)	Lie deep to the external intercostals (positioned on the inside)	Attach to the spaces between the ribs	Depress the rib cage which helps to move air out of the lungs when exhaling	Used during forced expiration (as in coughing)

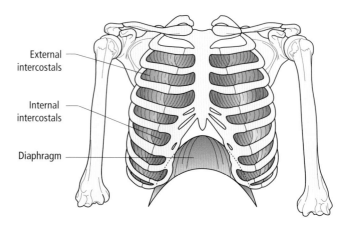

External intercostals

Internal intercostals

Diaphragm

Fig 4.13 The muscles of respiration

The muscles of the posterior aspect of the trunk

Name of muscle	Position	Attachments	Action/s	Key facts
Erector spinae (ee-**rek**-tor **spee**-nee)	Made up of separate bands of muscle that lie in the groove between the vertebral column and the ribs	Attaches to the sacrum and iliac crest at one end to the ribs, transverse and spinous processes of the vertebrae and the occipital bone at the other end of the ribs	Extension, lateral flexion and rotation of the vertebral column	A very important postural muscle as it helps to extend the spine

(*Continued*)

Name of muscle	Position	Attachments	Action/s	Key facts
Latissimus dorsi (la-**tis**-i-mus **door**-si)	Large sheet of muscle extending across the back of the thorax	Broad muscle that attaches to the posterior of the iliac crest and sacrum, lower six thoracic and five lumbar vertebrae at one end and the humerus at the other end	Extends, adducts and rotates the humerus medially	Often referred top as the 'swimmer's muscle' as it allows extension of the arm in water One of the major muscles implicated in lower back pain due to its pelvis attachments
Quadratus lumborum (**quad-dra-**tus **lum-bor-**um)	Deep muscle located medially either side of the lumbar vertebrae	Attaches to the top of the posterior of the iliac crest at one end and to the twelfth rib and transverse processes of the first four lumbar vertebrae at the other end	Lateral flexion (sidebending) of the lumbar vertebrae	Excessive bending to the side can strain and injure the quadratus lumborum muscle
Gluteus maximus (**gloo**-tee-us **max**-i-mus)	Large muscle covering the buttock	Attaches to the back of the ilium along the sacroiliac joint at one end, and into the top of the femur at the other	Extends the hip, abducts and laterally rotates thigh	Sometimes referred to as the 'speedskater's muscle' as it is powerful in extending, abducting and lateralling rotating the thigh Often implicated in postural defects
Gluteus medius (**gloo**-tee-us **meed**-ee-us)	Muscle is partly covered by the gluteus maximus	Attaches to the outer surface of the ilium at one end and the outer surface of the femur at the other end	Abducts thigh, medially rotates thigh	When this muscle becomes tight it can create postural distortions. It pulls and depresses the pelvis towards the thigh on that side, resulting in a 'functional short leg'
Gluteus mimimus (**gloo**-tee-us **min**-i-mus)	Lies beneath the gluteus medius	Attachments are the same as for gluteus medius: outer surface of the ilium at one end to the outer surface of the femur at the other end	Abducts thigh, medially rotates thigh	See above re gluteus medius
Piriformis (pi-ri-**for**-mis)	Deeply seated pelvic girdle muscle	Attaches to the anterior of the sacrum at one end and the top of the femur at the other	Lateral rotation and abduction of the hip	Largest lateral rotator of the hip. If it becomes tight, it can restrict mobility in the hip

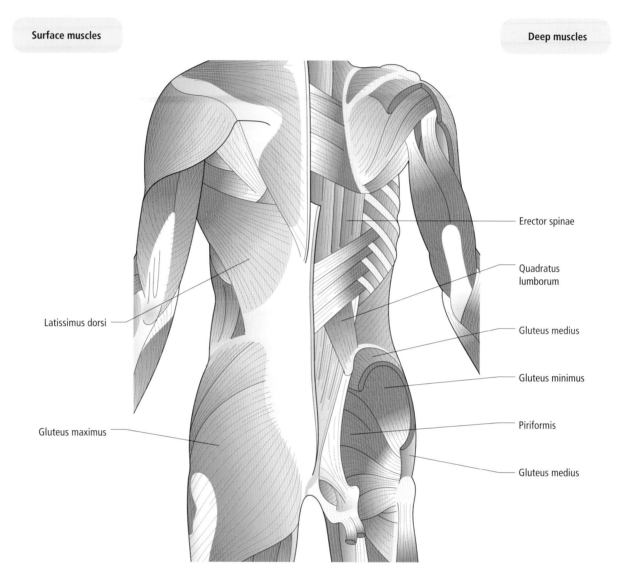

| Surface muscles | | Deep muscles |

Erector spinae

Quadratus lumborum

Gluteus medius

Gluteus minimus

Latissimus dorsi

Piriformis

Gluteus maximus

Gluteus medius

Fig 4.14 The muscles of the posterior of the trunk

Deep pelvic muscles

Name of muscle	Position	Attachments	Action/s	Key facts
Psoas (so-as)	Long, thick and deep pelvic muscle	Attaches to the anterior transverse processes of T12–L5 (twelfth thoracic to fifth lumbar vertebrae) to the inside of the top of the femur at the other end	Flexes the thigh	The iliacus and psoas muscles are often considered as one and may be referred to as iliopsoas

Both muscles are primary flexors of the thigh and therefore serve to advance the leg in walking |
| **Iliacus** (i-lee-**ak**-us) | Large, fan-shaped muscle deeply situated in the pelvic girdle | Attaches to the iliac crest at one end and to the inside of the top of the femur at the other end | Flexes and laterally rotates the femur | See above |

Fig 4.15 Deep pelvic muscles – psoas and iliacus

Student activity

Now complete Activity 4.2 in the resources for this book on Dynamic Learning Online.

Student activity

Now complete Activity 4.3 in the resources for this book on Dynamic Learning Online.

Surface muscles

Deep muscles

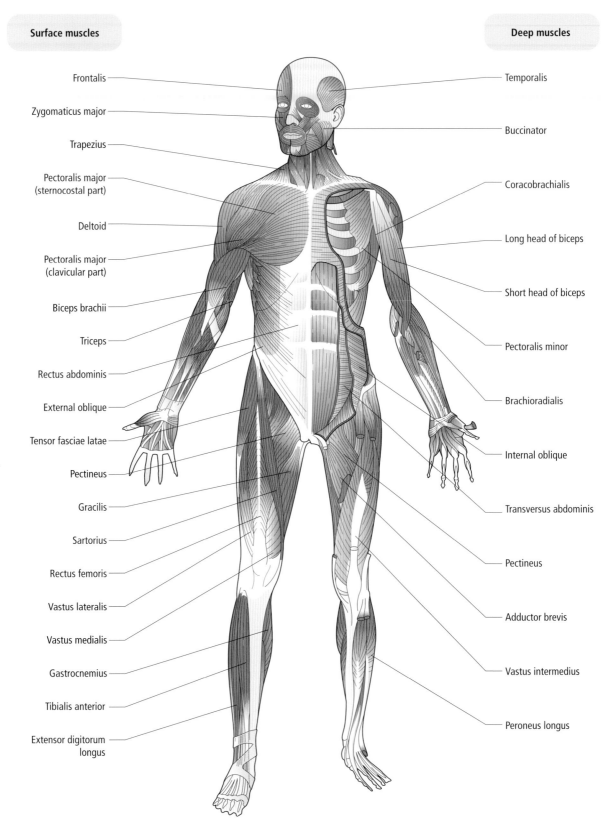

Frontalis

Zygomaticus major

Trapezius

Pectoralis major
(sternocostal part)

Deltoid

Pectoralis major
(clavicular part)

Biceps brachii

Triceps

Rectus abdominis

External oblique

Tensor fasciae latae

Pectineus

Gracilis

Sartorius

Rectus femoris

Vastus lateralis

Vastus medialis

Gastrocnemius

Tibialis anterior

Extensor digitorum
longus

Temporalis

Buccinator

Coracobrachialis

Long head of biceps

Short head of biceps

Pectoralis minor

Brachioradialis

Internal oblique

Transversus abdominis

Pectineus

Adductor brevis

Vastus intermedius

Peroneus longus

Fig 4.16 Anterior muscles of the body

Surface muscles

Deep muscles

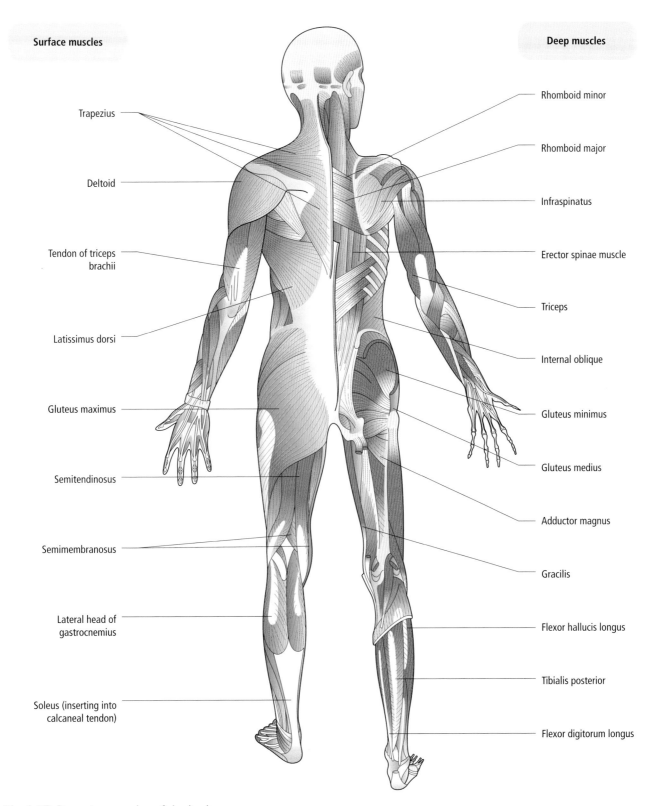

Trapezius

Deltoid

Tendon of triceps
brachii

Latissimus dorsi

Gluteus maximus

Semitendinosus

Semimembranosus

Lateral head of
gastrocnemius

Soleus (inserting into
calcaneal tendon)

Rhomboid minor

Rhomboid major

Infraspinatus

Erector spinae muscle

Triceps

Internal oblique

Gluteus minimus

Gluteus medius

Adductor magnus

Gracilis

Flexor hallucis longus

Tibialis posterior

Flexor digitorum longus

Fig 4.17 Posterior muscles of the body

Common pathologies of the muscular system

Atony

This is a state in which the muscles are floppy and lacking their normal degree of elasticity.

Atrophy

This is the wasting of muscle tissue due to undernourishment or lack of use and diseases such as poliomyelitis.

Carpal tunnel syndrome

This is characterised by pain and numbness in the thumb or hand resulting from pressure on the median nerve of the wrist. Pain and pins and needles sensation may radiate to the elbow. It is known to cause severe pain at night and can cause muscle wasting of the hand. There is a higher risk of this condition in occupations requiring repetitive strains of the wrist, such as massage therapists and secretaries.

Fibromyalgia

This is a chronic condition that produces musculo-skeletal pain. Predominant symptoms include widespread musculo-skeletal pain, lethargy and fatigue. Other characteristic features include a non-refreshing sleep pattern in which the patient experiences interrupted sleep, and wakes feeling exhausted and more tired than later in the day.

Other recognised symptoms include early morning stiffness, pins and needles sensation, unexplained headaches, poor concentration, memory loss, low mood, urinary frequency, abdominal pain, irritable bowel syndrome. Anxiety and depression are also common.

Fibrositis

Fibrositis is an inflammatory condition of the fibrous connective tissues, especially in the muscle fascia (also known as muscular rheumatism).

Myositis

This condition is the inflammation of a skeletal muscle.

Muscular atrophy

This is the wasting away of muscles due to poor nutrition, lack of use or a dysfunction of the motor nerve impulses.

Muscle fatigue

This is the loss of the ability of a muscle to contract efficiently due to insufficient oxygen, exhaustion of energy supply and the accumulation of lactic acid.

Muscle spasm

This is an increase in muscle tension due to excessive motor nerve activity resulting in a knot in the muscle.

IN PRACTICE

In the case of muscular disorders it is important to avoid any methods of treatment that could increase the inflammatory response in the acute stage of the condition.

IN PRACTICE

With carpal tunnel syndrome avoid localised massage to the wrist if there is acute inflammation present in the area. In a chronic state this condition can be helped by elevating the limb to encourage lymph drainage, localised massage to loosen scar tissue and passively moving the elbow, wrist and fingers in order to maintain the range of movement. Remedial exercises such as passive stretching of the flexors and extensors of the wrist can be helpful in aiding this condition.

IN PRACTICE

In the case of a client with fibromyalgia it is best to advise gentler treatment applications of a shorter duration.

Muscle cramp

This is an acute painful contraction of a single muscle or group of muscles. Cramp is often associated with a mineral deficiency, an irritated nerve or muscle fatigue.

Muscular dystrophy

This is a progressively crippling disease in which the muscles gradually weaken and atrophy. The cause is unknown.

Rupture

A rupture is the tearing of a muscle fascia or tendon.

Shin splints

This is a soreness in the front of the lower leg due to straining of the flexor muscles used in walking.

Spasticity

This is characterised by an increase in muscle tone and stiffness. In severe cases, movements may become uncoordinated and involve a nervous dysfunction. Spasticity involves muscles with excessive tone and is a condition often associated with nervous dysfunction.

Strain

A strain is an injury that is caused by excessive stretching or working of a muscle or tendon that results in a partial or complete tear. Symptoms include pain, swelling, tenderness and stiffness in the affected area. Muscle strains are more common in the lower back and the neck.

Sprain

This is a complete or incomplete tear in the ligaments around a joint. It usually follows a sudden, sharp twist to the joint that stretches the ligaments and ruptures some or all of its fibres. Sprains commonly occur in the ankle, wrist and the back where there is localised pain, swelling and loss of mobility.

Stress

Stress is excessive muscular tension resulting in tight, painful muscles and restricted joint movements.

Tendinitis

This is the inflammation of a tendon, accompanied by pain and swelling.

Tennis elbow

This condition is the inflammation of the tendons that attach the extensor muscles of the forearm at the elbow joint.

Torticollis

This is a condition in which the neck muscles (sternomastoids) contract involuntarily. It is commonly called 'wryneck'.

IN PRACTICE

In the case of a sprain or strain, direct work over an area is contra-indicated until all signs of inflammation have dissipated.

Interrelationships with other systems

The muscular system is linked to the following body systems.

Cells and tissues/histology

There are three types of muscle tissue in the body – skeletal or voluntary muscle, smooth and cardiac. Fascia, tendons and ligaments are all made from connective tissue and serve a function in muscle attachments.

Skeletal system

Bones and joints provide the leverage in a movement and the muscles provide the pull upon the bone to effect the movement.

Circulatory system

The circulatory system is responsible for delivering oxygen, glycogen and water to the working muscles. It also transports waste products, such as carbon dioxide and lactic acid, away from the muscles.

Respiratory system

The respiratory system provides the working muscles with vital oxygen which is transported in the blood to be combined with glycogen to release energy.

Nervous system

Muscles rely on nervous stimulation in order to function. Skeletal muscles are moved as a result of nervous stimulus which they receive from the brain via a motor nerve.

Digestive system

The energy needed for muscle contraction is obtained principally from carbohydrate digestion. Carbohydrates are broken down and glucose, which is not required immediately by the body, is converted into glycogen and stored in the liver and muscle.

Key words associated with the muscular system

skeletal/voluntary muscle	sarcomere	origin
tissue	motor nerve	insertion
cardiac muscle tissue	motor point	antagonists
smooth/involuntary muscle	neurotransmitter	agonist/prime mover
fasciculi	glycogen	synergists
epimysium	lactic acid	fixators
endomysium	muscle fatigue	isometric contraction
perimysium	muscle tone	isotonic contraction
myofibrils	tendon	concentric contractions
actin	ligament	eccentric contractions
myosin	fascia	

Revision summary of the muscular system

- The muscular system is comprised mainly of **skeletal** or **voluntary muscle tissue** that is primarily attached to bones.
- The other types of muscle tissue are **cardiac muscle tissue** found in the wall of the heart and **smooth muscle tissue** located in the wall of the stomach and small intestines.
- Through contraction, muscle performs three important functions – movement, maintaining posture and heat production.
- **Voluntary** or **skeletal muscle tissue** consists of muscle fibres held together by fibrous connective tissue and penetrated by numerous tiny blood vessels and nerves.
- Voluntary muscle tissue is made up of bands of elastic or contractile tissue bound together in bundles and enclosed by a connective tissue sheath.
- Each muscle fibre is enclosed in an individual wrapping of connective tissue called the **endomysium**.
- The muscle fibres are wrapped together in bundles, known as **fasciculi** and covered by the **perimysium** (fibrous sheath), which are then gathered to from the muscle belly (main part of the muscle) with its own sheath, the fascia **epimysium**.
- Each skeletal muscle fibre is made up of thin fibres called **myofibrils** which are made up of two different types of protein strands called **actin** and **myosin**. This gives skeletal muscle its striated or striped appearance.
- Muscle fibre contraction results from a sliding movement within the **myofibrils** in which **actin** and **myosin** filaments merge.
- Skeletal muscle is moved as a result of nervous stimulus received from the brain via a motor nerve.
- Each nerve fibre ends in a **motor point**, the end portion of the nerve, and is the part through which the stimulus is given to contract.
- The muscle cells in smooth or involuntary muscle are spindle shaped and tapered at both ends with each muscle cell containing one centrally located oval-shaped nucleus.
- **Smooth muscle** contracts or relaxes in response to nerve impulses, stretching or hormones.
- **Cardiac muscle** is found only in the heart and like skeletal muscle it is striated. However, it is branched in structure and has intercalated discs in between each muscle cell.
- The contraction of cardiac muscle is regulated by nerves and hormones.
- During muscular contraction a sliding movement occurs within the contractile fibres (**myobibrils**).
- The **actin** filaments move in towards the **myosin** and cause the muscle fibres to shorten and thicken.
- During relaxation the muscle fibres elongate and return to their original shape.
- The energy needed for muscle contraction comes from **glycogen** (stored in the liver and the muscles) and oxygen.
- If insufficient oxygen is available to a working muscle a waste product called **lactic acid** forms which can cause a muscle to ache.
- The term **muscle fatigue** is defined as the loss of ability of a muscle to contract efficiently due to insufficient oxygen, exhaustion of glucose and the accumulation of lactic acid.
- During exercise the circulatory and respiratory systems adjust to cope with the increased oxygen demands of the body. More blood is distributed to the working muscles and the rate and depth of breathing is increased.
- When muscle tissue is warm, muscle contraction will occur faster due to the increase in circulation and acceleration of chemical reactions.
- Conversely when muscle tissue is cooled, the chemical reactions and circulation slow down.
- The term **muscle tone** is the state of partial contraction of a muscle to help maintain body posture.
- Good muscle tone can be recognised by the muscles appearing firm and rounded.
- Poor muscle tone may be recognised by the muscles appearing loose and flattened.
- **Tendons** are tough bands of white fibrous tissue that link muscle to bone.
- Unlike muscle they are inelastic and therefore do not stretch.
- **Ligaments** are strong, fibrous, elastic tissues that link bones together and therefore stabilize joints.
- **Fascia** consists of fibrous connective tissue that envelops a muscle and provides a pathway for nerves, blood vessels and lymphatic vessels.
- **Fascia**, therefore, plays a key role in maintaining the 'health' of a muscle.
- Muscle attachments are known as **origin** and **insertion**.

- The **origin** is the end of the muscle closest to the centre of the body and the **insertion** is the furthest attachment.
- The **insertion** is generally the most movable point and is the point at which the muscle work is done.
- In movement coordination muscles work in pairs or groups.
- Muscles are classified by functions as **agonists** (prime movers), **antagonists**, **synergists** and **fixators** (stabilisers).
- **Antagonists** are two muscles or sets of muscles pulling in opposite directions to each other, with one relaxing to allow the other to contract.

- **Agonist/prime mover** is known as the main activating muscle.
- **Synergyst** refers to muscles on the same side of a joint that work together to perform the same movements.
- Muscular contractions can be **isometric** or **isotonic**.
- **Isometric contraction** is when the muscle works without actual movements (postural muscles).
- **Isotonic contraction** is when the muscles force is considered to be constant but the muscle length changes.
- There are two types of isotonic contraction – **concentric contractions** (towards the centre) and **eccentric contractions** (away from the centre).

1 Which of the following is not a function of the muscular system?
   a movement
   b production of heat
   c exchange of gases
   d maintenance of posture

2 A voluntary muscle will only contract if a stimulus is applied to it via a:
   a sensory nerve
   b mixed nerve
   c motor nerve
   d association nerve

3 A tendon attaches:
   a muscle to bone
   b muscle to ligament
   c bone to bone
   d bone to ligament

4 Where would you not find involuntary muscle tissue?
   a bladder
   b stomach
   c brain
   d heart

5 The fuel for muscle contraction is provided by:
   a ATP
   b pyruvic acid
   c glucose
   d actin and myosin

6 The state of continuous partial contraction of muscles is known as:
   a hypertrophy
   b muscle spasm
   c muscle tone
   d atrophy

7 An injury caused by excessive stretching or working of a muscle is known as a:
   a sprain
   b strain
   c spasm
   d spasticity

8 Which of the following is not associated with muscle cramp?
   a muscle fatigue
   b mineral deficiency
   c irritated nerve
   d poor nutrition

9 A chronic condition that produces musculo-skeletal pain, lethargy and fatigue is known as:
   a fibrositis
   b muscular dystrophy
   c myositis
   d fibromyalgia

10 The connective tissue that forms the outermost layer of the muscle is:
   a perimysium
   b epimysium
   c endomysium
   d endocardium

11 The muscle that closes the mouth is the:
   a orbicularis oculi
   b risorius
   c levator anguli oris
   d orbicularis oris

12 The muscle that turns the head to the opposite side is the:
   a platysma
   b sternocleidomastoid
   c frontalis
   d occipitalis

13 The action of the zygomaticus muscle is to:
   a draw the angle of the mouth upwards
   b draw the angle of the jaw upwards
   c raise the jaw
   d draw the angle of the mouth downwards

14 The facial expression associated with the mentalis muscle is:
   a smiling
   b laughing
   c pouting
   d all of the above

15 The position of the buccinator muscle is the:
   a corner of the mouth
   b in the cheek
   c chin
   d sides of the nose

16 The action of the rhomboid muscles is to:
   a adduct the scapula
   b elevate the scapula
   c adduct the humerus
   d abduct the humerus

17 Which of the following muscles does not flex the forearm?
   a biceps
   b brachialis
   c triceps
   d pronator teres

18 The action of the hamstring muscles is:
   a flexion of the knee and extension of the hip
   b flexion of the hip and knee
   c extension of the knee and flexion of the hip
   d adduction of the thigh and flexion of the hip

19 Which of the following muscles is not a plantar flexor of the foot?
   a gastrocnemius
   b peroneus longus
   c tibialis anterior
   d soleus

20 Which of the following muscles does not rotate the humerus?
   a subscapularis
   b supraspinatus
   c infraspinatus
   d teres minor

21 The deepest of the abdominal muscles is the:
   a rectus abdominus
   b external obliques
   c internal obliques
   d transversus abdominus

5 the cardiovascular system

Introduction

The cardiovascular system is the body's transport system and comprises blood, blood vessels and the heart. Blood provides the fluid environment for our body's cells and is transported in specialised tubes called blood vessels. The heart acts like a pump which keeps the blood circulating around the body in a constant circuit.

Objectives

By the end of this chapter, you will be able to recall and understand the following knowledge:

- the composition and functions of blood
- the structural and functional significance of the different type of blood cells
- the structural and functional differences between the different blood vessels
- major blood vessels of the heart
- the pulmonary and systemic blood circulation
- blood pressure and the pulse rate
- the interrelationships between the cardiovascular and other body systems
- common pathologies of the cardiovascular system

Blood

Blood is the fluid tissue or medium in which all materials are transported to and from individual cells in the body. Blood is, therefore, the chief transport system of the body.

The percentage composition of blood

Blood is composed of 55 per cent of fluid or plasma which is a clear, pale yellow, slightly alkaline fluid consisting of the following substances:

- 91 per cent of plasma is water
- 9 per cent remaining consists of dissolved blood proteins, waste, digested food materials, mineral salts and hormones
- 45 per cent of blood is made up of the blood cells erythrocytes, leucocytes and thrombocytes.

Functions of blood

There are four main functions of blood:

- transport
- defence
- regulation
- clotting.

Transport

Blood is the primary transport medium for a variety of substances that travel throughout the body.

- Oxygen is carried from the lungs to the cells of the body in red blood cells.
- Carbon dioxide is carried from the body's cells to the lungs.
- Nutrients such as glucose, amino acids, vitamins and minerals are carried from the small intestine to the cells of the body.
- Cellular wastes such as water, carbon dioxide, lactic acid and urea are carried in the blood to be excreted.
- Hormones, which are internal secretions that help to control important body processes, are transported by the blood to target organs.

Defence

White blood cells are collectively called leucocytes and they play a major role in combating disease and fighting infection.

Regulation

Blood helps to regulate heat in the body by absorbing large quantities of heat produced by the liver and the muscles. This is then transported around the body to help to maintain a constant internal temperature. Blood also helps to regulate the body's pH balance.

Clotting

Clotting is an effective mechanism in controlling blood loss from blood vessels when they have become damaged as in a cut. Specialised blood cells called thrombocytes, or platelets, form a clot around the damaged area to prevent the body from losing too much blood and to prevent the entry of bacteria.

Blood cells

There are three types of blood cells:

- **erythrocytes** – red blood cells
- **leucocytes** – white blood cells
- **thrombocytes** – platelets.

KEY FACTS

Red blood cells are called erythrocytes and they contain the red protein pigment haemoglobin that combines with oxygen to form oxyhaemoglobin. The pigment haemoglobin assists the function of the erythrocyte in transporting oxygen from the lungs to the body's cells and carrying carbon dioxide away.

KEY FACTS

White blood cells are known as phagocytes as they have the ability to engulf and ingest micro-organisms which invade the body and cause disease. Specialised white blood cells called lymphocytes produce antibodies to protect the body against infection.

Overview of the three types of blood cells

Type of blood cell	Description	Function
Erythrocyte	Disc-shaped structures Non-nucleated Red in colour due to protein haemoglobin	Transports the gases of respiration
Leucocytes	Largest of all the blood cells White due to lack of haemoglobin	Protect the body against infection and disease
Thrombocytes/platelets	Granular, disc-shaped, small fragments of cells	Blood clotting

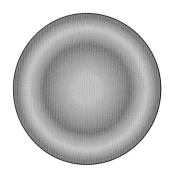

Fig 5.1 An erythrocyte

Erythrocytes

Erythrocytes are disc-shaped structures and make up more than 90 per cent of the formed elements in blood. They are formed in red bone marrow and contain the iron-protein compound haemoglobin.

Old and worn-out erythrocytes are destroyed in the liver and the spleen. The haemoglobin is broken down and the iron within it is retained for further haemoglobin synthesis. Erythrocytes have a life span of only about four months and, therefore, have to be continually replaced. The function of erythrocytes is to transport the gases of respiration (they transport oxygen to the cells and carry carbon dioxide away from the cells).

Leucocytes

Leucocytes are the largest of all the blood cells and appear white due to their lack of haemoglobin. They have a nucleus and are generally more numerous than erythrocytes. There are two main categories of leucocytes:

- **Granulocytes** – these account for about 75 per cent of white blood cells and can be further divided into **neutrophils, eosonophils** and **basophils**.
- **Agranulocytes** – these can be divided into **lymphocytes** which account for about 20 per cent of all white blood cells and **monocytes** which account for about 5 per cent of white blood cells.

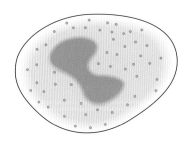

Fig 5.2 A leucocyte

Leucocytes usually survive for only a few hours, but in a healthy body some can live for months or even years. The main function of leucocytes is to protect the body against infection and disease in a process known as phagocytosis which means to engulf and ingest microbes, dead cells and tissue.

Thrombocytes

Fig 5.3 A thrombocyte

Thrombocytes are also known as **platelets**. These are small fragments of cells and are the smallest cellular elements of the blood. They are formed in bone marrow and are dics-shaped with no nucleus. Thrombocytes normally have a short life span of just five to nine days.

They are very significant in the blood clotting process as they initiate the chemical reaction that leads to the formation of a blood clot. Platelets stop the loss of blood from a damaged blood vessel in the following way:

- Platelets gather where a blood vessels is injured and red cells are flowing out.
- The first platelets to arrive form a plug across the opening and release chemicals that convert fibrinogen (a coagulation factor) to fibrin.
- Fibrin forms a mesh of needle-like fibres, that trap platelets and other blood cells, creating an insoluble clot.

Blood vessels

Blood flows round the body by the pumping action of the heart and is carried in vessels known as arteries, veins and capillaries.

Overview of arteries, veins and capillaries

Arteries	Carry blood away from heart
Veins	Carry blood towards the heart
Capillaries	Unite arterioles and venules, forming a network in the tissues

Key factors about blood vessels

External layer
Middle layer
Endothelium (internal layer)
Lumen

Fig 5.4 The structure of an artery

Arteries
- Arteries carry blood away from the heart.
- Blood is carried under high pressure.
- Arteries have thick muscular and elastic walls to withstand pressure.
- Arteries have no valves, except at the base of the pulmonary artery where they leave the heart.
- Arteries carry oxygenated blood, except the pulmonary artery, to the lungs.
- Arteries are generally deep-seated, except where they cross over a pulse spot.
- Arteries give rise to small blood vessels called arterioles which deliver blood to the capillaries.

Veins

External layer
Middle layer
Valve
Endothelium
(internal layer)

Fig 5.5 The structure of a vein

- Veins carry blood towards the heart.
- Blood is carried under low pressure.
- Veins have thinner muscular walls.
- Veins have valves at intervals to prevent the back flow of blood.
- Veins carry deoxygenated blood, except the pulmonary veins, from the lungs.
- Veins are generally superficial, not deep-seated.
- Veins form finer blood vessels called venules which continue from capillaries.

Capillaries

Fig 5.6 The structure of a capillary

- Capillaries are the smallest vessels.
- Capillaries unite arterioles and venules, forming a network in the tissues.
- The wall of a capillary vessel is only a single layer of cells thick. It is, therefore, sufficiently thin to allow the process of diffusion of dissolved substances to and from the tissues to occur.
- Capillaries have no valves.
- Blood is carried under low pressare but higher than in veins.
- Capillaries are responsible for supplying the cells and tissues with nutrients.

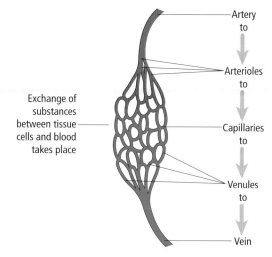

Fig 5.7 Blood flow from an artery to a vein

KEY FACTS

The key function of a capillary is to permit the exchange of nutrients and waste between the blood and tissue cells. Substances such as oxygen, vitamins, minerals and amino acids pass through to the tissue fluid to nourish the nearby cells, and substances such as carbon dioxide and waste are passed out of the cell. This exchange of nutrients can only occur through the semi-permeable membrane of a capillary as the walls of arteries and veins are too thick.

Oxygenated blood flowing through the arteries appears bright red in colour due to the oxygen pigment haemoglobin. As it moves through capillaries, it offloads some of its oxygen and picks up carbon dioxide. This explains why blood flow in veins appears darker.

The heart

The heart is a hollow organ made up of cardiac muscle tissue which lies in the thorax above the diaphragm and between the lungs.

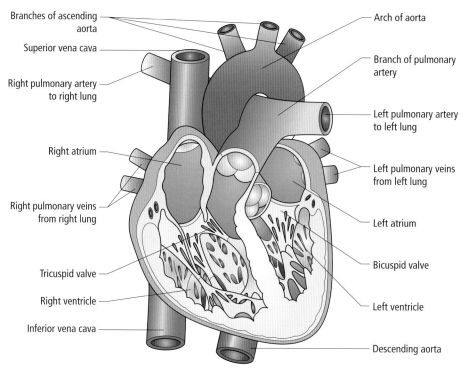

Fig 5.8 The structure of the heart

Composition of the heart

The heart is composed of three layers of tissue:

- **Pericardium: the outer layer.** This is a double-layered bag enclosing a cavity filled with pericardial fluid which reduces friction as the heart moves during its beating.
- **Myocardium: the middle layer.** This is a strong layer of cardiac muscle which makes up the bulk of the heart.
- **Endocardium: the inner layer.** This lines the heart's cavities and is continuous with the lining of the blood vessels. The heart is divided into a right and left side by a partition called a septum and each side is further divided into a thin-walled atrium above and a thick-walled ventricle below. The top chambers of the heart (the atria) take in blood from the body from the large veins and pump it to the bottom chambers. The lower chambers, the ventricles, pump blood to the body's organs and tissues.

There are four sets of valves that regulate the flow of blood though the heart:

The valves of the heart

Tricuspid valve	Found between the right atrium and the right ventricle
Bicuspid or **mitral valve**	Found between the left atrium and the left ventricle
Aortic valve	Found between the left ventricle and the aorta
Pulmonary valve	Found between the pulmonary artery and the right ventricle

The bicuspid and tricuspid valves (also known as the atrio-ventricular valves) help to maintain the direction of blood flow through the heart by allowing blood to flow into the ventricles but keeping it from returning to the atria.

The aortic and pulmonary valves are known as the semi-lunar valves. They control the blood flow out of the ventricles into the aorta and the pulmonary arteries and prevent any backflow of blood into the ventricles. These valves open in response to pressure generated when the blood leaves the ventricles. The heart muscle is supplied by the two coronary arteries (right and left) which originate from the base of the aorta.

Blood flow through the heart

Blood moves into and out of the heart in a well-coordinated and precisely timed rhythm.

BODY FACT

If either of the coronary arteries is unable to supply sufficient blood to the heart muscle, a heart attack occurs. The most common site of a heart attack is the anterior or inferior part of the left ventricle.

STUDY TIP

It is helpful when following the text in the boxes on page 156 to look at Figure 5.9 and follow the arrows, as these show the direction of blood flow through the heart. Also the colour blue indicates deoxygenated blood and red, oxygenated blood.

Remember that although arteries generally carry oxygenated blood and veins carry deoxygenated blood, there is always an exception to the rule (the pulmonary arteries which carry deoxygenated blood and the pulmonary veins which carry oxygenated blood).

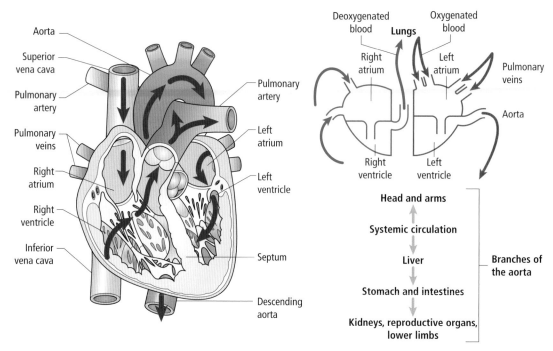

Fig 5.9 Blood flow through the heart

For descriptive purposes the blood flow can be divided into three stages:

Stage 1	Deoxygenated blood from the body enters the superior and inferior vena cava and flows into the right atrium. When the right atrium is full, it empties through the tricuspid valve into the right ventricle
Stage 2	When the right ventricle is full, it contracts and pushes blood through the pulmonary valve into the pulmonary artery. The pulmonary artery divides into the right and left branch and takes blood to both lungs where the blood becomes oxygenated. The four pulmonary veins leave the lungs carrying oxygen-rich blood back to the left atrium
Stage 3	This process takes place at the same time as the process described in stage 1. Oxygen-rich blood leaves the left atrium and passes through the left ventricle via the bicuspid or mitral valve. When the left ventricle is full it contracts, forcing blood through the aortic valve into the aorta and to all parts of the body (except the lungs). The walls of the left ventricle are thicker in order to provide the extra strength to push blood out of the heart and around the body

Student activity

Now complete Activity 5.1 in the resources for this book on Dynamic Learning Online.

Function of the heart

The function of the heart is to maintain a constant circulation of blood throughout the body. The heart acts as a pump and its action consists of a series of events known as the cardiac cycle.

The cardiac cycle

The cardiac cycle is the sequence of events between one heartbeat and the next and is normally less than a second in duration.

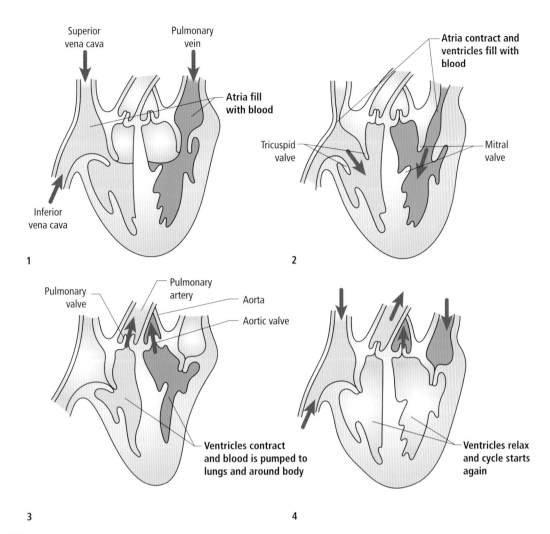

Fig 5.10 The cardiac cycle

- During a cardiac cycle the atria contract simultaneously and force blood into the relaxed ventricles.
- The ventricles then contract very strongly and pump blood out through the aorta and the pulmonary artery.
- During ventricular contraction the atria relax and fill up again with blood.

The heart rate can be determined by the number of cardiac cycles per minute. In an average healthy person this is likely to be between 60 and 70 cycles or beats per minute.

The heart has its own built-in rhythm. The coordinated rhythm of the heart is initiated by the built-in electrical system in the sinoatrial (SA) node which sets the pace of the heart rate. The signal originates in the right atrium and travels to the left atrium causing the atria to contract. At the precise moment the atria have completed their contraction, the signal travels through the atrioventricular (AV) bundle to the right ventricle and into the left ventricle causing the ventricles to contract.

Heart sounds

Heart sounds may be heard through a stethoscope. Closure of the heart valves produces two main sounds:

- The first is a low-pitched 'lubb' which is generated by the closing of the bicuspid and tricuspid valves.
- The second is a higher-pitched 'dubb' caused by the closing of the aortic and pulmonary valves.

Blood is transported as part of a double circuit and consists of two separate systems which are joined only at the heart.

The pulmonary circulation

The pulmonary circulation is the circulatory system's contribution to respiration. This consists of the circulation of deoxygenated blood from the right ventricle of the heart to the lungs via the pulmonary arteries. It becomes oxygenated here and is then returned to the left atrium by the pulmonary veins to be passed to the aorta for the general or systemic circulation.

The pulmonary circulation is essentially the circulatory system between the heart and the lungs where a high concentration of blood oxygen is restored and the concentration of carbon dioxide in the blood is lowered.

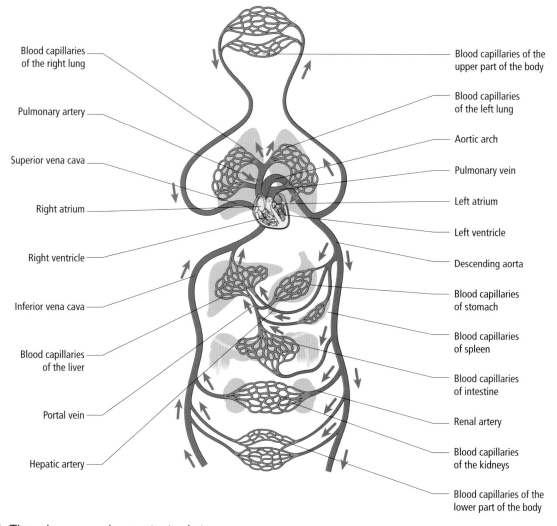

Fig 5.11 The pulmonary and systemic circulation

The general or systemic circulation

The systemic circuit is the largest circulatory system and carries oxygenated blood from the left ventricle of the heart through to the aorta. Oxygenated blood is then passed around the body through the various branches of the aorta. Deoxygenated blood is returned to the right atrium via the superior and inferior vena cava to be passed to the right ventricle to enter the pulmonary circuit. The function of the systemic circulation is to bring nutrients and oxygen to all systems of the body and carry waste materials away from the tissues for elimination.

The portal circulation

Located within the systemic circuit is the portal circulation which collects blood from the digestive organs (stomach, intestines, gall bladder, pancreas and spleen) and delivers this blood to the liver for processing, via the hepatic portal veins. As the liver has a key function in maintaining proper concentrations of glucose, fat and protein in the blood, the hepatic portal

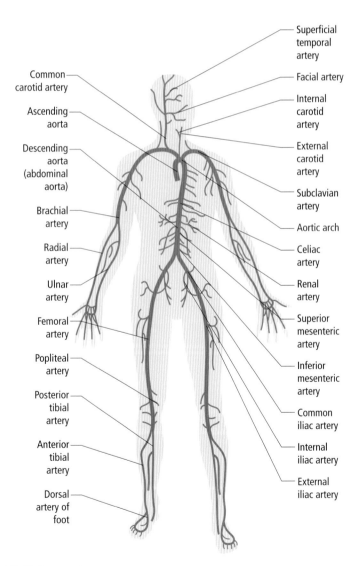

Fig 5.12 Main arteries

system allows the blood from the digestive organs to take a detour through the liver to process these substances before they enter the systemic circulation.

Main arteries

The aorta is the main artery of the systemic circuit which carries oxygenated blood around the body. It is divided into three main branches which subdivide into branches to supply the whole of the body:

- The ascending part has branches which supply the head, neck and the top of the arms.
- The descending thoracic part of the aorta has branches which supply organs of the thorax.
- The descending abdominal part has branches which supply the legs and organs of the digestive, renal and reproductive systems.

The names of most major arteries are derived from the anatomical structures they serve such as the femoral artery which is found close to the femur. Arteries generally lie deeply seated. They are found on both sides of the body and are identified as either right or left.

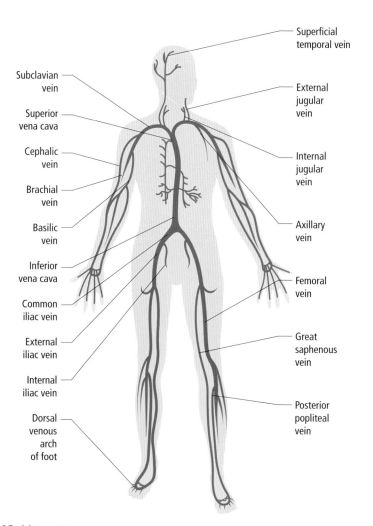

Fig 5.13 Main veins

Main veins

The major veins of the body are the **superior** and **inferior vena cava** which convey deoxygenated blood from the other veins to the right atrium of the heart.

- The **inferior vena cava** is formed by the joining of the right and left **iliac veins**. It receives blood from the lower parts of the body below the diaphragm.
- The **superior vena cava** originates at the junction of the two **innominate** (**briachiocephalic**) veins. It drains blood from the upper parts of the body (head, neck, thorax and arms).

Like arteries, veins are also named for their locations and have two branches (right and left). Veins are more superficially placed than arteries.

Blood vessels of the head and neck

Blood is supplied to parts within the neck, head and brain through branches of the **subclavian** and **common carotid arteries**. The **common cartoid artery** extends from the **brachiocephalic artery**. It extends on each side of the neck and divides at the level of the larynx into two branches:

- The **internal carotid artery** passes through the temporal bone of the skull to supply oxygenated blood to the brain, eyes, forehead and part of the nose.
- The **external carotid artery** is divided into branches (facial, temporal and occipital arteries) which supply the skin and muscles of the face, side and back of the head respectively. This vessel also supplies more superficial parts and structures of the head and neck. These include the salivary glands, scalp, teeth, nose, throat, tongue and thyroid gland.

The **vertebral arteries** is a main division of the **subclavian artery**. They arise from the **subclavian arteries** in the base of the neck near the tip of the lungs and pass upwards through the openings (foramina) of transverse

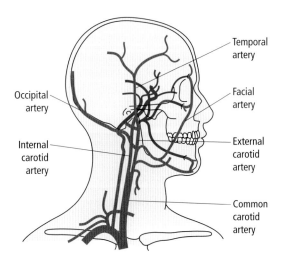

Fig 5.14 Blood flow to the head and neck

processes of the cervical vertebrae where they unite to form a single **basilar artery.** The **basilar artery** then terminates by dividing into two posterior **cerebral arteries** that supply the occipital and temporal lobes of the cerebrum.

The majority of blood draining from the head is passed into three pairs of veins:

- external jugular veins
- internal jugular veins
- vertebral veins.

Within the brain all veins lead to the internal jugular veins.

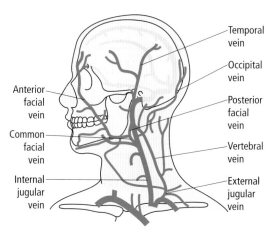

Fig 5.15 Venous drainage from the head and neck

The **external jugular veins** are smaller than the **internal jugular veins** and lie superficial to them. They receive blood from superficial regions of the face, scalp and neck. The **external jugular veins** descend on either side of the neck, passing over the sternomastoid muscles and beneath the platysma. They empty into the right and left **subclavian veins** in the base of the neck.

The **internal jugular veins** form the major venous drainage of the head and neck and are deep veins that parallel the **common carotid artery.** They collect deoxygenated blood from the brain, and pass downwards through the neck besides the **common carotid arteries** to join the **subclavian veins**.

The **vertebral veins** descend from the transverse openings (or foramina) of the cervical vertebrae and enter the **subclavian veins**. The **vertebral veins** drain deep structures of the neck such as the vertebrae and muscles.

Blood vessels of the arm and hand

The blood supply to the arm begins with the **subclavian artery** (a branch of the aorta). The subclavian artery becomes the axillary artery and then the **brachial artery** which runs down the inner aspect of the upper arm to about 1 cm below the elbow where it divides into the **radial** and **ulnar arteries**.

The **radial artery** runs down the forearm and continues over the carpals to pass between the first and second metacarpals into the palm. The **ulnar artery** runs down the forearm next to the ulnar bone, across the carpals into the palm of the hand. Together, the **radial** and **ulnar arteries** form two arches in the hand called the **deep** and **superficial arches**. From these arteries branch others to supply blood to the structures of the upper arm, forearm, hand and fingers.

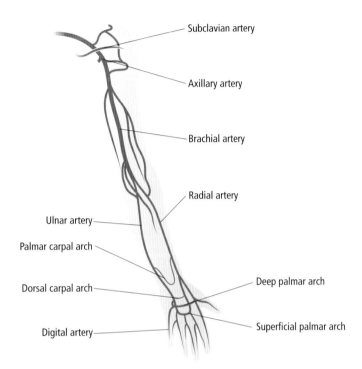

Subclavian artery

Axillary artery

Brachial artery

Radial artery

Ulnar artery

Palmar carpal arch

Dorsal carpal arch

Deep palmar arch

Superficial palmar arch

Digital artery

Fig 5.16 Arteries of the arm and hand

The venous return of blood from the hand begins with the **palmar arch** and **plexus** which is a network of capillaries in the palm. The veins that carry deoxygenated blood up the forearm are the **radial vein, ulnar vein** and **median vein**.

The **radial vein** runs parallel to the radius bone of the forearm, the ulnar vein runs parallel to the ulna bone of the forearm and the **median vein** runs up the middle of the forearm. Just above the elbow, the **radial** and **ulnar veins** join to become the **brachial vein** and the **median vein** joins the **basilic vein** which originates just below the elbow along with the **cephalic vein**.

As the veins continue over the elbow they link to form a network that eventually divides with the **basilic vein** joining the **brachial vein** which then becomes the **axillary vein**. The **cephalic vein** travels up the arm separately and becomes the **subclavian vein** in the upper chest.

Blood vessels of the thoracic and abdominal walls

The thoracic wall is supplied by branches of the **subclavian artery** and the **thoracic aorta**. The abdominal wall is supplied by branches of the **abdominal aorta**. The thoracic and abdominal walls are drained by

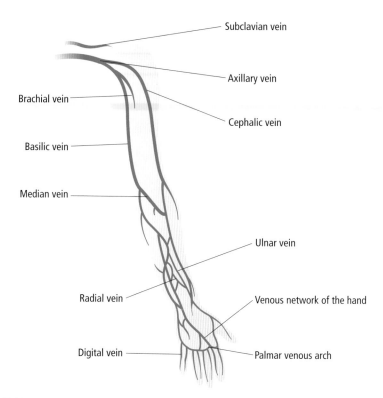

Fig 5.17 Veins of the arm and hand

branches of the **brachiocephalic veins.** Blood from the abdominal organs enters the **hepatic portal system** and the from the liver the blood is carried by the **hepatic veins** to the **inferior vena cava.**

Blood vessels of the leg and foot

The aorta travels down the length of the trunk to the lower abdomen where it divides into two arteries which supply either leg. The **femoral artery** is the artery in the thigh, named after the thigh bone. At the knee the **femoral**

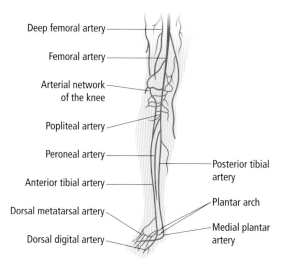

Fig 5.18 Arteries of the leg and foot

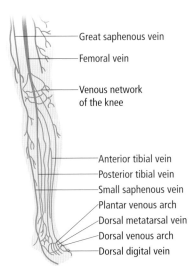

- Great saphenous vein
- Femoral vein
- Venous network of the knee
- Anterior tibial vein
- Posterior tibial vein
- Small saphenous vein
- Plantar venous arch
- Dorsal metatarsal vein
- Dorsal venous arch
- Dorsal digital vein

Fig 5.19 Veins of the leg and foot

artery becomes the **popliteal artery** which divides into two below the knee. One of these arteries runs down the front of the lower leg and is called the **anterior tibial artery**, while the other runs down the back and is called the **posterior tibial artery**. This artery divides at the inside of the ankle becoming the **medial plantar artery** on the inside of the foot and the **plantar arch** on the sole of the foot. The **anterior tibial artery** becomes the **doral metatarsal artery** on top of the foot.

There is a network of veins in the foot that become the **dorsal venous arch** on top of the foot. This travels the inside of the foot to the ankle where it becomes the **small saphenous vein**. It continues up the back of the whole leg to the thigh where it is known as the **great saphenous vein.**

Two small veins called the **anterior tibial veins** travel up the front of the lower leg, while two veins, the **posterior tibial veins**, run up the back. These four veins converge just below the knee to become the **popliteal vein** at the back of the knee and then eventually the **femoral vein** in the thigh. The **great saphenous vein** and the **femoral vein** join at the groin and return to the heart via the **inferior vena cava**.

Blood shunting

Along certain circulatory pathways, such as in the intestines, there are strategic points where small arteries have direct connection with veins. When these connections are open, they act as shunts which allow blood in the artery to have direct access to a vein.

These interconnections allow for sudden and major diversions of blood volume according to the physical needs of the body. In relation to circulation, this means that treatment should not be given after a heavy meal due to the increased circulation to the intestines, resulting in a diminished supply to other areas of the body.

Blood pressure

Blood pressure is the amount of pressure exerted by blood on an arterial wall due to the contraction of the left ventricle. The pressure in the arteries varies during each heartbeat. The maximum pressure of the heartbeat is known as the systolic pressure and represents the pressure exerted on the arterial wall during active ventricular contraction. Systolic pressure can, therefore, be measured when the heart muscle contracts and pushes blood out into the body through the arteries.

The minimum pressure, or diastolic pressure, represents the static pressure against the arterial wall during rest or pause between contractions. Therefore, the mimimum pressure is when the heart muscle relaxes and blood flows into the heart from the veins. Blood pressure may be measured with the use of a sphygmomanometer.

Factors affecting blood pressure

As blood pressure is the result of the pumping of the heart in the arteries, anything that makes the heart beat faster will raise the blood pressure. Factors affecting the blood pressure include:

BODY FACT

Blood pressure is regulated by sympathetic nerves in the arterioles. An increase in stimulation of the sympathetic nervous system, as in exercise, can therefore result in a temporary increase in blood pressure.

- excitement
- anger
- stress
- fright
- pain
- exercise
- smoking and drugs.

A normal blood pressure reading is between 100 and 140 mmHg systolic and between 60 and 90 mmHg diastolic. Blood pressure is measured in millimetres of mercury and is expressed as 120/80 mmHg.

The pulse

The pulse is a pressure wave that can be felt in the arteries which corresponds to the beating of the heart. The pumping action of the left ventricle of the heart is so strong that it can be felt as a pulse in arteries a considerable distance from the heart. The pulse can be felt at any point where an artery lies near the surface. The radial pulse can be found by placing two or three fingers over the radial artery below the thumb. Other sites where the pulse may be felt include the carotid artery at the side of the neck and over the brachial artery at the elbow.

The average pulse in an adult is between 60 and 80 beats per minute. Factors affecting the pulse rate include:

- exercise
- heat
- strong emotions such as grief, fear, anger or excitement.

Common pathologies of the circulatory system

Anaemia

This is a condition where the haemoglobin level in the blood is below normal. The main symptoms are excessive tiredness, breathlessness on exertion, pallor and poor resistance to infection. There are many causes of anaemia. It may be due to a loss of blood resulting from an accident or operation, chronic bleeding, iron deficiency or due to a blood disease such as leukaemia.

Aneurysm

Aneurysm is an abnormal balloon-like swelling in the wall of an artery. This may be due to degenerative disease (congenital defects, arteriosclerosis) or any condition which causes weakening of the arterial wall such as trauma, infections, hypertension.

Angina

This is a pain in the left side of the chest and usually radiating to the left arm caused by insufficient blood to the heart muscle, usually on exertion or

IN PRACTICE

In the case of clients with a circulatory disorder, always take a detailed history of the client's symptoms and medical/surgical treatment. It is important to seek advice from the client's GP before treating as this may determine the nature and duration of the proposed treatment.

excitement. The pain is often described as constricting or suffocating which can last for a few seconds or moments. Patient may become pale and sweaty. This condition indicates ischaemic heart disease.

Arteriosclerosis

Arteriosclerosis is a circulatory system condition characterised by a thickening, narrowing, hardening and loss of elasticity of the walls of the arteries.

High blood pressure

High blood pressure is when the resting blood pressure is above normal. The World Health Organisation defines high blood pressure as consistently exceeding 160 mmHg systolic and 95 mmHg diastolic. High blood pressure is a common complaint and if serious may result in a stroke or a heart attack, due to the fact that the heart is made to work harder to force blood through the system. Causes of high blood pressure include:

- smoking
- obesity
- lack of regular exercise
- eating too much salt
- excessive alcohol consumption
- too much stress.

High blood pressure can be controlled by:

- anti-hypertensive drugs which help to regulate and lower blood pressure
- decreasing salt and fat intake to prevent hardening of the arteries
- keeping weight down
- giving up smoking and cutting down on alcohol consumption
- relaxation and leading a less stressful life.

Low blood pressure

Low blood pressure is when the blood pressure is below normal and is defined by the World Health Organisation as a systolic blood pressure of 99 mmHg or less and a diastolic of less than 59 mmHg. Low blood pressure may be normal for some people in good health, during rest and after fatigue. The danger with low blood pressure is an insufficient supply of blood reaching the vital centres of the brain. Treatment may be by medication, if necessary.

Congenital heart disease

This is a defect in the formation of the heart which usually decreases its efficiency. Defects may be in the following forms:

- **Ventricular septal defects** – non-closure of the opening between the right and left ventricle
- **Atrial septal defect** – non-closure of the opening between the right and left atrium
- **Coarctation of the aorta** – narrowing of the aorta
- **Pulmonary stenosis** – narrowing of the pulmonary artery
- **Patent ductus arteriosus** – non-closure of the communication between the pulmonary artery and the aorta that exists in the foetus until delivery
- a combination of defects.

The symptoms may vary according to the severity of the defect.

Haemophilia

This is a hereditary disorder in which the blood clots very slowly due to deficiency of either of two coagulation factors – Factor VIII (the antihaemophiliac factor) or Factor IX (called the Christmas factor). They are both coagulation factors normally present in blood. Deficiency of either of these factors, which are inherited by males from their mothers, results in the inability of the blood to clot (haemophilia).

The patient may experience prolonged bleeding following an injury or wound and in severe cases there is spontaneous bleeding into the muscles and joints. Haemophilia is controlled by a sex-linked gene which means it is almost exclusively restricted to males. Women can carry the disease and pass it on to their sons without being affected themselves.

Haemorrhoids (piles)

This is an enlargement of the normal spongy blood-filled cushions in the walls of the anus. They usually form as a result of prolonged constipation.

Heart attack (myocardial infarction)

This is damage to the heart muscles which results from blockage of the coronary arteries. It can cause serious complications including heart failure.

Hepatitis

Hepatitis is an inflammation of the liver caused by viruses, toxic substances or immunological abnormalities.

- **Hepatitis A** – this is highly contagious and is transmitted by the faecal–oral route. It is transmitted by ingestion of contaminated food, water or milk. The incubation period is from 15 to 45 days.
- **Hepatitis B** – this is also known as serum hepatitis and is more serious than hepatitis A. It lasts longer and can lead to cirrhosis, cancer of the liver and a carrier state. It has a long incubation period of one and a half to two months. The symptoms may last from weeks to months. The virus is usually transmitted through infected blood, serum or plasma, however it can spread by oral or sexual contact as it is present in most body secretions.
- **Hepatitis C** – this can cause acute or chronic hepatitis and can also lead to a carrier state and liver cancer. It is transmitted through blood transfusions or exposure to blood products.

High cholesterol

Cholesterol is a fat-like material present in the blood and most tissues. A high level of cholesterol in the blood (due to a diet rich in animal fats and refined sugars) is often associated with the degeneration of the walls of the arteries and a predisposition to thrombosis.

Leukaemia

This term refers to any of a group of malignant diseases in which the bone marrow and other blood-forming organs produce an increased number of certain types of white blood cells. Overproduction of these white cells, which are immature or of abnormal form, suppresses the production of normal white cells, red cells and platelets which leads to increased susceptibility to infection. Other manifestations or signs include enlargement of the spleen, liver and the lymph nodes, spontaneous bruising and anaemia.

Pacemaker

This is an artificial electrical device implanted under the skin that stimulates and controls the heart rate by sending electrical stimuli to the heart. It is usually installed for heart block and mostly placed in one side of the upper chest.

Phlebitis

This condition is an inflammation of the wall of a vein, which is most commonly seen in the legs, as a complication of varicose veins. A segment of the vein becomes tender and painful and the surrounding skin may feel hot and appear red. Thrombosis may develop as a result of phlebitis (thrombophlebitis) with subsequent deep vein thrombosis (DVT). This can cause clots in the lungs or other organs with serious consequences.

Pulmonary embolism

A blood clot carried into the lungs where it blocks the flow of blood to the pulmonary tissue. This is a very serious condition and can be life-threatening. Clients who suffer this condition may require hospitalisation and measures to thin the blood, such as using warfarin. This condition presents with chest pain, cough and shortness of breath.

Raynaud's syndrome

This is a disorder of the peripheral arterioles characterised by spasm in the smooth muscle of the fingers and toes. It is generally brought on by cold or emotional upset. The effect is a pallor or discolouration of the skin due to the presence of poorly oxygenated haemoglobin. Extremities affected can become painful and uncomfortable and this is usually followed by redness and stiffness of the toes and fingers.

Stress

Stress can be defined as any factor which affects physical or emotional health. When the body is under stress the heart beats faster increasing the circulation of blood. Excessive or prolonged stress can lead to high blood pressure, coronary thrombosis and heart attacks.

Stroke

This is a blocking of blood flow to the brain by an embolus in a cerebral blood vessel. A stroke can result in a sudden attack of weakness affecting one side of the body, due to the interruption to the flow of blood to the brain. A stroke can vary in severity from a passing weakness or tingling in a limb to a profound paralysis and a coma if severe. Sometimes the term is used to describe cerebral haemorrhage when an artery or congenital cyst of blood vessels in the brain bursts, resulting in damage to the brain and causing similar signs to thrombus of cerebral vessels. Haemorrhage is usually associated with severe headaches and can cause neck stiffness.

Thrombosis

This is a condition in which the blood changes from a liquid to a solid state and produces a blood clot. Thrombosis in the wall of an artery obstructs the blood flow to the tissue it supplies. In the brain this is one of the causes of a stroke and in the heart, it results in a heart attack (coronary thrombosis). Thrombosis may also occur in a vein (deep vein thrombosis). The thrombus (blood clot) may be detached from its site of formation and be carried in the blood to lodge in another part. See pulmonary embolism.

Varicose veins

Veins are known as varicose when the valves within them lose their strength. As a result of this, blood flow may become reversed or static. Valves are concerned with preventing the back flow of blood. When their function is impaired they are unable to prevent the blood from flowing downwards, causing the walls of the affected veins to swell and bulge out and become visible through the skin. Varicose veins may be due to several factors:

- hereditary tendencies
- ageing
- obesity, such as excess weight, puts pressure on the walls of the veins
- pregnancy
- sitting or standing motionless for long periods of time, causing pressure to build up in the vein.

IN PRACTICE

Varicose veins can be extremely painful and great care needs to be taken. Treatment is, therefore, contraindicated in the area affecting the veins.

Interrelationships with other systems

The cradiovascular system links to the following body systems:

Integumentary
The circulatory system transports blood rich in nutrients and oxygen to the skin, hair and nails.

Skeletal
Red bone marrow is responsible for the development of blood cells.

Muscular
The heart is a muscular organ and contracts rhythmically and continuously to pump blood around the body.

Lymphatic
The lymphatic system assists the circulatory system in transporting additional waste products away from the tissues in order to maintain blood volume, pressure and prevent oedema.

Respiratory

The respiratory system oxygenates and deoxygenates blood in the lungs.

Digestive

Nutrients broken down by digestive processeses are transported by blood to the liver to be assimilated by the body.

Nervous

Blood pressure is regulated by sympathetic nerves in the arterioles.

Endocrine

Hormones are carried by blood to their target organs.

Key words associated with the cardiovascular system

blood	myocardium	cardiac cycle
erythrocyte	endocardium	pulmonary circulation
leucocyte	septum	systemic circulation
thrombocyte	atrium	blood pressure
clotting	ventricle	systolic
artery	superior vena cava	diastolic
vein	inferior vena cava	high blood pressure
capillary	pulmonary artery	low blood pressure
heart	pulmonary veins	pulse
pericardium	aorta	

Revision summary of the cardiovascular system

- **Blood** is a type of liquid connective tissue.
- Blood transports substances between the body cells and the external environment to help maintain a stable cellular environment.
- The percentage composition of blood is 55 per cent fluid or plasma and 45 per cent blood cells.
- There are three main types of blood cells – **erythrocytes, leucocytes** and **thrombocytes**.
- The function of an **erythrocyte** is transporting oxygen to the cells and carry carbon dioxide away.
- **Leucocytes** are designed to protect the body against infection.
- **Thrombocytes** are involved in the clotting process.
- There are four main functions of blood – transport, defence, regulation of heat and clotting.
- Blood is carried around the body in vessels known as **arteries, veins** and **capillaries**.
- **Arteries** carry oxygenated blood away from the heart. They have thick, muscular walls in order to withstand the high pressure of blood.
- **Veins** carry deoxygenated blood towards the heart. They have thinner muscular and elastic walls and blood is carried under lower pressure.
- **Capillaries** are the smallest vessels in the circulatory system.
- **Capillaries** unite **arterioles** and **venules**. Their walls are sufficiently thin to allow dissolved substances in and out of them.
- The **heart** lies in the **thorax** above the diaphragm and between the lungs.
- The heart is composed of three layers of tissue – an outer **pericardium**, middle layer **myocardium** and the inner layer **endocardium**.
- The heart is divided into a right and left side by a partition called a **septum**. Each side is divided into a thin-walled top chamber called an **atrium** and a thick-walled bottom layer called a **ventricle**.
- The **atria** (top chambers) take in blood from the large veins and pump it to the bottom chambers.
- The **ventricles** (bottom chambers) pump blood to the body's organs and tissues.
- Blood flows through the heart in three stages.
- In stage 1 deoxygenated blood is empties into the **right atrium** from the two main veins (**superior** and **inferior vena cava**). It then flows through the **right ventricle**.
- In stage 2 the **right ventricle** contracts and pushes blood into the **pulmonary artery** and up to the lungs to become oxygenated.

- In stage 3 (occurring at the same time as stage 1) oxygenated blood leaves the **left atrium**, passes through the **left ventricle** and then into the **aorta** amd around the body.
- The **cardiac cycle** is the sequence of events between one heart beat and the next.
- The duration of a **cardiac cycle** is less than a second.
- During a cardiac cycle the **atria** contract simultaneosuly and force blood into the relaxed ventricles.
- The **ventricles** contract strongly and push blood out through the aorta and the **pulmonary artery**.
- As the **ventricles** contract the **atria** relax and fill up with blood.
- Blood is transported as part of a double circuit.
- The **pulmonary circulation** is the circulatory system between the heart and the lungs. It consists of the circulation of deoxygenated blood from the **right ventricle** of the heart to the **lungs** via the **pulmonary arteries** to become oxygenated. Oxygenated blood is then returned to the **left atrium** by the **pulmonary veins**.
- The **systemic circulation** is the largest circualtory system and carries oxyegnated blood from the left ventricle of the heart to the aorta and around the body.
- **Blood pressure** is defined as the amount of pressure exterted by blood on a arterial wall due to the contraction of the **left ventricle**.
- The maximum pressure is called the **systolic** pressure and represents the pressure exerted on the arterial walls during ventricular contraction The lowest pressure is called the **diastolic** pressure and is when the heart muscle relaxes (ventricular relaxation) and blood flows into the heart from the veins.
- A normal blood pressure reading is between 100 and 140 mmHg **systolic** and between 60 and 90 mmHg **diastolic**.
- **High blood pressure** is when the resting blood pressure is above normal and when consistently exceeding 160 mmHg systolic and 95 mmHg diastolic.
- **Low blood pressure** is defined as a systolic pressure of 99 mmHg or less and diastolic of 59 mmHg.
- The **pulse** is a pressure wave that can be felt in the arteries, such as the carotid or brachial, and corresponds to the beating of the heart and the contraction of the left ventricle.
- An average **pulse** is between 60 and 80 beats per minute.

1 What makes up 55 per cent of the composition of blood?
   a hormones
   b haemoglobin
   c blood cells
   d plasma

2 The blood cell designed to protect the body against infection is:
   a leucocyte
   b erythrocyte
   c platelet
   d thrombocyte

3 The function of an artery is to:
   a carry blood towards the heart
   b carry deoxygenated blood
   c carry oxygenated blood
   d carry blood under low pressure

4 The function of a capillary is to:
   a prevent backflow of blood
   b supply cells and tissues with nutrients
   c carry only deoxygenated blood
   d carry only oxygenated blood

5 The blood vessel that carries deoxygenated blood from the heart to the lungs is the:
   a pulmonary vein
   b pulmonary artery
   c aorta
   d inferior vena cava

6 Oxygenated blood is carried around the body through the various branches of the:
   a superior vena cava
   b left ventricle
   c left pulmonary veins
   d aorta

7 The blood supply to the arm begins with the:
   a brachial artery
   b subclavian artery
   c ulnar artery
   d radial artery

8 The sounds created by the beating heart are due to:
   a blood moving from one heart chamber to another
   b compression from the respiring lungs
   c the closing of the heart's valves
   d contraction of the ventricles

9 The bicuspid valve of the heart is found between the:
   a left atrium and left ventricle
   b right atrium and right ventricle
   c pulmonary artery and right ventricle
   d left ventricle and aorta

10 An average pulse is between how many beats per minute?
   a 50 and 70
   b 60 and 80
   c 90 and 120
   d 40 and 50

11 Blood pressure may be defined as the amount of pressure exerted by blood on an arterial wall due to the contraction of the:
   a aortic valve
   b left atrium
   c vena cavae
   d left ventricle

12 A circulatory disorder in which there is hardening of the arteries is:
   a arteriosclerosis
   b aneurysm
   c angina
   d thrombosis

13 The main vessel that carries deoxygenated blood from the upper part of the body back to the heart is:
   a superior vena cava
   b inferior vena cava
   c internal jugular vein
   d brachiocephalic vein

14 The condition presenting with constricting pain in the left side of the chest radiating to the left arm is:
a anaemia
b angina
c stroke
d aneurysm

15 The portal circulation collects blood from the digestive organs and delivers it to which organ for processing?
a spleen
b pancreas
c stomach
d liver

16 Which of the following is **not** likely to raise blood pressure?
a stress
b relaxation
c pain
d heat

17 A heart attack is damage to the heart muscle resulting from the blockage of the:
a cephalic arteries
b coronary arteries
c carotid arteries
d iliac arteries

18 Which of the following is **not** part of the circulatory system to the leg and foot?
a peroneal artery
b basilic artery
c femoral artery
d great saphenous vein

19 Which of the following is a unique part of the structure of a vein?
a thick muscular wall
b valves
c thick elastic wall
d single cell layer thick

20 Which of the following is considered a normal blood-pressure reading in a healthy adult at rest?
a 120/80
b 160/90
c 140/100
d 180/90

6 the lymphatic system and immunity

Introduction

The lymphatic system is a one-way drainage system for the tissues. It helps to provide a circulatory pathway for tissue fluid to be transported as lymph from the tissue spaces of the body into the venous system, where it becomes part of the blood circulation. Through the filtering action of the lymphatic nodes, along with specific organs such as the spleen, the lymphatic system also helps to provide immunity against disease.

The human body is equipped with a variety of defence mechanisms that prevent the entry of foreign agents known as pathogens. This defence is called immunity. When working effectively, the immune system protects the body from most infectious micro-organisms. It does this both directly by cells attacking the micro-organisms and indirectly by releasing chemicals and protective antibodies.

Objectives

By the end of this chapter you will be able to recall and understand the following knowledge:

- the functions of the lymphatic system
- the definition of lymph and how it is formed
- the connection between blood and lymph
- the circulatory pathway of lymph
- the names and positions and drainage of the main lymphatic nodes of the head, neck and the body
- the immune response
- the interrelationships between the lymphatic and other body systems
- common pathologies of the lymphatic system.

Functions of the lymphatic system

Drainage of excess fluid from the tissues

The lymphatic system is important for the distribution of fluid and nutrients in the body because it drains excess fluid from the tissues and returns to the blood protein molecules which are unable to pass back through the blood capillary walls because of their size.

Fighting infection

The lymphatic nodes help to fight infection by filtering lymph and destroying invading micro-organisms. Lymphocytes are reproduced in the lymph node and following infection they generate antibodies to protect the body against subsequent infection. Therefore, the lymphatic system plays an important part in the body's immune system.

Absorbtion of products of fat digestion

The lymphatic system also plays an important part in absorbing the products of fat digestion from the villi of the small intestine. While the products of carbohydrate and protein digestion pass directly into the bloodstream, fats pass directly into the intestinal lymphatic vessels, known as lacteals.

What is lymph?

Lymph is a transparent, colourless, watery liquid which is derived from tissue fluid and is contained within lymphatic vessels. It resembles blood plasma in composition, except that it has a lower concentration of plasma proteins. This is because some large protein molecules are unable to filter through the cells forming the capillary walls so they remain in blood plasma. Lymph contains only one type of cell and these are called lymphocytes.

How is lymph formed?

As blood is distributed to the tissues some of the plasma escapes from the capillaries and flows around the tissue cells, delivering nutrients such as oxygen and water to the cell and picking up cellular waste such as urea and carbon dioxide. Once the plasma is outside the capillary and is bathing the tissue cells, it becomes tissue fluid. Some of the tissue fluid passes back into the capillary walls to return to the blood stream via the veins and some is collected by lymphatic vessels where it becomes lymph. Lymph is then taken through its circulatory pathway and is ultimately returned to the bloodstream.

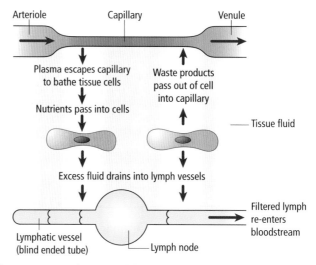

Fig 6.1 The connection between blood and lymph

The connection between blood and lymph

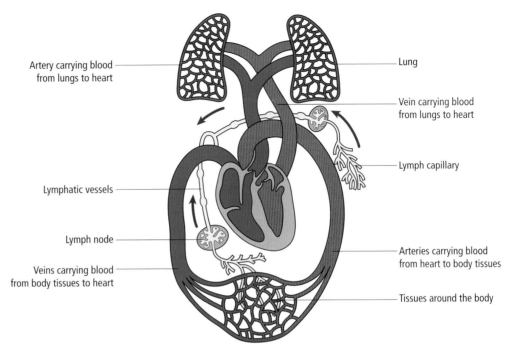

Artery carrying blood
from lungs to heart

Lung

Vein carrying blood
from lungs to heart

Lymph capillary

Lymphatic vessels

Lymph node

Arteries carrying blood
from heart to body tissues

Veins carrying blood
from body tissues to heart

Tissues around the body

Fig 6.2 How the lymphatic system works

The lymphatic system is, therefore, often referred to as a secondary circulatory system as it consists of a network of vessels that assist the blood in returning fluid from the tissues back to the heart. In this way, the lymphatic system is a complementary system for the circulatory system. After draining the tissues of excess fluid, the lymphatic system returns this fluid to the cardiovascular system. This helps to maintain blood volume, blood pressure and prevent oedema.

Structure of the lymphatic system

The lymphatic system contains the following structures:

- lymphatic capillaries
- lymphatic vessels
- lymphatic nodes
- lymphatic collecting ducts.

Overview of the structures of the lymphatic system

Structure	Description	Function
Lymphatic capillaries	Minute blind-end tubes, similar in structure to blood capillaries	Drain away excess fluid and waste products from the tissue spaces of the body
Lymphatic vessels	Similar in structure to veins; have one-way valves and thin, collapsible walls	Carry the lymph towards the heart

(Continued)

Structure	Description	Function
Lymphatic nodes	Oval or bean-shaped structures covered by a capsule of connective tissue. Made up of lymphatic tissue	Filter lymph of micro-organisms, cell debris or harmful substances
Lymphatic ducts (thoracic and right lymphatic)	The thoracic duct is the largest lymphatic vessel in the body and extends from second lumbar vertebra up through the thorax to the root of the neck The right lymphatic duct is very short in length. It lies in the root of the neck	Collect lymph from the whole body and return it to the blood via the subclavian veins

Lymphatic capillaries

Lymphatic vessels commence as lymphatic capillaries in the tissue spaces of the body as minute blind-end tubes, as lymph is a one-way circulatory pathway. The walls of the lymphatic capillaries are like those of the blood capillaries in that they are a single-cell-layer thick to make it possible for tissue fluid to enter them. However, they are permeable to substances of larger molecular size than those of the blood capillaries.

The lymphatic capillaries mirror the blood capillaries and form a network in the tissues, draining away excess fluid and waste products from the tissue spaces of the body. Once the tissue fluid enters a lymphatic capillary it becomes lymph and is gathered up into larger lymphatic vessels.

Lymphatic vessels

Lymphatic vessels are similar to veins in that they have thin, collapsible walls and their role is to transport lymph through its circulatory pathway. They have a considerable number of valves which help to keep the lymph flowing in the right direction and prevent backflow. Superficial lymphatic vessels tend to follow the course of veins by draining the skin, whereas the deeper lymphatic vessels tend to follow the course of arteries and drain the internal structures of the body. Networks or plexuses of lymphatic channels exist throughout the body. These intertwined channels are found in the following areas:

- **mammary plexus** – lymphatic vessels around the breasts
- **palmar plexus** – lymphatic vessels in the palm of the hand
- **plantar plexus** – lymphatic vessels in the sole of the foot.

The lymphatic vessels carry the lymph towards the heart under steady pressure and about two to four litres of lymph pass into the venous system every day. Once lymph has passed through the lymph vessels it drains into at least one lymphatic node before returning to the blood circulatory system.

Lymphatic nodes

At intervals along the lymphatic vessels lymphatic nodes occur. A lymphatic node is an oval or bean-shaped structure covered by a capsule of connective tissue. It is made up of lymphatic tissue and is divided into two regions: an outer cortex and an inner medulla.

There are more than 100 lymphatic nodes placed strategically along the course of lymphatic vessels. They vary in size between one to 25 mm in length and are massed in groups. Some are superficial and lie just under the skin, whereas others are deeply seated and are found near arteries and veins.

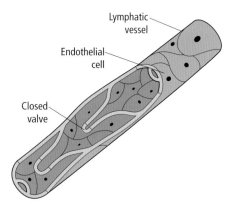

Lymphatic vessel

Endothelial cell

Closed valve

Fig 6.3 A lymphatic vessel

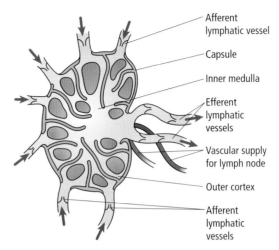

Afferent
lymphatic vessel

Capsule

Inner medulla

Efferent
lymphatic
vessels

Vascular supply
for lymph node

Outer cortex

Afferent
lymphatic
vessels

Fig 6.4 A lymphatic node

Each lymphatic node receives lymph from several afferent lymphatic vessels and blood from small arterioles and capillaries. Valves of the afferent lymphatic vessels open towards the node, therefore lymph in these vessels can only move towards the mode. Lymph flows slowly through the node moving from the cortex to the medulla, and leaves through an efferent vessel which opens away from the node. The afferent vessels enter a lymphatic node and the efferent vessels drain lymph from a node.

The function of a lymphatic node is to act as a filter of lymph to remove or trap any micro-organisms, cell debris or harmful substances which may cause infection so that when lymph enters the blood, it has been cleared of any foreign matter. When lymph enters a node, it comes into contact with two specialised types of leucocytes:

- **macrophages** – these are phagocytic in action. They engulf and destroy dead cells, bacteria and foreign material in the lymph
- **lymphocytes** – these are reproduced within the lymphatic nodes and can neutralise invading bacteria and produce chemicals and antibodies to help fight disease.

Once filtered the lymph leaves the node by one or two efferent vessels which open away from the node. Lymphatic nodes occur in chains so that the efferent vessel of one node becomes the afferent vessel of the next node in the pathway of lymph flow. Lymph drains through at least one lymphatic node before it passes into two main collecting ducts before it is returned to the blood.

Lymphatic ducts

From each chain of lymphatic nodes the efferent lymph vessels combine to form lymphatic trunks which empty into two main ducts – the thoracic and the right lymphatic ducts. These ducts collect lymph from the whole body and return it to the blood via the subclavian veins.

The thoracic duct is the main collecting duct of the lymphatic system. It is the largest lymphatic vessel in the body and extends from the second lumbar vertebra up through the thorax to the root of the neck. The thoracic duct collects lymph from the left side of the head and neck, left arm, lower limbs and abdomen, and drains into the left subclavian vein to return it to the bloodstream.

KEY FACT

If an area of the body becomes inflamed or otherwise diseased, the nearby lymph nodes will swell up and become tender, indicating that they are actively fighting the infection.

The right lymphatic duct is very short in length. It lies in the root of the neck and collects lymph from the right side of the head and neck and the right arm and drains into the right subclavian vein to be returned to the bloodstream.

Lymphatic drainage

Movement of lymph throughout the lymphatic system is known as lymphatic drainage and it begins in the lymphatic capillaries. The movement of lymph out of the tissue spaces and into the lymphatic capillaries is assisted by:

- The pressure exerted by the skeletal muscles against the vessels during movement.
- Changes in internal pressure during respiration.
- The compression of lymph vessels from the pull of the skin and fascia during movement.

Lymphatic drainage of the head and neck

The main groups of lymphatic nodes relating to the head and neck are as follows:

Fig 6.5 Lymphatic nodes of the head and neck

Name of lymphatic nodes	Position	Areas from which lymph is drained
Cervical nodes (deep)	Deep within the neck, located along the path of the larger blood vessels (carotid artery and internal jugular vein)	Drain lymph from the larynx, oesophagus, posterior of the scalp and neck, superficial part of chest and arm
Cervical nodes (superficial)	Located at the side of the neck, over the sternomastoid muscle	Drain lymph from the lower part of the ear and the cheek region
Submandibular nodes	Beneath the mandible	Drain chin, lips, nose, cheeks and tongue
Occipital nodes	At the base of the skull	Drain back of scalp and the upper part of the neck
Mastoid nodes (post auricular)	Behind the ear in the region of the mastoid process	Drain the skin of the ear and the temporal region of the scalp
Parotid nodes	At the angle of the jaw	Drain nose, eyelids and ear

Lymphatic drainage of the body

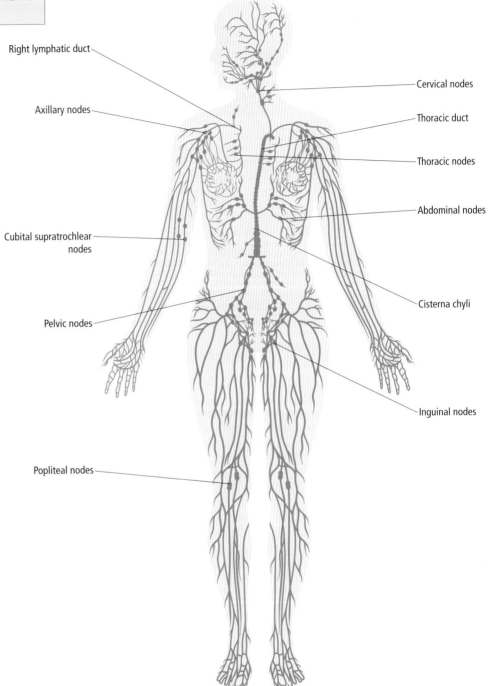

Right lymphatic duct

Axillary nodes

Cubital supratrochlear nodes

Pelvic nodes

Popliteal nodes

Cervical nodes

Thoracic duct

Thoracic nodes

Abdominal nodes

Cisterna chyli

Inguinal nodes

Fig 6.6 Lymphatic nodes of the body

Lymph nodes are mainly clustered at joints where they assist in pumping lymph through the nodes when the joint moves. The superficial lymph nodes are most numerous in the groin, axillae and neck. Most of the deep lymph nodes are found alongside blood vessels of the pelvic, abdominal and thoracic cavities. The main groups of lymphatic nodes relating to the body are as follows:

Name of lymphatic nodes	Position	Area from which lymph is drained
Cervical nodes (deep)	Deep within the neck, located along the path of the larger blood vessels	Drain lymph from the larynx, oesophagus, posterior of the scalp and neck, superficial part of chest and arm
Cervical nodes (superficial)	Located at the side of the neck over the sternomastoid muscle	Drain lymph from the lower part of the ear and cheek region
Axillary nodes	In the underarm region	Drain the upper limbs, wall of the thorax, breasts, upper wall of the abdomen
Supratrochlear/ cubital nodes	In the elbow region (medial side)	Upper limbs passing through the axillary nodes
Thoracic nodes	Within the thoracic cavity and along the trachea and bronchi	Organs of the thoracic cavity and from the internal wall of the thorax
Abdominal nodes	Within the abdominal cavity along the branches of the abdominal aorta	Organs within the abdominal cavity
Pelvic nodes	Within the pelvic cavity, along the paths of the iliac blood vessels	Organs within the pelvic cavity
Inguinal	In the groin	Lower limbs, external genitalia and lower abdominal wall
Popliteal	Behind the knee	The lower limbs through deep and superficial nodes

Student activity

Now complete Activity 6.2 in the resources for this book on Dynamic Learning Online.

Summary of the circulatory pathway of lymph

1	Plasma escapes blood capillary and bathes tissue cells
2	Excess fluid flows through a network of lymphatic capillaries
3	Tissue fluid enters lymph vessels where it becomes lymph
4	Larger lymphatic vessels lead to lymph nodes
5	Lymph passes through at least one lymphatic node where it is filtered
6	Filtered lymph is collected into lymphatic ducts
7	Collected lymph is drained into the venous system via the subclavian veins

Lymphatic organs

Lymphatic organs, whose functions are closely related to those of the lymph nodes, are the spleen, tonsils and thymus.

Spleen

The spleen is the largest of the lymphatic organs and is located on the left-hand side of the abdominal cavity between the diaphragm and the stomach. As the spleen is largely a mass of lymphatic tissue, it contains lymph nodes which produce lymphocytes and macrophages which are phagocytic.

The spleen:

- is a major site for filtering out worn out red blood cells and destroying micro-organisms in the blood.
- is concerned with protection from disease and the manufacture of antibodies. It functions with the lymphatic system by storing lymphocytes and releasing them as part of the immune response.
- serves as a blood reservoir and can release small amounts of blood into the circulation during times of emergency or blood loss.

Tonsils

The tonsils are composed of lymphatic tissue and are located in the oral cavity and the pharynx. There are three different sets of tonsils, all of which provide defence against micro-organisms that enter the mouth and nose. The palatine tonsils are the set commonly identified as the tonsils and are located at the back of the throat, one on each side. The pharyngeal tonsils are known as the adenoids and lie on the wall of the nasal part of the pharynx. The third set, the lingual tonsils, are found below the tongue.

Thymus

The thymus gland is a triangular-shaped gland composed of lymphatic tissue. It is located in the upper chest above the superior vena cava and below the thyroid where it lies against the trachea. The function of the thymus is important in the new-born baby in promoting the development and maturation of certain lymphocytes and in programming them to become T-cells (specialised types of lymphocytes of the immune system). The thymus gland begins to atrophy after puberty and becomes only a small remnant of lymphatic tissue in adulthood.

The immune system

The immune system is not a specific structural organ system but more of a functional system. It draws upon the structures and processes of each of the organs, tissues and cells of the body and the chemicals produced in them to eliminate any pathogen, foreign substance or toxic material that can be damaging to the body. Immunity can, therefore, be defined as the ability of the body to resist infection and disease by the activation of specific defence mechanisms.

The human body has a variety of different defence mechanisms. Some are non-specific in that they do not differentiate between one threat and another. Others are specific as the body mounts its defence specifically against a particular kind of threat.

Non-specific immunity

Non-specific immunity is programmed genetically in the human body from birth. The non-specific defences that are present from birth include:

- mechanical barriers
- chemicals
- inflammation
- phagocytosis
- fever.

Mechanical barriers

These are barriers such as the skin and mucous membrane that line the tubes of the respiratory, digestive, urinary and reproductive systems. As long as these barriers remain unbroken, many pathogens are unable to penetrate them.

The respiratory system is lined with mucous-secreting cells to help remove micro-organisms from the respiratory tract. The highly acidic environment in the stomach can help to kill pathogens, along with the production of saliva which has an antimicrobial effect. Urine helps to deter the growth of micro-organisms in the genito-urinary tract. The pH of the vagina protects against the multiplication and growth of microbes.

Chemicals

Chemicals are liberated by different cells that play an important role in immunity. There are many different types of chemicals involved in immunity including interferons, complements and histamine.

Interferons

These are proteins produced by cells infected by viruses. Interferon forms antiviral proteins to help protect uninfected cells and inhibit viral growth. There are three types of human interferon:

- **alpha** (from white blood cells)
- **beta** (from fibroblasts)
- **gamma** (from lymphocytes).

Complements

Complements are proteins found in blood that combine to create substances that phagocytise (ingest) bacteria.

Histamine

This is a chemical released by a variety of tissue cells. This includes mast cells, basophils (a type of white blood cell) and platelets. The release of histamine causes vasodilation to bring more blood to the area of injury or infection. It also increases vascular permeability to allow fluid to enter the damaged area and dilute the toxins released.

Inflammation

Inflammation is a sequence of events involving chemical and cellular activation that destroys pathogens and aids in the repair of tissues. It is a tissue response and symptoms include localised redness, swelling, heat and pain. The major actions that occur during an inflammation response include the following:

- The blood vessels dilate, resulting in an increase in blood volume (hyperaemia) to the affected area.
- Capillary permeability increases, causing tissues to become red, swollen, warm and painful.
- White blood cells invade the area and help to control pathogens by phagocytosis.
- In the case of bacterial infections, pus may form.
- Body fluids collect in the inflamed tissues. These fluids contain fibrinogen and other blood factors that promote clotting.
- Fibroblasts may appear and a connective tissue sac may be formed around the injured tissues.
- Phagocytic cells remove dead cells and other debris from the site of inflammation.
- New cells are formed by cellular reproduction to replace dead injured ones.

Phagocytosis

Neutrophils and monocytes are the most active phagocytic cells of the blood. Neutrophils are able to engulf and ingest smaller particles while monocytes can phagocytise larger ones. Moncoytes give rise to macrophages (large scavenger cells) which become fixed in various tissues and attached at the inner walls of the blood and lymphatic vessels.

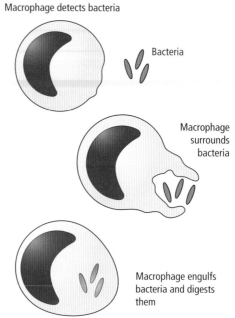

Fig 6.7 Phagocytosis

Fever

An individual is said to have a fever if their body temperature is maintained above 37.28°C (99°F). The increase in temperature during a fever tends to inhibit some viruses and bacteria. It also speeds up the body's metabolism and, thereby, increases the activity of defence cells.

Specific immunity

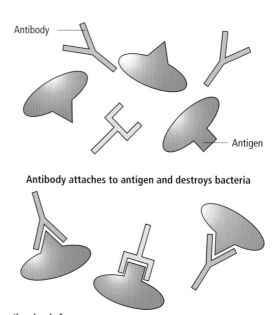

Fig 6.8 The antibody defence system

Immunity involves interaction between two types of molecule – an antigen and an antibody.

An antigen is any substance that the body regards as foreign or potentially dangerous and against which it produces an antibody. An antibody is a specific protein produced to destroy or suppress antigens.

Antibodies circulate in the blood and tissue fluid, killing germs or making them harmless. Antibodies also neutralise poisonous chemicals called toxins which germs produce. Specific immunity involves very specific responses to each identified foreign substance and calls on special memory cells to help if the invader reappears. This is the ability to recognise certain antigens and destroy them. The body must be able to identify which substances are capable of causing a threat before any type of response can be initiated.

How antibodies work

Antibodies work in many different ways. Some neutralise the antigens when they combine with them and prevent them from carrying out their effects. Others may lyse (destroy) the cell on which the antigen is present. When antibodies are bound to antigens on the surface of bacteria, they attract other white blood cells like macrophages to engulf them.

The key cells of specific immunity are a specialised group of white blood cells called lymphocytes. They are capable not only of recognising foreign agents but remembering the agents they have encountered and, therefore, are able to react more rapidly and with greater force if they encounter the agent again.

The immune response

There are two types of immune response produced by different types of lymphocytes:

- **Humoral immunity** – this involves the B-lymphocytes which produce free antibodies that circulate in the bloodstream.
- **Cell-mediated immunity** – this is effected by the helper T-cells, suppressor T-cells and natural killer (NK) cells that recognise and respond to certain antigens to protect the body against their effects.

Lymphocytes develop in the following three ways:

- T-cells begin in the bone marrow and grow in the thymus gland. They are able to recognise antigens and respond by releasing inflammatory and toxic materials. Specialised T-cells also regulate the immune response, either by amplifying the response (T4 cells) or by suppressing the body's response (T8 cells). Some T-cells develop into memory cells and handle secondary response on re-exposure to antigens that have already produced a primary response.
- B-cells grow and develop in the bone marrow. B-cells contain immunoglobulin, an antibody that responds to specific antigens. Some B-cells modify and become non-antigen specific which means that they have a greater ability to respond to bacterial and viral pathogens. Some B-cells become memory cells and are able to deal with re-exposure to antigens.
- A type of lymphocyte that does not develop the same structural or functional characteristics as the T-cells or B-cells are the natural killer cells (NK) cells. They also develop in the bone marrow and when mature can attack and kill tumour cells and virus-infected cells during their initial developmental stage before the immune system is activated.

Primary and secondary responses

The initial response of the body on first exposure to antigens is known as the primary response. It normally takes about two weeks after exposure to the antigen for antibody levels to peak. This is due to the fact that B-cells have to become converted to plasma cells that secrete antibodies specifically against the antigen.

If the individual is exposed to the antigen the second time, the presence of memory cells stimulates rapid production of antibodies and this is known as the secondary response. The antibody levels are much higher than the primary response and remain elevated for a very long time. Secondary response can occur even if many years have elapsed since the first exposure to the antigen.

Immunisation

The body may be artificially stimulated into producing antibodies and this is known as immunisation. This prepares the body to ward off infection in advance and is carried out by inoculating an individual with a vaccine (a liquid containing antigens powerful enough to stimulate antibody formation without causing harm). Vaccines have been developed against many diseases including diphtheria, polio, tetanus, whooping cough and measles.

Allergy

Under certain circumstances abnormal responses or allergic reactions may occur when a foreign substance, or antigen, enters the body. An allergic reaction can only occur if the person has already been exposed to the antigen at least once before and has developed some antibody to it.

The type and severity of an allergic reaction depends upon the strength and persistence of the antibody screen evoked by previous exposure to the antigen. These antibodies are located on the cells in the skin or mucous membranes of the respiratory and gastro-intestinal tracts. Typical antigens include pollen, dust, feathers, wool, fur, certain foods and drugs.

The reactions may cause symptoms of hay fever, asthma, eczema, urticaria and contact dermatitis. If there is much cellular damage, excessive amounts of histamine may be released causing circulatory failure (anaphylaxis). Anaphylactic shock is an extreme and generalised form of allergic reaction whose widespread release of histamine causes swelling (oedema), constriction of the bronchioles, heart failure, circulatory collapse and may even result in death.

Common pathologies of the lymphatic system

Acquired Immune Deficiency Syndrome (AIDS)

This is a condition contracted as a result of the Human Immunodeficiency Virus (HIV) which progressively destroys the immunity of the individual. The HIV virus suppresses the body's immune response, allowing the opportunist infections to take hold, and results in AIDS.

AIDS patients become vulnerable to infections that do not affect normal individuals. Infections that produce mild symptoms otherwise may produce severe symptoms in them. Patients may also be prone to usual cancers.

IN PRACTICE

In the case of Hodgkin's disease, advice from the client's consultant physician is necessary before undertaking any form of treatment. Caution is advised regarding the risk of spread of the disease through lymphatic drainage. Clients are vulnerable to infection due to reduced immunity. It is inadvisable to treat if the client is debilitated; however, clients may otherwise benefit from a gentle, relaxing treatment.

IN PRACTICE

In the case of lupus, care is required when handling as skin lesions may be tender and joint pain and tenderness may be present. Avoid contact if you are suffering from any infectious illness, as medication that clients may be taking for this condition can suppress immunity and clients are therefore prone to infections.

IN PRACTICE

Remember that lymphoedema is symptomatic of many disease processes (particularly cardiovascular disease) and therefore advice from the client's GP is essential before offering any form of treatment.

This syndrome is caused by contact with infected blood or body fluids. It is common in drug addicts using infected injection needles and syringes and having unprotected sexual intercourse.

Hodgkin's disease

This is a malignant disease of the lymphatic tissues, usually characterised by painless enlargement of one or more groups of lymph nodes in the neck, armpit, groin, chest or abdomen. The spleen, liver, bone marrow and bones may also be involved. Apart from the enlarging nodes there may also be weight loss, fever, profuse sweating at night and itching.

Lupus erythematosus

This is a chronic inflammatory disease of connective tissue affecting the skin and various internal organs. It is an auto-immune disease and can be diagnosed by the presence of abnormal antibodies in the bloodstream. Typical signs are a red scaly rash on the face, arthritis and progressive damage to the kidneys. Often the heart, lungs and brain are also affected by progressive attacks of inflammation, followed by the formation of scar tissue. It can also cause psychiatric illness due to direct brain involvement but the skin is affected in a milder form only.

Lymphoedema

This is an abnormal swelling of body tissues due to an accumulation of tissue fluid. It could be the result of heart failure, liver or kidney disease or due to chronic varicose veins. The resultant swelling of the tissues may be localised, as with an injury or inflammation or may be more generalised, as in heart or kidney failure. Subcutaneous oedema commonly occurs in the legs and ankles due to the influence of gravity, and is a common problem in women before menstruation and in the last trimester of pregnancy.

Interrelationships with other systems

The lymphatic system links to the following body systems.

Cells and tissues
Lymphatic tissue is a specialised type of tissue found in lymph nodes, spleen, tonsils, the adenoids, walls of the large intestine and glands in the small intestine.

Skin
Lymph vessels are numerous in the dermis of the skin. They form a network allowing the removal of waste from the skin's tissues.

Skeletal
Red bone marrow is responsible for the development of cells found in both blood and lymph.

Muscular
The action of skeletal muscles aids lymphatic drainage.

Circulatory
The lymphatic system aids the circulatory system in that it assists the blood in returning fluid from the tissues back to the heart.

Respiratory
Low pressure in the thorax created by breathing movements aids the movement of lymph.

Digestive
The lymphatic system plays an important part in absorbing the products of fat digestion from the villi of the small intestine.

Key words associated with the lymphatic system

lymph	parotid nodes	tonsils
oedema	axillary nodes	thymus
lacteals	supratrochlear nodes	immunity
lymphatic capillaries	thoracic nodes	specific immunity
tissue (interstitial) fluid	abdominal nodes	non-specific immunity
lymphatic vessels	pelvic nodes	antigen
lymphatic nodes	inguinal nodes	antibody
deep cervical nodes	popliteal nodes	humoral immunity
superficial cervical nodes	thoracic duct	cell-mediated immunity
submandibular nodes	right lymphatic duct	immunisation
occipital nodes	subclavian veins	allergic reaction
mastoid nodes	spleen	

Revision summary of the lymphatic system

- The lymphatic system is closely associated with the cardiovascular system.
- The lymphatic system assists the blood by draining the tissues of excess fluid and returning the fluid from the tissues back to heart. This helps to maintain blood volume, blood pressure and prevent **oedema** (waterlogging of the tissues).
- The lymphatic system also plays an important role in the body's immune system as the lymph nodes fight infection and generate antibodies.
- The lymphatic system also absorbs the products of fat digestion through the intestinal lymph vessels called the **lacteals**.
- **Lymph** is a clear, colourless, water fluid derived from tissue fluid and contained within lymph vessels.
- Lymph is similar in composition to blood except that it has a lower concentration of plasma proteins.
- The circulatory pathway of lymph begins with **lymphatic capillaries** which lie in the tissue spaces between the cells.
- **Tissue (interstitial) fluid** drains into **lymphatic capillaries** and the excess fluid becomes **lymph**.
- **Lymphatic capillaries** merge to form larger vessels called **lymphatic vessels** which convey lymph in and out of structures called **lymph nodes**.
- The main groups of lymph nodes relating to the head and neck include **deep cervical, superficial cervical, submandibular, occipital, mastoid and parotid nodes**.
- The main group of lymph nodes relating to the body include **superficial cervical, deep cervical, axillary, suptratrochlear, thoracic, abdominal, pelvic, inguinal** and **popliteal nodes**.
- Lymph passes through at least one node where it is filtered of cell debris, micro-organisms and harmful substances.
- Once filtered, the lymph is collected into two main ducts – **thoracic duct** (the largest duct) which collects lymph from the left side of the head and neck, left arm, lower limbs and abdomen and the **right lymphatic duct** which collects lymph from the right side of the head and neck and the right arm.
- The collected lymph is then drained into the venous system via the right and left **subclavian veins**.
- Other lymphatic organs include the **spleen, tonsils** and **thymus gland**.
- **Immunity** is the ability of the body to resist infection and disease by the activation of specific defence mechanisms.
- There are two types of **immunity** – specific and non-specific.
- **Non-specific immunity** is programmed genetically from birth and includes mechanical barriers (skin and mucous membrane), chemicals, inflammation, phagocytosis and fever.
- **Specific immunity** involves interaction between an **antigen** and an **antibody**.
- An **antigen** is any substance that the body regards as foreign or potentially dangerous, and against which it produces an antibody.
- An **antibody** is a specific protein produced to destroy or suppress antigens.
- There are two types of immune response produced by different types of lymphocytes – **humoral immunity** involving B-lymphocytes which produce free antibodies that circulate in the bloodstream and **cell-mediated immunity** effected by helper T-cells, suppressor T-cells and natural killer (NK) cells that recognise and respond to certain antigens to protect the body against their effects.
- **Immunisation** is when the body is artificially stimulated into producing antibodies.
- An **allergic reaction** may occur when a foreign substance, or antigen, enters the body.
- An allergic reaction can only occur if the person has already been exposed to the antigen at least once before and has developed some antibody to it.
- **Antibodies** are located on the cells in the skin or mucous membranes of the respiratory and gastro-intestinal tracts. Typical antigens include pollen, dust, feathers, wool, fur, certain foods and drugs.

The lymphatic system and immunity
Multiple-choice questions

1 Lymph is derived from:
  a plasma proteins
  b tissue fluid
  c blood plasma
  d lymphocytes

2 Lymph is similar in composition to blood except it has a lower concentration of:
  a water
  b protein
  c waste
  d hormones

3 Lymphatic capillaries are:
  a similar in structure to veins
  b oval shaped structures
  c similar in structure to arteries
  d minute blind-end tubes

4 Which of the following is not a function of the lymphatic system?
  a prevention of oedema
  b production of heat
  c production of lymphocytes
  d absorption of fat

5 The lymphatic system has a close relationship to which other system?
  a nervous
  b respiratory
  c urinary
  d circulatory

6 In order to be cleansed of foreign matter lymph must pass through at least one:
  a lymphatic node
  b lymphatic vessel
  c lymphatic capillary
  d lymphatic duct

7 Which of the following nodes drains lymph from the lower limbs?
  a axillary
  b cervical
  c popliteal
  d supratrochlear

8 Which of the following drains lymph from the back of the scalp and the upper part of the neck?
  a parotid
  b occipital
  c deep cervical
  d superficial cervical

9 The axillary nodes are situated in the:
  a neck
  b underarm
  c groin
  d elbow

10 Which of the following nodes drains lymph from the chin, lips, nose, cheeks and tongue?
  a parotid
  b mastoid
  c submandibular
  d occipital

11 The two main lymphatic ducts are:
  a thoracic and left subclavian
  b thoracic and right lymphatic
  c right and left subclavian
  d right and left lymphatic

12 The largest of the lymphatic organs is the:
  a tonsils
  b liver
  c thymus
  d spleen

13 Which duct collects the majority of lymph?
  a thoracic duct
  b left lymphatic duct
  c right lymphatic duct
  d cisterna chyli

14 Collected lymph is drained into the venous system via the:
  a subclavian arteries
  b superior vena cava
  c subclavian veins
  d brachiocephalic veins

15 In the context of immunity a foreign substance is otherwise known as an:
   a antibody
   b antigen
   c allergy
   d interferon

16 The viral infection which progressively destroys immunity in an individual is:
   a AIDS
   b lupus erythematosus
   c myalgic encephalomyelitis
   d Hodgkin's disease

17 Lymph nodes vary in size between:
   a 1 and 25 mm in length
   b 5 and 25 mm in length
   c 15 and 20 mm in length
   d 20 and 25 mm in length

18 Which of the following is **not** a cause of generalised oedema?
   a heart failure
   b respiratory disease
   c liver disease
   d kidney disease

19 The spleen is located in the:
   a right-hand side of the abdominal cavity
   b superior to the thymus
   c left-hand side of the abdominal cavity
   d behind the intestines

20 Proteins produced by cells infected by viruses are called:
   a complements
   b histamine
   c interferons
   d pathogens

7 the respiratory system

Introduction

The respiratory system consists of the nose, naso-pharynx, pharynx, larynx, trachea, bronchi and lungs, which provide the passageway for air, in and out of the body. Oxygen is needed by every cell of the body for survival. Respiration is the process by which the living cells of the body receive a constant supply of oxygen and remove carbon dioxide and other gases. Our respiratory system serves us in many ways, exchanging oxygen and carbon dioxide, detecting smell, producing speech and regulating pH.

Objectives

By the end of this chapter you will be able to recall and understand the following knowledge:

- the functions of the respiratory system
- the structure and functions of the main structures of the respiratory system
- the process of the interchange of gases in the lungs
- the mechanism of breathing
- the theory of olfaction
- the importance of correct breathing
- the interrelationships between the respiratory and other body systems
- common pathologies of the respiratory system.

Functions of the respiratory system

- **Exchange of gases** – oxygen and carbon dioxide exchange is the primary function of the respiratory system in order to sustain life.
- **Olfaction** – specialised nerve endings embedded in the nasal cavity send impulses for the sense of smell to the brain.
- **Speech** – the vocal cords in the larynx aid in producing speech.
- **Homeostasis** – the respiratory system helps to maintain homeostasis by maintaining oxygen levels in the blood and through the elimination of wastes such as carbon dioxide and heat.

The structures of the respiratory system

Naso-pharynx (nasal cavity) — Pharynx

Epiglottis — Oesophagus

Larynx — Trachea

Right lung — Left lung

Bronchus — Ribs

Bronchioles — Pleural cavity

Intercostal muscles — Pleural membranes

Fig 7.1 Structures of the respiratory system

Overview of the structures of the respiratory system

Structure	Description	Function
Nose	Lined with cilia and mucous membrane	Inhales air Moistens, warms and filters the air Senses smell
Naso-pharynx	Upper part of the nasal cavity behind the nose lined with mucous membrane	Continues to filter, warm and moisten the incoming air
Pharynx	Large muscular tube lined with mucous membrane lies behind the mouth and between the nasal cavity and the larynx	Acts as a passageway for air, food and drink Resonating chamber for sound
Larynx	Short passage connecting the pharynx to the trachea	Provides a passageway for air between the pharynx and the trachea Produces sound
Trachea	Tube anterior to the oesophagus and extends from the larynx to the upper chest, composed of smooth muscle and up to 20 C-shaped rings of cartilage	Transports air from the larynx into the bronchi

Structure	Description	Function
Bronchi	Two short tubes (similar in structure to the trachea) which lead to each lung	Carry air into the lungs
Lungs	Cone-shaped spongy organs situated in the thoracic cavity on either side of the heart	Facilitate the exchange of the gases oxygen and carbon dioxide

BODY FACT

Due to the close proximity of the throat to the eustachian tube, throat infections can easily spread to the ear via the eustachian tubes.

KEY FACTS

The sinuses are air-filled spaces located within the maxillary, frontal, ethmoid and sphenoid bones of the skull. These spaces open into the nasal cavity and are lined with mucous membrane that are continuous with the lining of the nasal cavity. Consequently, mucous secretions can drain from the sinuses into the nasal cavity. If this drainage is blocked by membranes that are inflamed and swollen because of nasal infections or allergic reactions, the accumulating fluids may cause increasing pressure within a sinus and a painful sinus headache.

BODY FACT

The larynx grows rapidly in males during puberty, creating an increased prominence of the Adam's apple. The elongated vocal cords vibrate with a lower frequency, resulting in a deeper voice.

The nose

The nose is divided into the right and left cavities. It is lined with tiny hairs called cilia which begin to filter the incoming air, and mucous membrane which secretes a sticky fluid called mucus to prevent dust and bacteria from entering the lungs. The nose moistens, warms and filters the air and is an organ which senses smell.

The naso-pharynx

The naso-pharynx is the upper part of the nasal cavity behind the nose and is lined with mucous membrane. The eustachian tubes from the middle ears open into the naso-pharynx so that air pressure inside the ear can be adjusted to prevent damage to the eardrum. At the back of the naso-pharynx there is lymphoid tissue such as the adenoids. The function of the naso-pharynx is to continue to filter, warm and moisten the incoming air.

The pharynx

The pharynx or throat is a large muscular tube lined with mucous membrane which lies behind the mouth and between the nasal cavity and the larynx. The tonsils are found at the back of the pharynx. The pharynx serves as an air and food passage but cannot be used for both purposes at the same time, otherwise choking would result. The air is also warmed and moistened further as it passes through the pharynx.

The larynx

The larynx (voice box) is a short passage connecting the pharynx to the trachea. The larynx is a box-like cavity with rigid walls which contain the vocal cords and stiff pieces of cartilage, such as the Adam's apple, which prevent collapse and obstruction of the airway. The vocal cords are bands of elastic ligaments that are attached to the rigid cartilage of the larynx by skeletal muscle. When air passes over the vocal cords they vibrate and produce sound. The opening into the larynx from the pharynx is called the glottis. During the process of swallowing, the glottis is covered by a flap of tissue called the epiglottis which prevents food from 'going down the wrong way'. The larynx provides a passageway for air between the pharynx and the trachea.

The trachea

The trachea or windpipe is a tube anterior to the oesophagus and extends from the larynx to the upper chest. It is composed of smooth muscle and up to 20 C-shaped rings of cartilage which serve a dual purpose. The incomplete section of the ring allows the oesophagus to expand into the trachea when a food bolus is swallowed and the rings help to keep the trachea permanently open. The trachea passes down into the thorax and connects the larynx with the bronchi which pass into the lungs.

The bronchi

The bronchi are two short tubes similar in structure to the trachea which lead to and carry air into each lung. They are lined with mucous membrane and ciliated cells and, like the trachea, contain cartilage to hold them open. The mucus traps solid particles and cilia move them upwards, preventing dirt from entering the delicate lung tissue. The bronchi subdivide into bronchioles in the lungs. These subdivide yet again and finally end in minute air-filled sacs called alveoli.

The lungs

The lungs are paired cone-shaped spongy organs situated in the thoracic cavity on either side of the heart. The left lung has two lobes and the right lung has three lobes. The right lung is thicker and broader than the left and is also slightly shorter than the left, as the diaphragm is higher on the right side to accommodate the liver which lies below it. Internally, the lungs consist of millions of tiny air sacs called alveoli which are arranged in lobules and resemble bunches of grapes. The function of the lungs is to facilitate the exchange of the gases oxygen and carbon dioxide. In order to carry this out efficiently, the lungs have several important features:

- a very large surface area (about 1,000 square foot) provided by approximately 300 million alveoli
- thin permeable membrane surrounding the walls of the alveoli
- a thin film of water lining the alveoli which is essential for dissolving oxygen from the alveoli air
- thin-walled blood capillaries forming a network around the alveoli which absorb oxygen from the air breathed into the lungs and release carbon dioxide into the air breathed out of the alveoli.

The structures enclosed within the lungs are bound together by elastic and connective tissue. On the outside the lungs have two layers of a serous membrane called pleura, an outer parietal layer that lines the thoracic cavity and an inner visceral layer that is attached to the surface of the lungs. Between the visceral and parietal pleurae is the pleural cavity which contains a lubricating fluid secreted by the membranes and reduces friction between the lungs and the chest wall.

The diaphragm

The diaphragm is the chief muscle of respiration and is a dome-shaped muscular partition that separates the thoracic cavity from the abdominal cavity. During contraction the diaphragm is pulled down creating a vacuum in the chest cavity which sucks air into the lungs. Relaxation of the

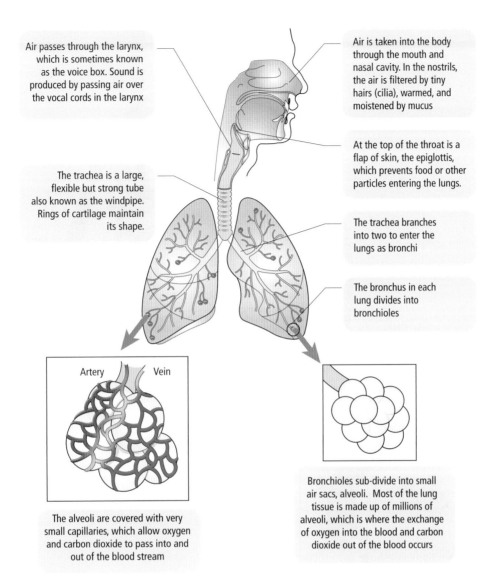

Air passes through the larynx, which is sometimes known as the voice box. Sound is produced by passing air over the vocal cords in the larynx

Air is taken into the body through the mouth and nasal cavity. In the nostrils, the air is filtered by tiny hairs (cilia), warmed, and moistened by mucus

At the top of the throat is a flap of skin, the epiglottis, which prevents food or other particles entering the lungs.

The trachea is a large, flexible but strong tube also known as the windpipe. Rings of cartilage maintain its shape.

The trachea branches into two to enter the lungs as bronchi

The bronchus in each lung divides into bronchioles

Artery   Vein

The alveoli are covered with very small capillaries, which allow oxygen and carbon dioxide to pass into and out of the blood stream

Bronchioles sub-divide into small air sacs, alveoli. Most of the lung tissue is made up of millions of alveoli, which is where the exchange of oxygen into the blood and carbon dioxide out of the blood occurs

Fig 7.2 The respiratory system

diaphragm causes it to rise, allowing the lungs to deflate and air is pushed out of the lungs as a result.

The interchange of gases in the lungs

Oxygen and carbon dioxide exchange is the primary function of the respiratory system. Oxygen is needed by every cell of the body and delivery is accomplished by way of the bloodstream. The respiratory and circulatory systems, therefore, both participate in this process. The interchange of gases in the lungs involves the absorption of oxygen from the air in exchange for carbon dioxide which is released by the body as a waste product of cell metabolism.

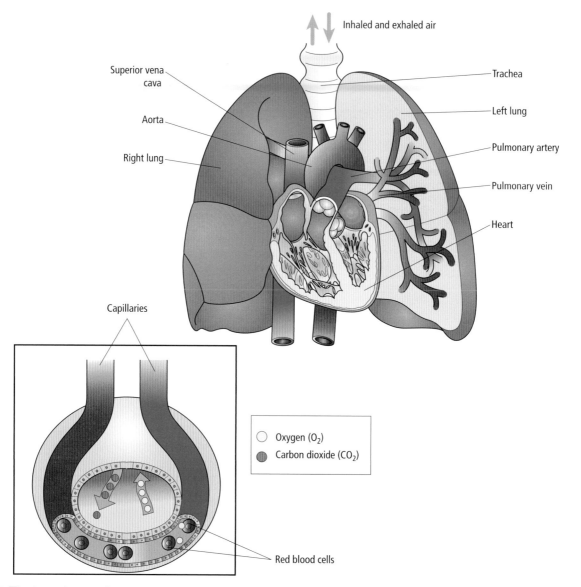

Fig 7.3 The interchange of gases

External respiration

This refers to gas exchange in the lungs between the blood and air in the alveoli that came from the external environment. The respiration process is as follows:

During inhalation oxygen is taken in through the nose and mouth. It flows along the trachea and bronchial tubes to the alveoli of the lungs where it diffuses through the thin film of moisture lining the alveoli
Oxygen diffuses from the air inside the alevoli across the alveolar walls and into the blood capillaries. The oxygen binds to the haemoglobin inside erythrocytes and is then transported to the cells throughout the body
Carbon dioxide is transported by the blood in the opposite direction from the cells of the body to the capillaries attached to the alveoli
The carbon dioxide then diffuses from the blood across the alveolar walls into the air inside the alveoli which will then be exhaled through the nose and mouth
Oxygen and carbon dioxide exchange across the wall of the alveoli at the same time

Internal/tissue respiration

This is the gas exchange between the blood and the tissues throughout the body. Oxygen diffuses from the blood into the cells and carbon dioxide diffuses from the cells into the bloodstream.

The mechanism of respiration

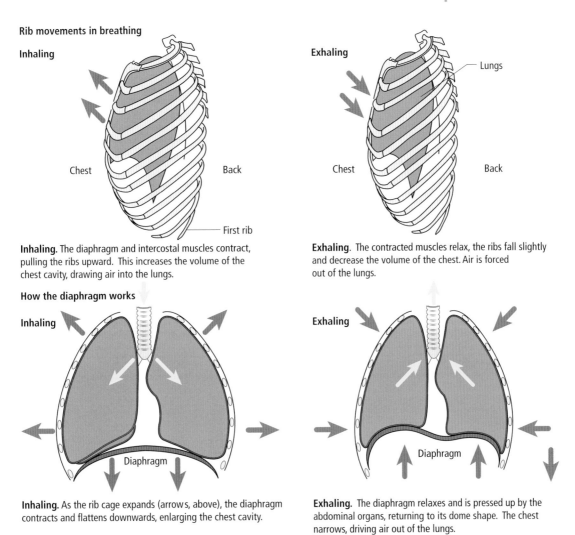

Rib movements in breathing

Inhaling

Chest   Back

First rib

Inhaling. The diaphragm and intercostal muscles contract, pulling the ribs upward. This increases the volume of the chest cavity, drawing air into the lungs.

Exhaling

Lungs

Chest   Back

Exhaling. The contracted muscles relax, the ribs fall slightly and decrease the volume of the chest. Air is forced out of the lungs.

How the diaphragm works

Inhaling

Diaphragm

Inhaling. As the rib cage expands (arrows, above), the diaphragm contracts and flattens downwards, enlarging the chest cavity.

Exhaling

Diaphragm

Exhaling. The diaphragm relaxes and is pressed up by the abdominal organs, returning to its dome shape. The chest narrows, driving air out of the lungs.

Fig 7.4 The mechanism of respiration

The major muscle of respiration is the diaphragm. The mechanism of respiration is the means by which air is drawn in and out of the lungs. It is an active process where the muscles of respiration contract to increase the volume of the thoracic cavity.

STUDY TIP

When studying inhaling and exhaling it may be helpful to consider the following summary in brief:

- Inhaling – as you breathe in, the diaphragm flattens to make more space. The intercostal muscles between your ribs move up and out. The lungs can now expand and air rushes in to fill the space.
- Exhaling – when you breathe out, the diaphragm and intercostal muscles relax. The diaphragm raises and the ribs move down and in. As there is now less space, air is forced out.

BODY FACT

Other accessory muscles which assist in inspiration include the sternomastoid, serratus anterior, pectoralis minor, pectoralis major and the scalene muscles in the neck.

KEY FACTS

Breathing is a relatively passive process. However, when more air needs to be exhaled, such as when coughing or playing a wind instrument, the process of expiration becomes active. This is assisted by muscles such as the internal intercostals which help to depress the ribs. Abdominal muscles, such as the external and internal obliques, rectus abdominus and transversus abdominus, help to compress the abdomen and force the diaphragm upwards, thus assisting expiration and squeezing more air out of the lungs.

Summary of the mechanism of respiration

Air is moved in and out of the lungs by the combined action of the diaphragm and the intercostal muscles
During inspiration the dome-shaped diaphragm contracts and flattens, increasing the volume of the thoracic cavity
The diaphragm is responsible for bringing approximately 75 per cent of the volume of air into the lungs
The external intercostal muscles are also involved in respiration and upon contraction they increase the depth of the thoracic cavity by pulling the ribs upwards and outwards. The external intercostal muscles are responsible for bringing approximately 25 per cent of the volume of air into the lungs
The combined contraction of the diaphragm and the external intercostals increases the thoracic cavity which then decreases the pressure inside the thorax so that air from outside of the body enters the lungs
During normal respiration the process of expiration is passive and is brought about by the relaxation of the diaphragm and the external intercostal muscles, along with the elastic recoil of the lungs. This increases the internal pressure inside the thorax so that air is pushed out of the lungs

Breathing rate

The normal breathing rate is 12 to 15 breaths per minute although this may increase during exercise and stress, and decrease during sleep. Breathing takes place rhythmically, with insipration lasting for about two seconds and expiration for approximately three seconds.

Regulation of breathing

Breathing, like the beating of the heart, occurs continuously and rhythmically without conscious thought. The basic pattern of breathing can be modified by voluntary intervention but the underlying mechanism is essentially automatic. It continues when we are asleep and unconscious.

Nervous control

Breathing is controlled by a group of neurons in the parts of the brain called the medulla oblongata and the pons, known as the respiratory centre. Nerve cells, called chemoreceptors, found in the aorta and the carotid arteries send impulses to the respiratory centre in the medulla oblongata of the brain with messages about the levels of oxygen and carbon dioxide in the blood. When the levels of carbon dioxide and oxygen need adjusting, a nerve impulse is sent to the respiratory muscles and as a result, cellular needs for an adequate supply of oxygen and removal of carbon dioxide are met. The medulla oblongata controls the rate and depth of respiration and the pons moderates the rhythm of the switch from inspiration to expiration.

Olfaction

Olfaction is a special sense which is capable of detecting different smells and evoking emotional responses due to its close link with the endocrine system. The process of olfaction is assisted by the nervous system as smells received by the nose are transmitted by nerve impulses to be perceived by the brain.

The structure of the olfactory system

The special features of the olfactory system are as follows:

- **Nose** – this is the organ of olfaction or smell.
- **Mucous membrane** – this lines the nose, moistens the air passing over it and helps to dissolve the odorous gas passing through the nasal cavity. The mucous membrane has a very rich blood supply, and warmth from the blood flowing through the tiny capillaries in the nose raises the temperature of the air as it passes through the nose.
- **Cilia** – these are the tiny hairs inside the nose which are covered in mucous. They are highly sensitive and are extensions of nerve fibres connecting with the olfactory cells.
- **Olfactory cells** – these lie embedded in the mucous in the upper part of the nasal cavity. These nerve cells are sensory and are specially adapted for sensing smell. Each olfactory cell has a long nerve fibre called an axon, leading out of the main body of the cell which picks up information received and passes it on to the brain.
- **Olfactory bulb** – this is the area of the brain situated in the cerebral cortex, which perceives smell.

The theory of olfaction

Olfaction is a special sense in that odour perception is transmitted directly to the brain. The process of olfaction may be summarised as follows.

Reception

The volatile particles of an essential oil evaporate on contact with air.
Some volatile molecules pervade the air and some enter the nose.
The odiferous particles of the essential oil dissolve in the mucous, which lines the inner nasal cavity, prior to their stimulation at the receptor sites.

Transmission

The captivated aromatic molecules are picked up by the cilia which protrude from the olfactory receptor cells located at the top of the nasal cavity.
The olfactory receptor cells have a long nerve fibre called an axon and an electrochemical message of the aroma is transmitted along the axons of receptor cells to join the olfactory nerves.
The fibres of the olfactory nerves pass through the cribriform plate of the ethmoid bone in the roof of the nose to reach the olfactory bulb, where the odorant signal is chemically converted before being relayed to the brain.

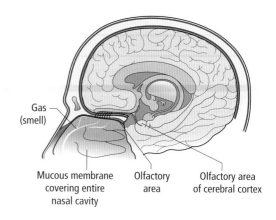

Labels: Gas (smell), Mucous membrane covering entire nasal cavity, Olfactory area, Olfactory area of cerebral cortex

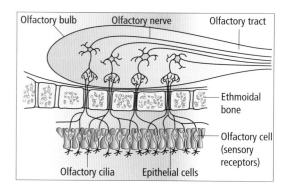

Labels: Olfactory bulb, Olfactory nerve, Olfactory tract, Ethmoidal bone, Olfactory cell (sensory receptors), Olfactory cilia, Epithelial cells

Fig 7.5 Olfaction

Perception

Once the message reaches the olfactory bulb, the olfactory impulses pass into the olfactory tract and pass directly to the cerebral cortex where the smell is perceived.
The temporal lobe of the brain contains the primary olfactory area which is directly connected to the limbic area, which is concerned with emotions, memory and sex drive.
The olfactory bulb also connects closely with the hypothalamus, the nerve centre which governs the endocrine system.

BODY FACT

In most nerves in the body the transmission of a nerve impulse is achieved through the spinal cord and then on to the brain. However, in the case of the olfactory cells the nerve fibres connect directly with the olfactory bulb of the brain and therefore have a powerful and immediate effect on the emotions.

The importance of correct breathing

Exercise increases the rate and depth of breathing due to the muscle cells requiring more oxygen. The breathing rate can more than double during vigorous exercise. Correct breathing is very important as it ensures that all the body's cells receive an adequate amount of oxygen and dispose of enough carbon dioxide to enable them to function efficiently. It is important to note that breathing affects both our physiological and psychological state. Deep breathing exercises can help to increase the vital capacity and function of the lungs.

IN PRACTICE

In the case of a client with asthma, always obtain a detailed history during the consultation stage, specifically the triggers that bring on an attack. If the client has a history of allergies then ensure they are not allergic to any preparations or substances you may be proposing to use. Position the clients according to their individual comfort, usually in a semi-reclined position. It is advisable for the client to have their required medications handy, in the event of an attack.

Common pathologies of the respiratory system

Asthma

This condition presents as attacks of shortness of breath and difficulty in breathing due to spasm or swelling of the bronchial tubes. This is caused by hypersensitivity to allergens such as pollens of various plants, grass, flowers, pet hair, dust mites and various proteins in foodstuffs such as shellfish, eggs and milk. Asthma may be exacerbated by exercise, anxiety, stress or smoking. It can run in families and may also be associated with hay fever and eczema.

Bronchitis

This is a chronic or acute inflammation of the bronchial tubes. Chronic bronchitis is common in smokers and may lead to emphysema which is caused by damage to the lung structure. Acute bronchitis can result from a recent cold or flu.

Cancer of the lung

This may be caused by chronic inhalation of cancer-producing air and industrial pollutants such as cigarette smoke and asbestos fibres. Usually there are no symptoms initially and it is often detected only in the advanced stages. Late symptoms include chronic cough, hoarseness, difficulty in breathing, chest pain, blood in sputum, weight loss and weakness.

Emphysema

This is a chronic obstructive pulmonary disease in which the alveoli of the lungs become enlarged and damaged, reducing the surface area for the exchange of oxygen and carbon dioxide. Severe emphysema causes breathlessness which is made worse by infection. It is commonly associated with chronic bronchitis, smoking and advancing age.

Hay fever

This is an allergic reaction involving the mucous passages of the upper respiratory tract and the conjunctiva of the eyes, caused by pollen or other allergens. It causes nose blockages, sneezing and watery eyes.

Pleurisy

This is an inflammation of the pleura of the lung. It presents as an intense stabbing pain over the chest on breathing deeply. There is difficulty in breathing, respiration is shallow and rapid and fever is present. Pleurisy may develop as a complication of pneumonia, tuberculosis or trauma to the chest.

Pneumonia

Pneumonia is the inflammation of the lung caused by bacteria in which the alveoli become filled with inflammatory cells and the lung becomes solid. Symptoms include fever, malaise and headache, together with a cough and chest pain.

Rhinitis

This condition is the inflammation of the mucous membrane of the nose, causing a blocked, runny and stuffy nose. It may be caused by a virus infection such as a cold, or an allergic reaction.

Sinusitis

This condition involves inflammation of the paranasal sinuses. It is usually caused by a viral or bacterial infection or may be associated with a common cold or allergy. The congestion of the nose results in a blockage in the opening of the sinus into the nasal cavity and a build-up of pressure in the sinus. The condition presents with nasal congestion followed by a mucous discharge from the nose. The pain is located in specific areas depending on the sinuses affected. If the frontal sinuses are affected, a major symptom is a headache over one or both eyes. If the maxillary sinuses are affected, one or both cheeks will hurt and it may feel as if there is a toothache in the upper jaw.

Stress

Stress can be defined as any factor which affects physical or emotional health. Examples of excessive stress on the respiratory system include exacerbation of asthma and the development of frequent colds.

Tuberculosis (TB)

This infectious disease is caused by the bacillus (bacteria) *mycobacterium tuberculosis*. The main transportation of tuberculosis is via droplet infection and hence the most common site for the bacilli to spread to is the lungs. The bacilli can also result from drinking unpasteurised milk from infected cows. It is characterised by the formation of nodules in the body tissues. Symptoms include coughing, sneezing, night sweats, fever, weight loss and the spitting of blood. Enlarged lymph nodes can also be an indication of TB. Prevention of the disease is available through the BCG vaccine.

Interrelationships with other systems

The respiratory system links to the following body systems.

Cells and tissues
Squamous and ciliated are examples of types of simple epithelium that line the respiratory system.

Integumentary
Oxygen absorbed through the respiratory process is carried to the skin via its capillaries to facilitate cell renewal.

Skeletal
The bones of the thorax (sternum, ribs and 12 thoracic vertebrae) provide vital protection for the organs of respiration (heart and lungs).

Muscular

The mechanism of respiration is created by the combined action of the diaphragm and the intercostal muscles.

Circulatory

Blood transports oxygen breathed into the lungs around the body to the cells and transports carbon dioxide from the cells to the lungs to be exhaled.

Nervous

Breathing is an involuntary response that results from the stimulation of the respiratory centre in the medulla and the pons of the brain.

Endocrine

The hormone adrenalin, produced by the adrenal glands, is released into the bloodstream to change the rate of breathing when the body is under stress.

Digestive

The mouth and the pharynx link the respiratory and digestive systems.

Key words associated with the respiratory system

nose	bronchioles	olfactory cells
naso-pharynx	lungs	olfactory bulb
pharynx	alveoli	diaphragm
larynx	diffusion	intercostal muscles
trachea	cilia	inspiration
bronchi	mucous membrane	expiration

Revision summary of the respiratory system

- The respiratory organs include the **nose, naso-pharynx, pharynx, larynx, trachea, bronchi, bronchioles** and **lungs**.
- The respiratory organs act with the cardiovascular system to supply oxygen and remove carbon dioxide from the blood.
- The **nose** is lined with **cilia** and **mucous membrane** and is adapted for warming, moistening and filtering air, and senses smell.
- Smell is perceived by specialised **olfactory cells** which connect directly with the olfactory bulb in the brain.
- The **pharynx** or throat connects the nasal cavity to the larynx.
- As well as providing an air passage between the nasal cavity and **larynx**, the **pharynx** also serves as a food passage for the digestive system.
- The **larynx** is a short passage that connects the pharynx with the trachea and contains the vocal cords.
- The **trachea** or windpipe is made up mainly of cartilage and passes down into the thorax to connect the larynx with the bronchi which pass into the lungs.
- The **lungs** are situated in the thoracic cavity on either side of the heart.
- Internally the lungs consist of tiny air sacs called **alveoli** which provide a very large surface area for the exchange of gases oxygen and carbon dioxide.

- The interchange of gases occurs as a result of simple **diffusion**.
- During **inhalation** oxygen in taken in through the **nose** and **mouth**, along the **trachea** and **bronchi** to the **lungs**, where it diffuses through a thin film of moisture lining the **alveoli**.
- Oxygen then diffuses across the permeable membrane surrounding the **alveoli** to be taken up by the red blood cells, and oxygen-rich blood is carried to the heart and pumped to the cells of the body.
- Carbon dioxide, collected from respiring cells, diffuses from the capillary walls into the **alveoli**, passes through the **bronchi** and **trachea**, and is exhaled through the **nose** and **mouth**.
- Air is moved in and out of the lungs by the combined action of the **diaphragm** and the **intercostal muscles**.
- During **inspiration** the combined contraction of the **diaphragm** and the **external intercostals** increase the volume of the **thoracic cavity** which decreases the pressure inside the thorax so that air enters the lungs.
- The process of **expiration** is passive and is brought about by the relaxation of the **diaphragm** and the **external intercostals** and the elastic recoil of the lungs.

The respiratory system
Multiple-choice questions

1 Which of the following is **not** a function of the respiratory system?
   a producing speech
   b detecting smell
   c regulating blood
   d exchanging oxygen and carbon dioxide

2 Which of the following acts as a passageway for air, food and drink?
   a larynx
   b trachea
   c pharynx
   d naso-pharynx

3 Another name for the throat is the:
   a larynx
   b epiglottis
   c pharynx
   d bronchioles

4 The windpipe is a common name for the:
   a trachea
   b pharynx
   c larynx
   d bronchi

5 The tiny air sacs in the lungs which provide a large surface area for diffusion are:
   a alveoli
   b surfactants
   c pleura
   d bronchioles

6 The trachea is made up of mainly:
   a spongy tissue
   b mucous membrane
   c cilia
   d cartilage

7 The part of the respiratory system extending from the larynx to the upper chest is the:
   a larynx
   b bronchi
   c trachea
   d pharynx

8 The normal breathing rate is:
   a 10 to 12 breaths per minute
   b 12 to 15 breaths per minute
   c 15 to 20 breaths per minute
   d 20 to 25 breaths per minute

9 During gas exchange, oxygen and carbon dioxide diffusion occurs in the:
   a body tissues
   b alveoli
   c venules
   d red blood cells

10 When oxygen passes through the alveoli into the bloodstream it binds with haemoglobin to form:
   a red blood cells
   b carbon dioxide
   c oxyhaemoglobin
   d nitrogen

11 Involuntary breathing results from stimulation of the respiratory centre in the:
   a medulla oblongata and pons
   b cerebellum
   c thalamus
   d hypothalamus

12 Chronic bronchitis may lead to which other respiratory disorder?
   a pleurisy
   b pneumonia
   c tuberculosis
   d emphysema

13 The conditon asthma is best described as:
   a a viral infection associated with a common cold
   b attacks of shortness of breath
   c an intense stabbing pain in the chest
   d nasal congestion and mucous discharge

14 The process of inspiration is brought about by:
a combined relaxation of the diaphragm and internal intercostals
b combined contraction of the diaphragm and external intercostals
c combined relaxation of the diaphragm and external intercostals
d combined contraction of the diaphragm and internal intercostals

15 The eustachian tube opens into the:
a pharynx
b trachea
c naso-pharynx
d larynx

16 The tonsils are found at the back of the:
a pharynx
b larynx
c nose
d naso-pharynx

17 Which receptors detect changes in the levels of carbon dioxide in the blood?
a baroreceptors
b thermoreceptors
c olfactory receptors
d chemoreceptors

18 Which of the following is responsible for bringing approximately 75 per cent of the volume of air into the lungs?
a diaphragm
b external intercostals
c internal intercostals
d transversus abdominis

19 Olfactory cells lie embedded in the mucous in the:
a lower part of the nasal cavity
b upper part of the nasal cavity
c olfactory bulb
d cerebral cortex

20 Sinusitis is usually caused by a:
a hypersensitivity to allergens
b swelling of the bronchial tubes
c genetic predisposition
d viral or bacterial infection

8

the nervous system

Introduction

The anatomical structures of the nervous system include the brain, spinal cord and nerves, which together form the main communication system for the body. The nervous system is the body's control centre or 'head office' and is, therefore, responsible for receiving and interpreting information from inside and outside the body.

The nervous system receives, interprets and integrates all stimuli to effect a response. It is also responsible for all mental processes and emotional responses and works intimately with the endocrine system to help regulate body processes.

Objectives

By the end of this chapter you will be able to recall and understand the following knowledge:

- the functions of the nervous system
- the organisation of the nervous system
- the characteristics of nervous tissue
- the structure and function of different types of neurones
- the transmission of nerve impulses
- an outline of the principal parts of the nervous system
- the interrelationships between the nervous and other body systems
- common pathologies of the nervous system.

Functions of the nervous system

The nervous system has three main functions:

1 It senses changes both within the body (the internal environment) and outside the body (the external environment).
2 It analyses the sensory information, stores some aspects and makes decisions as to how to respond. This is called integration.
3 It may respond to stimuli by initiating muscular contractions or glandular secretions.

Organisation of the nervous system

The nervous system has two main parts which both possess unique structural and functional characteristics:

- **central nervous system (CNS)** – this is the main control system that consists of the brain and the spinal cord
- **peripheral nervous system (PNS)** – this system can be subdivided into the **somatic nervous system** and the **autonomic nervous system**.

Somatic nervous system

This contains 31 pairs of spinal nerves and 12 pairs of cranial nerves and governs the impulses from the CNS to the skeletal muscles.

Automatic nervous system

This supplies impulses to smooth muscles, cardiac muscle, skin, special senses, proprioceptors (sensory nerve endings located in muscles and tendons that transmit information to coordinate muscular activity), organs and glands. The autonomic nervous system consists of a sympathetic and parasympathetic division.

Nervous tissue

There are two types of nervous tissue – **neuroglia** and **neurones**.

Neuroglia or glial cells are a special type of connective tissue of the central nervous system that is designed to support, nourish and protect the neurones. Glial cells are smaller and more numerous than neurones. They are unable to transmit impulses and never lose their ability to divide by mitosis.

The functional unit of the nervous system is a **neurone** which is a specialised nerve cell, designed to receive stimuli and conduct impulses. The nervous system contains billions of interconnecting neurones which are the basic impulse-conducting cells of the nervous system. Neurones have two major properties:

- **excitability** – the ability to respond to a stimulus and convert it to a nerve impulse
- **conductability** – the ability to transmit the impulses to other neurones, muscles and glands.

Neurones also occur in groups called ganglia outside the central nervous system and as single cells, known as a ganglion, in the walls of organs.

Parts of a neurone

Although neurones vary in their shape and size they all have three basic parts:

- **Cell body** – this has a central nucleus and is surrounded by cytoplasm and contains standard organelles such as mitochondria and a golgi body.
- **Dendrites** – these are highly branched extensions of the nerve cell. These neural extensions receive and transmit stimuli towards the cell body.
- **Axon** – this is long, single nerve fibre extending from the cell body. The function of an axon is to transmit impulses away from the cell body.

BODY FACT

Over 50 per cent of the brain is made up of glial cells and most brain tumours are, therefore, made up of glial cells.

BODY FACT

Nerve cells have the highest metabolic rate in the body and are easily damaged by toxins or lack of oxygen which leads to their destruction.

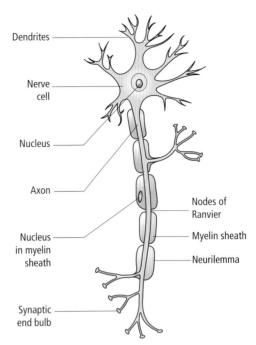

Fig 8.1 The structure of a nerve cell

Other parts of a neurone's structure include the following.

Myelin sheath
This is a fatty insulating sheath that covers the axon. Its function is to insulate the nerve and accelerate the conduction of nerve impulses along the length of the axon. The myelin sheath is produced by Schwann cells (large flat cells containing a nucleus and cytoplasm) which wrap themselves around the axon in a spiral fashion layer after layer.

Neurilemma
This is a fine delicate membrane that surrounds the axon and consists of a layer of one or more Schwann cells enclosing the myelin sheath. The neurilemma plays an important role in the regeneration of PNS nerve fibres.

Nodes of Ranvier
The myelin sheath has gaps at intervals of 2–3 mm along the length of the axon which are called the nodes of Ranvier. During neural activity impulses jump from one node to another, resulting in an increased rate of conduction.

Synapse
This is the minute gap across which nerve impulses pass from one neurone to the next at the end of a nerve fibre. Reaching a synapse causes the release of a neurotransmitter which diffuses across the gap and triggers an electrical impulse in the next neurone.

Synaptic end bulb/feet
The ends of the axon terminals have bulb-like structures containing sacs called synaptic vesicles that store the transmitters. These are chemicals that facilitate, arouse or inhibit the transmission of impulses between neurones across synapses.

KEY FACT

A thicker myelinated nerve fibre will enable nervous signals to be transmitted very quickly, such as pain fibres, whereas hot and cold receptor fibres are non-myelinated and their signals are transmitted more slowly.

There are three types of neurones:

Sensory/afferent neurones	Receive stimuli from sensory organs and receptors and transmit the impulse to the spinal cord and brain. Sensations transmitted by the sensory neurones include heat, cold, pain, taste, smell, sight and hearing
Motor/efferent neurones	Conduct impulses away from the brain and the spinal cord to muscles and glands in order to stimulate them into carrying out their activities
Association (mixed) neurones	Link sensory and motor neurones, helping to form the complex pathways that enable the brain to interpret incoming sensory messages, decide on what should be done and send out instructions in response along motor pathways to keep the body functioning properly

Fig 8.2 A simple nerve pathway

The transmission of nerve impulses

Neurones are responsible for neurotransmission, the conduction of electrochemical impulses throughout the nervous system. Neurone activity is provoked by:

- **mechanical** stimuli – touch and pressure
- **thermal** stimuli – heat and cold
- **chemical** stimuli – from external chemicals or from a chemical released by the body such as histamine.

Nerve impulses are caused by chemical changes in the cell body. Chemical compounds generate electrical charges called ions. Inside the nerve cell body there are potassium ions which cause a negative charge in the cell but outside of the cell are sodium ions which are positively charged.

Whenever there is a change of pressure, temperature or a chemical stimuli a section of the nerve membrane becomes permeable to sodium and the positively charged ions flow in, leaving the outside of the membrane negative. The combination of the negative potassium ions and the positive sodium ions causes an electrical charge which creates the impulse along the length of the nerve cell.

Nerve impulses are the signals of the nervous system that travel along the neurone from dendrite to axon. The function of a neurone is to transmit impulses from their origin to destination. The nerve fibres of a neurone are not actually joined together and, therefore, there is no anatomical continuity between one neurone and another.

The junction where nerve imulses are transmitted from one neurone to another is called a synapse. This is the junction between two neurones or between a neurone and a muscle or gland where they connect to transmit information.

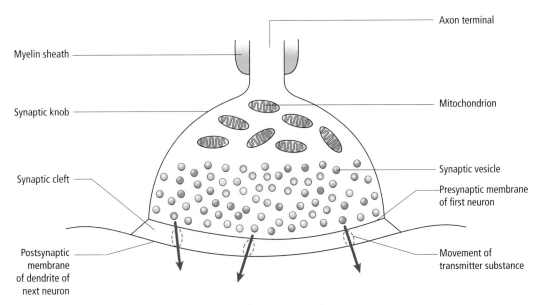

Fig 8.3 The conduction of a nerve impulse across a synapse

Impulses are relayed from one neurone to another by a chemical transmitter substance which is released by the neurone to carry impulses across the synapse to stimulate the next neurone. Synapses cause nerve impulses to pass in one direction only and are important in coordinating the actions of neurones. A special kind of synapse occurs at the junction between a nerve and a muscle and is known as a motor point, which is the point where the nerve supply enters the muscle.

KEY FACT

KEY FACT

An important neurotransmitter is **acetylcholine** which is vital to muscle contraction.

The conduction of a motor impulse in the contraction of skeletal muscle

Motor impulse initiated in brain

↓

Motor stimuli travel along length of the axon to the effector such as the muscle

↓

Motor impulse reaches motor point of muscle fibres

↓

Nerve impulse is passed across the neuromuscular junction

↓

Chemical transmitter substance released across synapse

↓

Muscle fibres contract and effect movement desired

The central nervous system

The central nervous system, consisting of the brain and spinal cord, is covered by a special type of connective tissue called the **meninges**. The meninges has three layers:

- **dura mater** – this is the outer protective fibrous connective tissue sheath covering the brain and spinal cord
- **pia mater** – this is the innermost layer which is attached to the surface of organs and is richly supplied with blood vessels to nourish the underlying tissues
- **arachnoid mater** – this provides a space for the blood vessels and circulation of cerebrospinal fluid.

Cerebrospinal fluid

This is a clear fluid derived from the blood and secreted into the inner cavities of the brain. It carries some nutrients to the nerve tissue and carries waste away but its main function is to protect the central nervous system by acting as a shock absorber for the delicate nervous tissue.

The brain

The brain is an extremely complex mass of nervous tissue lying within the skull. It is the main communication centre of the nervous system and its function is to coordinate the nerve stimuli received and effect the correct responses. The main parts of the brain include the cerebrum, thalamus, cerebellum and the brain stem.

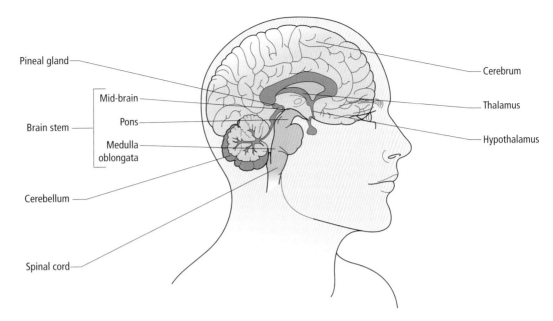

Fig 8.4 Principal parts of the brain

Overview of the principal parts of the brain

Part of brain	Location	Function
Cerebrum	Largest part of brain Makes up front and top part of brain	Intelligence Emotions
Thalamus	Lies either side of forebrain	Relays sensory impulses to the cerebral cortex
Hypothalamus	Small structure lies beneath the thalamus	Governs many important homeostatic functions (hunger, thirst, temperature regulation, anger, aggression, hormones, sexual behaviour, sleep patterns and consciousness)
Pineal gland	Pea-sized mass of nervous tissue attached by a stalk in the central part of the brain Attached to the upper portion of the thalamus	Secretes melatonin Regulation of circadian rhythms
Cerebellum	Cauliflower-shaped structure located at the posterior of the cranium, below the cerebrum	Coordination of skeletal muscles, posture and balance
Brain stem	Enlarged continuation of the spinal cord	Connects the brain with the spinal cord Contains control centres for heart, lungs and intestines

Cerebrum

This is the largest portion of the brain and makes up the front and top part of the brain. It is divided into two large cerebral hemispheres. Each cerebral hemisphere is divided into four lobes – **frontal**, **temporal**, **parietal** and **occipital**, named according to the skull bones that lie over them.

A mass of nerve fibres known as the **corpus callosum** bridges the hemispheres, allowing communication between corresponding centres in each hemisphere. The surface of the cerebrum is made up of convolutions called gyri and creases called sulci.

The outer layer of the cerebrum is called the **cerebral cortex** and is the region where the main functions of the cerebrum are carried out. The cortex is concerned with all forms of conscious activity such as vision, touch, hearing, taste and smell, as well as control of voluntary movements, reasoning, emotion and memory. The cortex of each cerebral hemisphere has a number of functional areas:

Sensory areas	Receive impulses from sensory organs all over the body. There are separate sensory areas for vision, hearing, touch, taste and smell
Motor areas	These have motor connections through motor nerve fibres with voluntary muscles all over the body
Association areas	In these areas association takes place between information from the sensory areas and remembered information from past experiences Conscious thought then takes place and decisions are made which often result in conscious motor activity controlled by motor areas

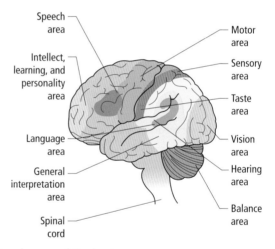

Fig 8.5 Functional areas of the brain

Thalamus

Lying deep in the cerebral hemispheres in each side of the forebrain are one of two egg-shaped masses of grey matter called the thalami. The thalami are relay and interpretation stations for the sensory messages (except olfaction) that enter the brain before they are transmitted to the cortex.

Hypothalamus

This small structure lies beneath the thalamus and governs many important homeostatic functions. It regulates the autonomic nervous and endocrine systems by governing the pituitary gland. It controls hunger, thirst, temperature regulation, anger, aggression, hormones, sexual behaviour, sleep patterns and consciousness.

Pineal gland

This is a pea-sized mass of nerve tissue attached by a stalk in the central part of the brain. It is located deep between the cerebral hemispheres where it is attached to the upper portion of the thalamus. The pineal gland secretes a hormone called melatonin which is synthesised from serotonin. The pineal gland is involved in the regulation of circadian rhythms. These are patterns of repeated activity that are associated with the environmental cycles of day and night such as sleep/wake rhythms. The pineal gland is also thought to influence mood.

Cerebellum

The cerebellum is a cauliflower-shaped structure located at the posterior of the cranium, below the cerebrum. It is the brain's second largest region. Like the cerebrum, it has two hemispheres and has an outer cortex of grey matter and an inner core of white matter. The cerebellum is concerned with muscle tone, the coordination of skeletal muscles and balance.

Brain stem

The brain stem contains three main structures:

- **Mid-brain** – this contains the main nerve pathways connecting the cerebrum and the lower nervous system. It also contains certain visual and auditory reflexes that coordinate head and eye movements with things seen and heard.
- **Pons** – this is below the mid-brain and relays messages from the cerebral cortex to the spinal cord and helps regulate breathing.
- **Medulla oblongata** – this is often considered the most vital part of the brain.

It is an enlarged continuation of the spinal cord and connects the brain with the spinal cord. Control centres within the medulla oblongata include those for the heart, lungs and intestines. The medulla also controls gastric secretions and reflexes such as sweating, sneezing, swallowing and vomiting.

Blood–brain barrier

The blood–brain barrier is a selective semipermeable wall of blood capillaries with a thick basement membrane. It prevents, or slows down, the passage of some drugs and other chemical compounds and keeps disease-causing organisms such as viruses from travelling into the central nervous system via the bloodstream.

Spinal cord

This is an extension of the brain stem which extends from an opening at the base of the skull down to the second lumbar vertebra.

It forms a two-way information pathway between the brain and the rest of the body via the spinal nerves. It is protected by three layers of tissues called the meninges and by cerebospinal fluid. Its function is to relay impulses to and from the brain. Sensory tracts conduct impulses to the brain and motor tracts conduct impulses from the brain.

The spinal cord provides the nervous tissue link between the brain and other organs of the body and is the centre for reflex actions which provide a fast response to external or internal stimuli.

Student activity

Now complete Activity 8.1 in the resources for this book on Dynamic Learning Online.

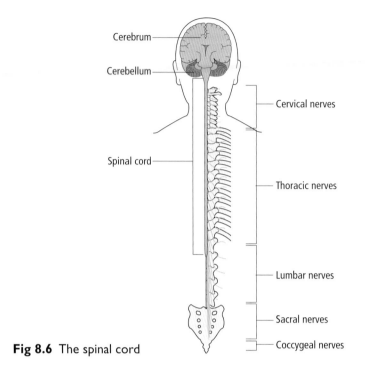

Fig 8.6 The spinal cord

Reflex action

A reflex action is a rapid and automatic response to a stimulus without any conscious thought of the brain.

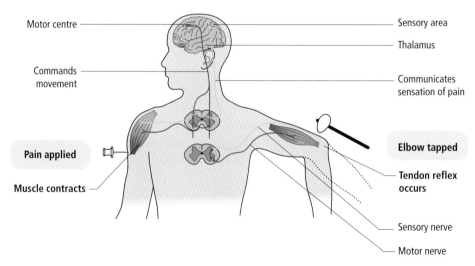

Fig 8.7 A reflex action

Reflexes are essentially designed to protect the body. A reflex action, sometimes called a reflex arc, is a neural relay cycle for quick motor response to a harmful sensory stimulus. It requires a sensory (afferent) neurone and a motor (efferent) neuron.

Instead of the sensory impulses going all of the way to the brain where it can be analysed and the correct response selected, a reflex allows a shorter and quicker response. A typical example of a reflex action is a hand touching a hot object which involves sensory and motor nerves being coordinated through the spinal cord. The stimulus triggers a sensory impulse which travels along the dorsal root to the spinal cord.

Two synaptic transmissions occur at the same time. One synapse continues the impulse along a sensory neurone to the brain, the other immediately relays the impulse to an interneuron which transmits it to a motor neurone.

The motor neurone delivers the impulse to a muscle or gland, producing an immediate response and in this case withdrawing the hand from the hot object.

The peripheral nervous system

The peripheral nervous system contains all the nerves outside of the central nervous system. It consists of cable-like nerves that link the central nervous system to the rest of the body. The peripheral nervous system can be sub-divided into the somatic nervous system and the autonomic nervous system.

The somatic nervous system contains:

- **31 pairs of spinal nerves** (nerves originating from the spinal cord)
- **12 pairs of cranial nerves** (nerves originating from the brain).

31 pairs of spinal nerves

These nerves pass out of the spinal cord and each has two thin branches which link it with the autonomic nervous system. Spinal nerves receive sensory impulses from the body and transmit motor signals to specific regions of the body, thereby providing two-way communication between the central nervous system and the body.

Each of the spinal nerves are numbered and named according to the level of the spinal column from which they emerge. There are:

- 8 cervical nerves
- 12 thoracic nerves
- 5 lumbar nerves
- 5 sacral nerves
- 1 coccygeal spinal nerve.

Each spinal nerve is divided into several branches forming a network of nerves or plexuses which supply different parts of the body:

Nerve plexus	Location	Area/s of the body it supplies
Cervical	Neck	Skin and muscles of the head, neck and upper region of the shoulders
Brachial	Top of shoulder	Skin and muscles of the arm, shoulder and upper chest
Lumbar	Between waist and hip	Front and sides of the abdominal wall and part of the thigh
Sacral	Base of the abdomen	Skin and muscles and organs of the pelvis
Coccygeal	Base of spine	Skin in the area of the coccyx and the muscles of the pelvic floor

12 pairs of cranial nerves

These nerves connect directly to the brain. Between them they provide a nerve supply to sensory organs, muscles and skin of the head and neck. Some of the nerves are mixed containing both motor and sensory nerves, while others are either sensory or motor.

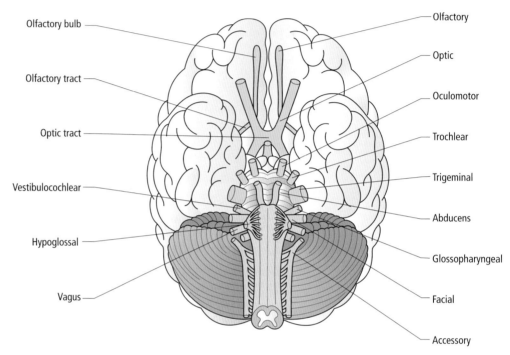

Fig 8.8 The cranial nerves

Cranial nerve	Type of nerve	Description
Olfactory	Sensory	Nerve of olfaction
Optic	Sensory	Nerve of vision
Oculomotor	Mixed nerve	Innervates both internal and external muscles of the eye and a muscle of the upper eyelid
Trochlear	Motor nerve	Smallest of the cranial nerves Innervates the superior oblique muscle of the eyeball which helps you look upwards
Abducens	Mixed nerve	Innervates only the lateral rectus muscle of the eye which helps you look to the side
Facial	Mixed nerve	Conducts impulses to and from several areas in the face and neck The sensory branches are associated with the taste receptors on the tongue, and the motor fibres transmit impulses to the muscles of facial expression
Vestibulocochlear	Sensory nerve	Transmits impulses generated by auditory stimuli and stimuli related to equilibrium, balance and movement

Cranial nerve	Type of nerve	Description
Glossopharyngeal	Mixed nerve	Supplies motor fibres to part of the pharynx and to the parotid salivary glands, and sensory fibres to the posterior third of the tongue and the soft palate
Vagus	Mixed	Has branches to numerous organs in the thorax and abdomen as well as the neck Supplies motor nerve fibres to the muscles of swallowing and to the heart and organs of the chest cavity Sensory fibres carry impulses from the organs of the abdominal cavity and the sensation of taste from the mouth
Accessory	Motor	Innervating muscles in the neck and upper back, such as the trapezius and the sternomastoid, as well as muscles of the palate, pharynx and larynx
Hypoglossal	Motor	Innervates the muscles of the tongue
Trigemenal has three main branches: • the **ophthalmic** branch carries sensations from the eye, nasal cavity and skin of the forehead, upper eyelid, eyebrow and part of the nose • the **maxillary** branch carries sensations from the lower eyelid, upper lip, gums, teeth, cheek, nose, palate and part of the pharynx • the **mandibular** branch carries sensations from the lower gums, teeth, lips, palate and part of the tongue	Mixed	Containing motor and sensory nerves that conduct impulses to and from several areas in the face and neck Also controls the muscles of mastication (the masseter, temporalis and pterygoids)

The autonomic nervous system

This is the part of the nervous system that controls the automatic body activities of smooth and cardiac muscle and the activities of glands. It is divided into the sympathetic and parasympathetic divisions, which possess complementary responses.

Effects of the sympathetic and parasympathetic nervous systems

Part of body	Effects of sympathetic stimulation	Effects of parasympathetic stimulation
Heart	Increases heart rate	Slows down heart rate
Lungs	Dilates bronchi to increase respiration	Slows down breathing rate
Blood vessels	Dilates blood vessels	Constricts blood vessels

(Continued)

Part of body	Effects of sympathetic stimulation	Effects of parasympathetic stimulation
Adrenal glands	Stimulates release of adrenalin	
Sweat glands	Stimulates/increases the secretion of sweat	
Digestive	Reduces peristalsis	Increases peristalsis
Liver	Increases conversion of glycogen to glucose by liver	Increases conversion of glucose to glycogen
Bladder	Relaxes bladder	Contracts bladder
Skin	Contricts arterioles so less blood flows near skin surface (skin looks pale)	
Eyes	Dilates pupils	Constricts pupils

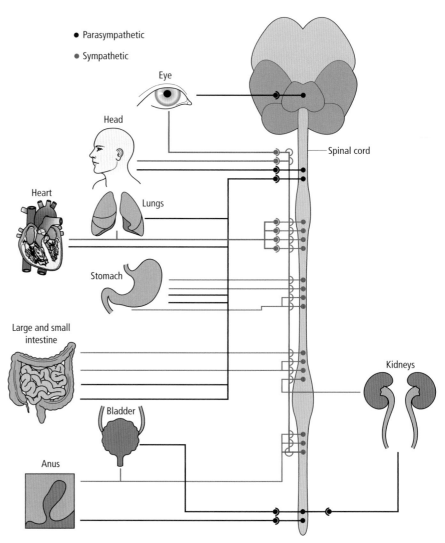

Fig 8.9 The autonomic nervous system

The sympathetic system

The activity of the sympathetic system is to prepare the body for expending energy and dealing with emergency situations.

Part of body	Effects of sympathetic stimulation	Body response
Heart	Increases rate of contraction of cardiac muscle	Heart rate increases
Lungs	Dilates bronchi	Breathing rate increases
Blood vessels	Dilates blood vessels	Increases body's ability to move
Adrenal glands	Stimulates release of adrenalin and noradrenaline	Body prepared for 'fight or flight' response
Sweat glands	Stimulates/increases the secretion of sweat	Sweaty palms and nervousness
Salivary glands	Decreases secretion of saliva	Dry mouth
Digestive	Reduces peristalsis	May feel constipated
Liver	Increases conversion of glycogen to glucose by liver	Provides extra glucose for tissues (may get 'sugar high')
Bladder	Relaxes bladder and closes sphincter muscles	Body can go long periods without urinating
Skin	Contricts arterioles	Less blood flows near skin surface (skin looks pale)
Eyes	Dilates pupils	Improves vision

KEY FACT

The sympathetic stimulation of the autonomic nervous system is increased by the release of the hormone adrenaline from the adrenal medulla. This is an example of the nervous and endocrine systems working synergistically.

The parasympathetic system

This balances the action of the sympathetic division by working to conserve energy and create the conditions needed for rest and sleep. It slows down the body processes except digestion and the functions of the genito-urinary system. In general, the actions of the parasympathetic system oppose those of the sympathetic system and the two systems work together to regulate the internal workings of the body. Effects of the parasympathetic nervous system include:

Part of body	Effects of parasympathetic stimulation	Body response
Heart	Slows down rate of contraction of cardiac muscle	Heart rate slows down, blood pressure reduces
Lungs	Constricts bronchi	Breathing rate slows down and becomes deeper
Blood vessels	Constricts blood vessels	Increases ability to sit still
Adrenal glands	No effect	
Sweat glands	No effect	

(Continued)

Part of body	Effects of parasympathetic stimulation	Body response
Salivary glands	Increases secretion of saliva	Stimulates digestion
Digestive	Increases peristalsis	May digest food better
Liver	No effect	
Bladder	Contracts bladder and relaxes sphincter muscles	More frequent bowel movements
Skin	No effect	
Eyes	Constricts pupils	

The sympathetic and parasympathetic nervous systems are finely balanced to ensure the optimum functioning of organs of the body.

Sense organs

The sense organs include the following:

- **Nose** (olfaction) – the specialised chemoreceptor olfactory nerve cells in the nose pick up information of an incoming odour and pass it to the olfactory bulb in the brain to be analsyed.
- **Tongue** (taste) – chemosensitive receptors are concentrated on the projections on the tongue called papillae. Within the papillae lie the tiny taste buds which are round in structure and form bundles of cell bodies and nerve endings of the seventh, ninth and tenth cranial nerves. The taste hairs are stimulated by food and drink that is placed in the mouth, sending messages in the form of electrical impulses to the taste area in the cerebrum for interpretation.
- **Eyes** (sight) – vision uses photoreceptors that are located in the eye. Light enters the eye through the pupil and strikes the retina. There are two types of photoreceptors located on the retina: rods and cones. These light sensitive cells convert the incoming light into nerve impulses and send them to the optic nerve to interpret what is being seen.
- **Ears** (hearing) – the ears are associated with the sensory functions of hearing and balance which are detected by mechanoreceptors. Sound waves are picked up in the ear and transmitted to the cerebrum via the eighth cranial nerve for interpretation. The ears send messages via the eighth cranial nerve to the cerebrum and cerebellum to detect changes in the position of the head. The messages are interpreted and the skeletal muscles are instructed to maintain balance and posture.
- **Skin** (touch) – there are numerous sensory nerve endings in the skin that are sensitive to touch, pain and changes in temperature (see Chapter 2).

Common pathologies of the nervous system

Anxiety

This can be defined as fear of the unknown but as an illness it can vary from a mild form to panic attacks and severe phobias that can be disabling socially, psychologically and at times physically.

It presents with a feeling of dread that something serious is likely to happen and is associated with palpitations, rapid breathing, sweaty hands, tremor (shakiness), dry mouth, general indigestion, feeling of butterflies in the stomach, occasional diarrhoea and generalised aches and pains in the muscles. It can present with similar features of mild-to-moderate depression of the agitated type. The causes of anxiety can be related to personality with some genetic and behavioural predisposition, a traumatic experience or physical illness such as hyperthyroidism.

Bell's palsy

This is a disorder of the seventh cranial nerve (facial nerve) that results in paralysis on one side of the face. The disorder usually comes on suddenly and is commonly caused by inflammation around the facial nerve as it travels from the brain to the exterior. It may be caused by pressure on the nerve due to tumours, injury to the nerve, infection of the meninges or inner ear or dental surgery. Diabetes, pregnancy and hypertension are other causes.

The condition may present with a drooping of the mouth on the affected side due to flaccid paralysis of the facial muscles and there may be difficulty in puckering the lips due to paralysis of the orbicularis oris muscle. Other symptoms include:

- Taste may be diminished or lost if the nerve has been affected proximal to the branch which carries taste sensations.
- It may be difficult to close the eye tightly and crease the forehead.
- The buccinator muscle is affected which prevents the client from puffing the cheeks and is the cause of food getting caught between the teeth and cheeks.
- There is excessive tearing from the affected eye.
- Pain may be present near the angle of the jaw and behind the ear.

Between 80 and 90 per cent of individuals recover spontaneously and completely in around one to eight weeks. Corticosteriods may be used to reduce the inflammation of the nerve.

Cerebral palsy

This condition is caused by damage to the central nervous system of the baby during pregnancy, delivery or soon after birth. The damage could be due to bleeding, lack of oxygen or other injuries to the brain. The signs and symptoms of this condition depend on the area of the brain affected. Symptoms include the following:

- Speech is impaired in most individuals and there may be difficulty in swallowing.
- There may or may not be mental retardation.
- Muscles may increase in tone to become spastic, making coordinated movements difficult. The muscles are hyperexcitable and even small movements, touch, stretch of muscle or emotional stress can increase the spasticity.
- The posture is abnormal due to muscle spasticity and the gait is also affected. Some may have abnormal involuntary movements of the limbs that may be exaggerated on voluntarily performing a task. Weakness of muscles may also be associated with the condition, along with seizures.
- There may be problems with hearing and vision.

Depression

This combines symptoms of lowered mood, loss of appetite, poor sleep, lack of concentration and interest, lack of sense of enjoyment, occasional constipation and loss of libido. There are occasions when there is suicidal thinking, death wish or active suicide attempts.

Depression can be the result of chemical imbalance, usually related to serotonin and noradrenalin. The cause of depression could be endogenous where there is no cause for depression but is thought to be linked to genetic predisposition, the result of physical illness or loss of a close relative, object, limb or a relationship. A depressed person looks miserable, hunchbacked, downcast and will usually avoid eye contact.

The severity can be variable but may become severe enough to become psychotic, manifested by hallucinations, delusions, paranoia or thought disorders.

Epilepsy

This is a neurological disorder which makes the individual susceptible to recurrent and temporary seizures. Epilepsy is a complex condition and classifications of types of epilepsy are not definitive. Types of epilepsy are as follows:

- **Generalised** – this may take the form of major or tonic-clonic seizures (formerly known as *grand mal*) in which at the onset the patient falls to the ground unconscious with their muscles in a state of spasm (tonic phase). This is then replaced by convulsive movements (clonic phase) when the tongue may be bitten and urinary incontinence may occur. Movements gradually cease and the patient may rouse in a state of confusion, complaining of a headache or may fall asleep.
- **Partial** – this may be idiopathic or a symptom of structural damage to the brain. In one type of partial idiopathic epilepsy, often affecting children, seizures may take the form of absences (formerly known as *petit mal*), in which there are brief spells of unconsciousness lasting for a few seconds. The eyes stare blankly and there may be fluttering movements of the lids and momentary twitching of the fingers and mouth. This form of epilepsy seldom appears before the age of three or after adolescence. It often subsides spontaneously in adult life but may be followed by the onset of generalised or partial epilepsy.

- **Focal** – this is partial epilepsy due to brain damage (either local or due to a stroke). The nature of the seizure depends on the location of the damage in the brain. In a Jacksonian motor seizure the convulsive movements may spread from the thumb to the hand, arm and face.
- **Psychomotor** – this type of epilepsy is caused by a dysfunction of the cortex of the temporal lobe of the brain. Symptoms may include hallucinations of smell, taste, sight and hearing. Throughout an attack the patient is in a state of clouded awareness and afterwards may have no recollection of the event.

Headache

This is a pain affecting the head excluding facial pain. It can result from diseases affecting ear, nose and throat such as sinusitis, as well as eye problems which could be corrected by glasses. Types of headaches include:

- **Simple headache** – this may occur at times of stress, during mensruation, the day after heavy alcohol consumption and part of cold and flu symptoms. These are transient and would normally settle spontaneously or require simple analgesia.
- **Chronic headaches** – these are daily headaches and tension headaches. The pain can be severe and disabling and can affect the whole head, behind the eyes or may be just a frontal headache. The client can describe the pain as like a band around the head.
- **Cervical spines (cervicalgia)** – this is normally in the back and sides of the head and can present with neck pain.
- **Migraine headache** – this is a specific form of headache, usually unilateral (one side of the head), associated with nausea or vomiting and visual disturbances such as scintillating light waves or zigzag fashion.
- **Intracranial (inside brain) diseases** – these are headaches caused by diseases such as a brain tumour, can present with nausea and vomiting and may cause other neurological signs and symptoms.

Herpes zoster (shingles)

This is a painful infection along the sensory nerves by the virus that causes chicken pox. Lesions resemble herpes simplex with erythema and blisters along the lines of the nerves. Areas affected are mostly on the back or upper chest wall. This condition is very painful due to acute inflammation of one or more of the peripheral nerves. Severe pain may persist at the site of shingles for months or even years after the apparent healing of the skin.

Meningitis

This is an inflammation of the meninges due to infection by viruses or bacteria. Meningitis presents with an intense headache, fever, loss of appetite, intolerance to light and sound and rigidity of muscles, especially those in the neck. In severe cases there may be convulsions, vomiting and delirium, leading to death. The different types of meningitis are as follows:

- **Meningocccal meningitis** – this involves a characteristic haemorrhagic rash anywhere on the body. The symptoms appear suddenly and the bacteria can cause widespread meningococcal infection culminating in meningococcal septicaemia. Unless treated rapidly death can occur within a week.
- **Bacterial meningitis** – this is treated with large doses of antibiotics.
- **Viral meningitis** – this does not respond to drugs but normally has a relatively benign prognosis.

Migraine

This is a specific form of headache, usually unilateral (one side of the head), associated with nausea or vomiting, visual disturbances such as scintillating light waves or zigzag fashion. The client may experience a visual aura before an attack actually happens. This is usually called a classical migraine. There are other types of migraine:

- **Ophthalmoplegic migraine** – this causes painful, red and watery eyes.
- **Neuropathic migraine** – it causes one-sided paralysis and weakness of the face and body.
- **Abdominal migraine** – this can affect children with recurring attacks of abdominal pain, sometimes accompanied by nausea and vomiting.

Migraines can be treated with simple analgesia or more specialised anti-migraine medication.

Motor neurone disease

This is a progressive degenerative disease of the motor neurones of the nervous system. It tends to occur in middle age and causes muscle weakness and wasting.

Multiple sclerosis

This is a disease of the central nervous system in which the myelin (fatty) sheath covering the nerve fibres is destroyed and various functions become impaired, including movement and sensations. Multiple sclerosis is characterised by relapses and remissions. It can present with blindness or reduced vision and can lead to severe disability within a short period. It can also cause incontinence, loss of balance, tremor and speech problems. Depression and mania can happen.

Myalgic encephalomyelitis (Chronic fatigue syndrome)

This condition is characterised by extreme disabling fatigue that has lasted for at least six months and is made worse by physical or mental exertion and is not resolved by bed rest. The symptom of fatigue is often accompanied by some of the following: muscle pain or weakness, poor coordination, joint pain, slight fever, sore throat, painful lymph nodes in the neck and armpits, depression, inability to concentrate and general malaise.

IN PRACTICE

Avoid therapy during acute migraine attacks and remember that stress and tension can increase frequency and likelihood of attacks. Remember that women are likely to have more attacks during premenstrual periods, when they are taking contraceptive pill, during the menopause or when starting HRT.

IN PRACTICE

Be aware of tenderness in the muscle and joints. Relaxation may help clients to cope, but be aware they tire easily and therefore it is best to keep treatment short and light.

It can happen in any age group, but recently children and adolescents are noticed to have a higher incidence.

Neuralgia

Neuralgia presents as attacks of pain along the entire course or branch of a peripheral sensory nerve. A common example is trigemenal neuralgia affecting the trigeminal nerve in the face.

Neuritis

This is an inflammation/disease of a single or several nerves with different causes such as infection, injury or poison. It causes pain along the length of the nerve and/or loss of the use of structures supplied by the nerve.

Parkinson's disease

This disease is caused by damage to the grey matter of the brain known as basal ganglia. It causes involuntary tremors of limbs with stiffness, rigidity and a shuffling gait. The face lacks expression and movements are slow. Clients may suffer from depression, confusion and anxiety.

Sciatica

This is lower back pain which can affect the buttock and thigh. On occasions it radiates to the leg and foot. In severe cases it can cause numbness and weakness of the lower limb. It can result from prolapse of the discs between the spinal vertebrae, tumour or blood clot (thrombosis). Diabetes or heavy alcohol intake can also produce symptoms of sciatica. This condition tends to recur and may require strong analgesia or surgery in severe cases.

Stress

Stress can be defined as any factor that affects physical or emotional well-being. Signs of stress affecting the nervous system include anxiety, depression, irritability, headaches, back pain and excessive tiredness.

IN PRACTICE

In the case of a client with sciatica, avoid unnecessary manipulation and check couch for comfort. Be aware that climbing or lying on the couch can produce pain. Relaxation and massage can be helpful and the aim in treatments should be to relax muscles and prevent spasms.

Interrelationships with other systems

The nervous system links to the following body systems.

Cells and tissues
Nervous tissue is a specialised type of tissue which can pick up and transmit electrical signals by converting stimuli into nerve impulses.

Skin
The skin is a highly sensitive organ and has many sensory nerve endings which respond to touch, temperature and pressure.

Skeletal
The skeleton provides protection for the spinal cord and the brain.

Muscular

The brain sends impulses to muscles via motor nerves in order to effect movement.

Circulatory

Blood transports vital oxygen to the nerve cells. The medulla oblongata in the brain is the control centre for the heart. The sympathetic nervous system prepares the body for activity by increasing the heart rate. The parasympathetic nervous system encourages the resting heart rate.

Respiratory

Oxygen inhaled into the body is carried to the nerve cells to enable them to function properly. Without oxygen nerve cells become damaged and die, causing irreversible damage. The sympathetic nervous system prepares the body for activity by increasing the respiration rate. The parasympathetic nervous system encourages the resting respiratory rate.

Endocrine

The endocrine system works closely with the nervous system in order to maintain homeostasis in the body.

Digestive

The nervous system influences the actions of the digestive system. The sympathetic nervous system effects include increased conversion of glycogen to glucose by the liver and decreased secretion of saliva. The parasympathetic nervous system effects include increased gastro-intestinal activity and stimulated salivation.

Key words associated with the nervous system

central nervous system	spinal nerves	meninges
brain	cervical	cerebrum
spinal cord	thoracic	thalamus
peripheral nervous system	lumbar	hypothalamus
somatic nervous system	sacral	pineal gland
cranial nerves	coccygeal	cerebellum
olfactory	plexuses	brain stem
optic	autonomic nervous system	pons
oculomotor	neurone	medulla oblongata
trochlear	neuroglia	spinal cord
trigeminal	cell body	reflex action
abducens	dendrites	sense organs
facial	axon	nose
vestibulocochlear	sensory neurone	eyes
glossopharyngeal	motor neurone	ears
vagus	mixed neurone	tongue
accessory	synapse	skin
hypoglossal	chemical transmitter substance	

Revision summary of the nervous system

- The nervous system helps regulate homeostasis and integrate all body activities by sensing changes, interpreting them and reacting to them.
- The **central nervous system** (CNS) consists of the brain and the spinal cord.
- The **peripheral nervous system** (PNS) consists of the somatic nervous system consisting of the cranial and spinal nerves and the autonomic (involuntary) nervous system.
- There are two types of nervous tissue.
- **Neurone** – this is a functional unit of the nervous system. This neurone is designed to receive stimuli and conduct impulses.
- **Neuroglia** – this is a specialised type of connective tissue that supports, nourishes and protects neurones.
- Neurones have two major properties – excitability and conductibility.
- Most **nerve cells**, or neurones, consist of a cell body, many dendrites and usually a single axon.
- There are three main types of neurones – sensory, motor and mixed.
- **Sensory neurones** conduct impulses from receptors to the CNS.
- **Motor neurones** conduct impulses to effectors (muscles).
- **Mixed neurones** conduct impulses to other neurones.
- The junction where nerve impulses are transmitted from one neurone to another is called a **synapse**.
- **Impulses** are relayed from one neurone to another by a chemical transmitter substance which is released by the neurone to carry impulses across the synapse to stimulate the next neurone.
- The **central nervous system** (brain and spinal cord) is covered by a special protective type of connective tissue in three layers called the **meninges**.
- The parts of the brain include the **cerebrum, thalamus, hypothalamus, pituitary gland, pineal gland, cerebellum** and the **brain stem**.
- The **cerebrum** is the largest part of the brain and is concerned with all forms of conscious activity. It has sensory areas which control vision, touch, hearing, taste and smell, also motor areas which control voluntary movements and association areas which control reasoning, memory and emotions.
- The **thalamus** is a relay and interpretation centre for all sensory impulses, except olfaction.

- The **hypothalamus** controls hunger, thirst, temperature regulation, anger, aggression, hormones, sexual behaviour, sleep patterns and consciousness.
- The **pineal gland** is involved in the regulation of circadian rhythms and is thought to influence mood.
- The **cerebellum** is concerned with the coordination of skeletal muscles, muscle tone and balance.
- The **brain stem** contains the mid-brain, pons and medulla oblongata.
- The **mid-brain** contains certain visual and auditory reflexes that coordinate head and eye movements with things seen and heard. The **pons** relays messages from the cerebral cortex to the spinal cord and helps regulate breathing.
- The **medulla oblongata** contains control centres for the heart, lungs and intestines.
- The **spinal cord** is an extension of the brain stem and its function is to relay impulses to and from the brain.
- A **reflex action** is a rapid and automatic response to a stimulus without any conscious action of the brain.
- The **peripheral nervous system** contains all the nerves outside of the central nervous system and can be subdivided into the **somatic nervous system** and the **autonomic nervous system**.
- The **somatic nervous system** contains **31 pairs of spinal nerves** (nerves originating from the spinal cord) and **12 pairs of cranial nerves** (nerves originating from the brain).
- The 31 pairs of spinal nerves are **8 cervical, 12 thoracic, 5 lumbar, 5 sacral** and **1 coccygeal**.
- Each **spinal nerve** is divided into several branches, forming a network of nerves or **plexuses** which supply different parts of the body.
- The 12 pairs of cranial nerves connect directly to the brain. They are **olfactory, optic, oculomotor, trochlear, trigeminal, abducens, facial, vestibulocochlear, glossopharyngeal, vagus, accessory** and **hypoglossal**.
- The **autonomic nervous system** is the part of the nervous system that controls the automatic body activities of smooth and cardiac muscle and the activities of glands. It is divided into the **sympathetic** and **parasympathetic** divisions.

- The activity of the **sympathetic** system is to prepare the body for expending energy and dealing with emergency situations.
- The **parasympathetic** system balances the action of the sympathetic division by working to conserve energy and create the conditions needed for rest and sleep. It slows down the body processes except digestion and the functions of the genito-urinary system.
- The **sense organs** include the **nose** (olfaction), **tongue** (taste), **eyes** (sight), **ears** (hearing) and **skin** (touch).

The nervous system
Multiple-choice questions

1 The two major divisions of the nervous system are:
   a the central nervous system and autonomic nervous system
   b the brain and the spinal cord
   c the central nervous system and peripheral nervous system
   d the peripheral nervous system and the brain

2 The components of the central nervous system include:
   a the spinal cord and cranial nerves
   b the brain and spinal cord
   c the sympathetic and parasympathetic nervous systems
   d the spinal cord and spinal nerves

3 The three basic parts of a neurone are:
   a cell body, axon and dendrites
   b cell body, nucleus and axon
   c cell body, sensory and afferent nerves
   d cell body, motor and efferent nerves

4 The fine, delicate membrane that surrounds the axon is called the:
   a neuroglia
   b nodes of Ranvier
   c neurilemma
   d synaptic knob

5 A sensory nerve is responsible for sending messages:
   a from the brain and spinal cord
   b to the brain and spinal cord
   c to and from the brain and spinal cord
   d from the brain only

6 The part of the brain that houses the thalamus and hypothalamus is the:
   a cerebellum
   b cerebrum
   c brain stem
   d medulla oblongata

7 The region of the brain concerned with the coordination of skeletal muscle is the:
   a mid-brain
   b cerebellum
   c pons
   d cerebrum

8 The part of the brain concerned with all forms of conscious activity is the:
   a cerebrum
   b thalamus
   c medulla oblongata
   d hypothalamus

9 Nerve impulses are the signals of the nervous system that travel along the neurone from:
   a dendrite to axon
   b axon to dendrite
   c axon to synapse
   d dendrite to synapse

10 The part of the neurone that covers the axon, insulating and accelerating the conduction of nerve impulses along the length of the axon is:
   a dendrite
   b motor end plate
   c myelin sheath
   d nodes of Ranvier

11 The part of the brain that contains vital control centres for the heart, lungs and intestines is the:
   a hypothalamus
   b medulla oblongata
   c cerebellum
   d mid-brain

12 Which of the following nerve plexuses supplies the front and sides of the abdominal wall and part of the thigh?
   a brachial
   b lumbar
   c sacral
   d coccygeal

13 The junction where nerve impulses are transmitted from one neurone to another is a:
   a synapse
   b dendrite
   c axon
   d neurotransmitter

14 The central nervous system is covered by a special type of connective tissue called:
  a meninges
  b neuroglia
  c cerebrospinal fluid
  d dendrites

15 Which of the following is **not** controlled by the hypothalamus?
  a hunger
  b thirst
  c taste
  d sexual behaviour

16 The spinal cord is an extension of which part of the brain?
  a medulla oblongata
  b mid-brain
  c pons
  d brain stem

17 Which of the following is **not** one of the cranial nerves?
  a trigeminal
  b facial
  c cervical
  d optic

18 Which of the following is an effect of the sympathetic nervous system?
  a increased heart rate
  b pupil constriction
  c decreased breathing rate
  d contraction of the bladder

19 Which of the following is **not** an effect of the parasympathetic nervous system?
  a increased peristalsis
  b decreased heart rate
  c contraction of the bladder
  d dilation of blood vessels

20 The disease of the central nervous system in which the myelin sheath covering the nerve fibres is destroyed is:
  a cerebral palsy
  b multiple sclerosis
  c Bell's palsy
  d motor neurone disease

9 the endocrine system

Introduction

The endocrine system comprises a series of internal secretions called hormones which help to regulate body processes by providing a constant internal environment. Hormones are chemical messengers and act as catalysts in that they affect the physiological activities of other cells in the body. The endocrine system works closely with the nervous system. Nerves enable the body to respond rapidly to stimuli whereas the endocrine system causes slower and longer-lasting effects.

IN PRACTICE

It is important for therapists to have a comprehensive knowledge of the endocrine system in order to understand the action of hormones and their significance in the healthy functioning of the body. Over or under secretion of certain hormones may result in disorders and disease in the body. For instance, hypersecretion of the hormone testosterone in women can lead to hair growth in the male sexual pattern.

◉ Objectives

By the end of this chapter you will be able to recall and understand the following knowledge:

- the functions of the endocrine system
- the definition of a hormone
- the location of the main endocrine glands of the body
- the principal hormone secretions from the main endocrine glands and their effects on the body
- the natural glandular changes that occur in the body such as puberty, menstruation, pregnancy and menopause
- the interrelationhips between the endocrine and other body systems
- common pathologies of the endocrine system.

Functions of the endocrine system

The functions of the endocrine system are:

- producing and secreting hormones which regulate body activities such as growth, development and metabolism
- maintaining the body during times of stress
- contributing to the reproductive process.

What is a hormone?

A hormone is a chemical messenger or regulator, secreted by an endocrine gland which reaches its destination by the bloodstream and has the power of influencing the activity of other organs. Some hormones have a slow action over a period of years such as the growth hormone from the anterior pituitary, while others have a quick action such as adrenaline from the adrenal medulla. Hormones, therefore, regulate and coordinate various functions in the body.

The endocrine glands are ductless glands, as the hormones they secrete pass directly into the bloodstream to influence the activity of another organ or gland. The main endocrine glands are as follows:

- pituitary gland
- thyroid gland
- parathyroid glands
- adrenal glands
- islets of Langerhans in the pancreas
- ovaries in the female
- testes in the male.

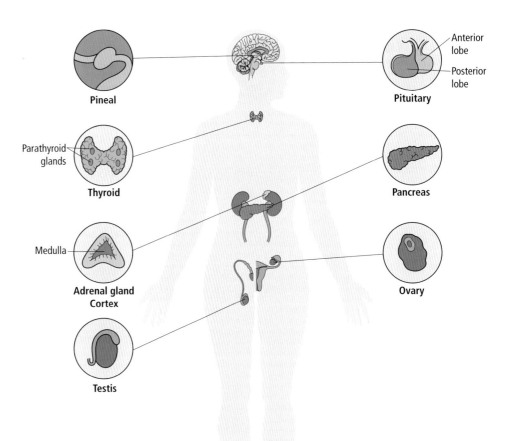

Fig 9.1 The endocrine glands

Overview of the endocrine glands

Endocrine gland	Location
Pituitary gland	Attached by a stalk to the hypothalamus of the brain
Thyroid gland	In the neck on either side of the trachea
Parathyroid glands	Four small glands situated on the posterior of the thyroid gland
Adrenal glands	Two triangular-shaped glands which lie on top of each kidney
Pancreas	Situated behind the stomach between the duodenum and the spleen
Ovaries	Situated in the lower abdomen below the kidneys
Testes	Situated in the groin in a sac called the scrotum

Student activity

Now complete Activity 9.1 in the resources for this book on Dynamic Learning Online.

STUDY TIP

When studying the endocrine system, it is helpful to think of not only where the hormone is secreted from but also the target organ it has an effect on. Sometimes this information may be apparent from the name of the hormone/s, for example thyroid-stimulating hormone (TSH) is secreted by the anterior lobe of the pituitary gland and the target it has an effect on is the growth and activity of the thyroid gland.

Pituitary gland

This is a lobed structure attached by a stalk to the hypothalamus of the brain. For many years the pituitary gland has been referred to as the 'master' endocrine gland because it secretes several hormones that control other endocrine glands. However, the pituitary itself has a master – the hypothalamus.

The hypothalamus is a small region of the brain that is the major integrating link between the nervous and endocrine systems. Hormones of the pituitary are controlled by releasing or inhibiting hormones produced by the hypothalamus.

The hypothalamus initiates the process by producing its own set of hormones (releasing or inhibiting hormones) as a result of stimulation in the brain. This has a cascading effect on the pituitary which in turn produces its own hormones that stimulate other glands. An example is thyrotrophin releasing hormone from the hypothalamus that promotes the pituitary to secrete thyroid-stimulating hormone which controls the growth and activity of the thyroid gland.

The pituitary gland consists of two main parts – an anterior and a posterior lobe.

Anterior lobe

The principal hormones secreted by the anterior lobe of the pituitary are as follows:

Growth hormone	Controls the growth of long bones and muscles
Thyroid-stimulating hormone (TSH)	Controls the growth and activity of the thyroid gland
Adrenocorticothrophic hormone (ACTH)	Stimulates and controls the growth and hormonal output of the adrenal cortex

(Continued)

Gonadotrophic hormones	Control the development and growth of the ovaries and testes
The gonads or sex hormones include: **a) Follicle-stimulating hormone**	In women this stimulates the development of the graafian follicle in the ovary which secretes the hormone oestrogen In men it stimulates the testes to produce sperm
b) Luteinising hormone	In women this helps to prepare the uterus for the fertilised ovum In men it acts on the testes to produce testosterone
Prolactin	Stimulates the secretion of milk from the breasts following birth
Melanocyte-stimulating hormone (MSH)	Stimulates the production of melanin in the basal cell layer of the skin

Fig 9.2 The pituitary and its master control

Posterior lobe

The posterior lobe of the pituitary secretes two hormones which are manufactured in the hypothalamus but are stored in the posterior lobe:

Anti-diuretic hormone (ADH)	Increases water reabsorption in the renal tubules of the kidneys
Oxytocin	Stimulates the uterus during labour and stimulates the breasts to produce milk

BODY FACT

Endocrine glands in the body have a feedback mechanism which is coordinated by the pituitary gland. This gland is influenced by the hypothalamus and will increase its output of releasing factors if other glands start to fail or will decrease its output if the level of the hormone in the bloodstream starts to rise.

Pineal gland

This is a pea-sized mass of nerve tissue attached by a stalk in the central part of the brain. It is located deep between the cerebral hemispheres where it is attached to the upper portion of the thalamus.

The pineal gland functions as a gland and secretes a hormone called **melatonin** which synthesises from serotonin. This gland is involved in the regulation of circadian rhythms, patterns of repeated activity that are associated with the environmental cycles of day and night such as sleep and wake rhythms. It is also thought to influence moods.

Thyroid gland

The thyroid gland is found in the neck, situated on either side of the trachea and is controlled by the anterior lobe of the pituitary.

The principal secretions of the thyroid gland are:

triodothyronine (T3)	Both T3 and T4 regulate growth and development and also influence mental, physical and metabolic activities
thyroxine (T4)	
calcitonin	Controls the level of calcium in the blood

The functions of the thyroid gland are as follows:

- controls the metabolic rate by stimulating metabolism
- influences growth and cell division
- influences mental development
- is responsible for the maintenance of healthy skin and hair
- stores the mineral iodine which it needs to manufacture thyroxin
- stimulates the involuntary nervous system and controls irritability.

The thyroid gland is controlled by a feedback mechanism. It will increase to meet the demand for more thyroid hormones at various times such as during the menstrual cycle, pregnancy and puberty.

Parathyroid glands

These are four small glands situated on the posterior of the thyroid gland. Their principal secretion is the hormone **parathormone** which helps to regulate calcium metabolism by controlling the amount of calcium in blood and bones.

Adrenal glands

These are two triangular-shaped glands which lie on top of each kidney. They consist of two parts – an outer cortex and an inner medulla.

Adrenal cortex

The principal hormones secreted by the adrenal cortex are as follows:

Hormone/s secreted	Effects
Glucocorticoids (cortisone and hydrocortisone)	• Influence the metabolism of protein and carbohydrates and utilise fats. They are important in maintaining the level of glucose in the blood so that blood glucose levels are increased at times of stress
Mineral corticoids (aldosterone)	• Act on the kidney tubules, retaining salts in the body, excreting excess potassium and maintaining the water and electrolyte balance
Sex corticoids testosterone, oestrogen and progesterone	• Control the development of the secondary sex characteristics and the function of the reproductive organs

BODY FACT

When the ovaries and testes mature, they produce the sex hormones themselves, therefore the production of sex corticoids in the adrenal cortex is important up to puberty.

KEY FACT

The effects described above are those felt when the body is under stress such as a pounding heart, increased ventilation rate, dry mouth and 'butterflies' in the stomach. Levels of stress hormones are broken down slowly so that effects on the sympathetic nervous system are long-lasting. Over the long term, if levels of these hormones remain elevated, they perpetuate factors for stress-related disorders.

Adrenal medulla

The principal hormones secreted by the adrenal medulla are adrenaline and noradrenaline. They are under the control of the sympathetic nervous system and are released at times of stress. The reponses of these hormones are fast due to the fact that they are governed by nervous control.

The effects of these stress hormones are similar, although **adrenaline** has a primary influence on the heart, causing an increase in heart rate, whereas **noradrenaline** has a greater effect on peripheral vasoconstriction which raises blood pressure.

A summary of the effects of **adrenaline** is as follows:

dilates the arteries, increasing blood circulation and the heart rate
dilates the bronchial tubes, increasing oxygen intake and the rate and depth of breathing
raises the metabolic rate
constricts the blood vessels to the skin and intestines, diverting blood from these regions to the muscles and brain to effect action

The effects of **noradrenaline** are similar to those of adrenalin and include:

vasoconstriction of small blood vessels leading to an increase in blood pressure
increase in the rate and depth of breathing
relaxation of the smooth muscle of the intestinal wall

Pancreas

The pancreas is known as a dual organ as it has an endocrine and an exocrine function.

Exocrine function of pancreas	secretion of pancreatic juice to assist with digestion
Endocrine function of pancreas	secretion is the hormone **insulin**, secreted by the islets of Langerhans cells in the pancreas

Sex glands

Testes

The testes are situated in the groin in a sac called the scrotum. They have two functions:

the secretion of the hormone testosterone, which controls the development of the secondary sex characteristics in the male at puberty (influenced by the luteinising hormone)
the production of sperm (influenced by the follicle-stimulating hormone from the anterior pituitary)

Ovaries

The ovaries are situated in the lower abdomen below the kidneys. The two ovaries are the sex glands in the female, each is attached to the upper part of the uterus by broad ligaments. The ovaries have two distinct functions:

production of ova at ovulation
production of the female sex hormones oestrogen and progesterone

Oestrogen is concerned with the development and maintenance of the reproductive system and the development of the secondary sex characteristics. Progesterone is produced by the ovaries after ovulation. It helps to prepare the uterus for the implantation of the fertilized ovum, develops the placenta and prepares the breasts for milk secretion.

The ovaries also secrete the following hormones in addition to oestrogen and progesterone:

- **Inhibin** – this hormone inhibits the secretion of the follicle-stimulating hormone (FSH) towards the end of the menstrual cycle.
- **Relaxin** – this hormone dilates the cervix and assists the pelvis in widening during childbirth.

Natural glandular changes

Puberty

This is the time at which the onset of sexual maturity occurs and the reproductive organs become functional. Changes in both sexes occur with the appearance of the secondary sexual characteristics such as the deepening of the voice in a boy and growth of breasts in girls. These changes are brought about by an increase in sex hormone activity, due to stimulation of the ovaries and testes by the pituitary gonadotrophic hormones.

The average age for girls to reach puberty is between ten and fourteen, although it can occur as early as eight or nine years of age. In boys, the average age is 13 to 16.

In girls the ovaries are stimulated by the gonadotrophic hormones – the follicle-stimulating hormone (FSH) and luteinising hormone (LH). The effects of puberty in girls include:

- the onset of ovulation and the menstrual cycle
- the female reproductive organs becoming functional
- the growth of pubic and axillary hair
- development of breast tissue
- increase in the amount of subcutaneous fat.

In boys the same gonadotrophoic hormones (FSH and LH) stimulate the testes to produce testosterone. The effects of puberty in boys include:

- voice breaking and larynx enlarging
- the growth of muscle and bone
- noticeable height increase
- the development of sexual organs
- the growth of pubic, facial, axillary, abdominal and chest hair
- the onset of sperm production.

The menstrual cycle

Starting at puberty, the female reproductive system undergoes a regular sequence of monthly events, known as the menstrual cycle. The ovaries undergo cyclical changes in which a certain number of ovarian follicles develop. When one ovum completes the development process, it is released into one of the fallopian tubes. If fertilisation does not occur, the developed ovum disintegrates and a new cycle begins.

The menstrual cycle lasts approximately 28 days, although it can be longer or shorter than this. There are three stages of the menstrual cycle:

- **profilterative** (first) phase – days 7 to 14 of the cycle
- **secretory** (second) phase – days 14 to 28 of the cycle
- **menstrual** (third) phase – days 1 to 7 of the cycle.

Profilerative phase

At the beginning of the cycle an ovum develops within an ovarian follicle in the ovary. This is in response to a hormone released by the anterior lobe of the pituitary gland called the follicle-stimulating hormone (FSH) which stimulates the follicles of the ovaries to produce the hormone oestrogen. Oestrogen stimulates the endometrium to promote the growth of new blood vessels and mucus-producing cells. When mature, it bursts from the follicle and travels along the fallopian tube to the uterus. This occurs about 14 days after the start of the cycle and is known as ovulation.

Secretory phase

A temporary endocrine gland, the corpus luteum, develops in the ruptured follicle in response to stimulation from the luteinising hormone (LH) secreted by the anterior lobe of the pituitary gland. The corpus luteum secretes the hormone progesterone which together with oestrogen causes the lining of the uterus (endometrium) to become thicker and richly supplied with blood in preparation for pregnancy.

Fig 9.3 The menstrual cycle

After ovulation, the ovum can only be fertilised during the next eight to 24 hours. If fertilisation does occur, the fertilised ovum becomes attached to the endometrium and the corpus luteum continues to secrete progesterone. Pregnancy then begins. The corpus luteum continues to secrete progesterone until the fourth month of pregnancy by which time the placenta has taken over this function.

Menstrual phase

If the ovum is not fertilised, the cycle continues and the corpus luteum shrinks and the endometrium is shed. This is called menstruation. Over a period of about five days, the muscles of the wall of the uterus contract to expel the unfertilised egg, pieces of endometrial tissue and some tissue fluid.

As soon as levels of progesterone drop, due to the breakdown of the endometrium and the corpus luteum, the pituitary gland starts producing progesterone again and hence stimulates the ovaries to produce another follicle and a new ovum. The cycle then begins again.

Pregnancy

Pregnancy takes approximately nine calendar months and is divided into three trimesters:

- The first trimester is the most important to the developing baby and is a time of radical hormonal changes. During this phase all of the body systems develop.
- The second trimester consists of rapid foetal growth and the completion of systemic development. Blood volume for the mother increases as additional workload is placed on all physiological functions. Cardiac output, breathing rate and urine production increase in response to foetal demands. The uterus enlarges greatly during pregnancy, along with the size of the breasts. Appetite increases in response to the foetal need for increasing amounts of nutrients.
- The third trimester is mostly a weight-gaining and maturing process, preparing the baby for life outside of the womb. Posture changes are evident at this stage as the mother gains more weight and internal organs are compressed. The body's connective tissue structure alters by softening, to allow for the expansion needed for the birth.

Hormonal changes that occur during pregnancy

During a typical menstrual cycle, the corpus luteum degenerates about two weeks after ovulation. Consequently, the levels of oestrogen and progesterone decline rapidly and the lining of the uterus (endometrium) is not maintained and is cast off as menstrual flow.

If this occurs after implantation the embryo becomes spontaneously aborted (miscarries). The mechanism that usually prevents this occurring involves a hormone called human chorionic gonadotrophic hormone (HCG) which is secreted by a layer of embryonic cells that surround the developing embryo. HCG causes the corpus luteum to be maintained in order to establish the pregnancy.

The maintenance of the corpus luteum is important for the first three months, after which the placenta is usually well developed and is able to secrete sufficient oestrogen and progesterone.

The secretion of the hormones oestrogen and progesterone is important during pregnancy as they:

- maintain the uterine wall
- inhibit the secretion of the gonadotrophic hormones FSH and LH
- stimulate development of the mammary glands
- inhibit uterine contractions until birth
- cause enlargement of the reproductive organs.

The ovaries and placenta produce inhibin which inhibits the secretion of the follicle-stimulating hormone (FSH) from the anterior lobe of the pituitary, thus preventing the development of ova during pregnancy.

At the end of the gestation period the levels of progesterone fall. Labour cannot begin until the levels of progesterone fall as progesterone inhibits uterine contractions. Oxytocin, secreted by the posterior lobe of the pituitary, stimulates uterine contractions and the ovaries and placenta secrete relaxin which helps to dilate the cervix and relaxes the ligaments and joints to assist labour.

Mood, sleep and energy levels are all affected during pregnancy due to the hormonal changes that occur during this period. Some women may report extreme tiredness at the start of their pregnancy and experience a surge of energy towards the end. Sleep patterns may be affected due to the activity of the growing foetus and hormone levels may promote tearfulness and emotional disturbances.

Menopausal women are often treated with hormone replacement therapy (HRT) in order to alleviate some of the unpleasant side effects. HRT usually involves administering oestrogens, along with progesterone.

Menopause

After puberty the menstrual cycle normally continues to occur at regular intervals into approximately the late forties or early fifties (most commonly between 45 and 55). At this time there are marked changes in which the cycle becomes increasingly irregular until the cycle ceases altogether. This period in a woman's reproductive life is called the menopause (female climacteric).

During the menopause there is a change in the balance of the sex hormones. The ovaries cease responding to the follicle-stimulating hormone (FSH) and this decline in function results in lower levels of oestrogen and progesterone secretion. As a result of reduced oestrogen concentration and lack of progesterone, the female's secondary sexual characteristics undergo varying degrees of change which may include a decrease in the size of the vagina, uterus and uterine tubes, as well as atrophy of the breasts.

Other changes that occur commonly in response to low oestrogen concentration include an increased loss of bone matrix, increasing the risk of osteoporosis, thinning of the skin and dryness of the mucous membrane lining the vagina.

Some women of menopausal age experience unpleasant vasomotor symptoms including sensations of heat in the face, neck and upper body, known as 'hot flushes'. Menopausal women may also experience varying degrees of headache, backache and fatigue, as well as emotional disturbances.

Common pathologies of the endocrine system

Addison's disease

Hyposecretion of corticosteroid hormones is responsible for the condition known as Addison's disease. Symptoms include loss of appetite, weight loss, brown pigmentation around joints, low blood sugar, low blood pressure, tiredness and muscular weakness. This disease is treatable by replacement hormone therapy.

Cretinism

Hyposecretion of thyroxine leads to cretinism in children which is a congential deficiency causing impaired mentality, small stature, coarsening of the skin and hair and deposition of fat on the body.

Cushing's syndrome

Hypersecretion of the glucocorticoids can lead to a condition known as Cushing's syndrome. This condition results from an excess amount of corticosteroid hormones in the body. Symptoms include weight gain, reddening of the face and neck, excess growth of facial and body hair, raised blood pressure, loss of mineral from bone and sometimes mental disturbances.

Diabetes mellitus

Hyposecretion can lead to a condition called diabetes mellitus. This condition is due to a deficiency or absence of insulin. The symptoms associated with diabetes include an increased thirst, increased output of urine, weight loss, thin skin with impaired healing capacity, increased tendency to develop minor skin infections and decreased pain threshold when insulin levels are low. There are two types of diabetes mellitus:

- **Insulin dependent diabetes** (early onset) – this occurs mainly in children and young adults and the onset is usually sudden. The deficiency or absence of insulin is due to the destruction of the islet cells in the pancreas. The causes are unknown but there is a familial tendency, suggesting genetic involvement.
- **Non-insulin dependent diabetes** (late onset): This type of diabetes occurs later in life and its causes are unknown. Insulin secretion may be below or above normal. Deficiency of glucose inside the body cells may occur where there is hyperglycaemia and a high insulin level. This may be due to changes in cell walls which block the insulin-assisted movement of glucose into cells. This type of diabetes can be controlled by diet alone, or diet and oral drugs.

Diabetes insipidus

Hyposecretion of the anti-diuretic hormone by the posterior lobe of the pituitary leads to the disease diabetes insipidus. Symptoms include dehydration, increased thirst and increased output of urine.

Dwarfism

Hyposecretion of the growth hormone during childhood leads to stunted growth, a condition known as dwarfism.

Gigantism

Hypersecretion of the growth hormone secreted by the anterior pituitary leads to gigantism in children, a disease marked by the rapid growth of the body to extremely large proportions (seven to eight feet). If the overproduction occurs in adulthood, then there is an abnormal enlargement of the hands and feet and coarsening of the facial features, due to the continued growth of tissues. This condition is known as acromegaly.

Gynaecomastia

Hypersecretion of oestrogen and progesterone in the male can lead to muscle atrophy and breast development.

Hirsutism

This is hair growth in the male sexual pattern due to hypersecretion of the hormone testosterone in women and an overproduction of androgens.

Hypoglycaemia

Hypoglycaemia (low blood sugar level) can lead to muscular weakness and incoordination, mental confusion and sweating. If severe it may lead to a hypoglycaemic coma.

IN PRACTICE

Always take a detailed history and liaise with the client's GP regarding the type of diabetes the client is suffering from. It is important for the therapist to be aware that feedback may be inadequate in those with decreased sensation, therefore pressure used in treatments should be carefully monitored. Caution should be exercised, as diabetic clients may have acute complications such as hypoglycaemia resulting in dizziness, weakness, pallor, rapid heart beat and excessive sweating. Always ensure that the client's glucose and other medications are available with the client when they come for treatment.

Myxoedema

Hyposecretion of thyroxine in an adult leads to myxoedema which is characterised by the slowing down of physical and mental activity resulting in lethargy, hair becoming brittle, skin becoming coarse and dry and a slow metabolism.

Polycystic ovary syndrome

Hyopsecretion of the hormones oestrogen and progesterone in the female can lead to polycystic ovary syndrome which is characterised by cysts on the ovaries, cessation of periods, obesity, atrophy of the breasts, hirsutism and sterility.

Seasonal affective disorder (SAD)

Hyposecretion of the hormone melatonin is thought to be associated with the condition seasonal affective disorder (SAD). Symptoms include depression (typically with the onset of winter), a general slowing down of mind and body and excessive sleeping and overeating.

Stress

Stress can be defined as any factor which affects physical or emotional health. Effects of short-term physical stress are associated with the hormone adrenaline and include an increased heart beat, rapid breathing, increased sweating, tense muscles, dry mouth, frequency of urination and a feeling of nausea. Stress can become negative stress when excess adrenaline is left in the bloodstream, following a short-term stress signal. Examples of possible symptoms of excessive stress on the endocrine system include amenorrhea (absence or stopping of periods), loss of libido and infertility.

IN PRACTICE

It is helpful to remember that clients with hyperthyroidism are intolerant of heat and those with hypothyroidism are intolerant of cold.

Thyrotoxicosis (Hyperthyroidism)

Hypersecretion of thyroxine leads to a condition known as thyrotoxicosis or Graves' disease. Thyrotoxicosis results in an increased metabolic rate, weight loss, sweating, restlessness, increased appetite, sensitivity to heat, raised temperature, frequent bowel action, anxiety and nervousness. When the thyroid gland produces and secretes an excessive amount of thyroxine, it may produce a goitre (an enlargement of the thyroid gland).

Tetany

When there is a deficiency (hyposecretion) of calcium in the blood a condition known as tetany occurs which is characterised by muscular twitchings particular to the hands and feet. These symptoms are quickly relieved by administering calcium.

Virilism

Hypersecretion of the hormone testosterone in women can lead to virilism (masculinisation) causing an overproduction of androgens.

Interrelationships with other systems

The endocrine system links to the following body systems.

Cells and tissues

Meiosis is the form of cell division involving the formation of sperm in the male amd ova in the female.

Skin

MSH (melanocyte-stimulating hormone) produced by the central lobe of the pituitary gland stimulates the production of melanin in the basal cell layer (stratum germinativium) of the skin.

Skeletal

The hormones calcitonin from the thyroid gland and parathormone from the parathyroid glands help to maintain the calcium levels in the blood for strength and flexibility.

Muscular

Muscles receive additional blood flow in response to the secretion of the hormone adrenalin at times of stress.

Circulatory

Hormones are secreted and carried in the blood stream to their target organs.

Respiratory

The adrenal glands increase the breathing rate in times of stress to provide more oxygen as fuel for the muscles.

Nervous

The endocrine system works closely with the nervous system in order to maintain homeostasis in the body. The endocrine system is linked to the nervous system by the hypothalamus and the pituitary gland.

Digestive

The production of insulin and glucagon in the pancreas helps to regulate blood sugar levels.

Urinary

The anti-diuretic hormone (ADH) helps to regulate fluid balance in the body.

Key words associated with the endocrine system

ductless glands	dwarfism	pancreas
hormone	diabetes insipidus	insulin
pituitary	melanocyte-stimulating	hypoglycaemia
thyroid	hormone (MSH)	diabetes mellitus
parathyroids	pineal gland	testosterone
adrenals	melatonin	oestrogen
islets of Langerhans	triodothyronine (T3)	progesterone
ovaries	thyroxine (T4)	virilism
testes	calcitonin	hirsutism
growth hormone	thyrotoxicosis/Graves'	amenorrhea
thyroid-stimulating hormone	disease	gynaecomastia
(TSH)	cretinism	polycystic ovary syndrome
adrenocorticotrophic	myxoedema	puberty
hormone (ACTH)	tetany	menstrual cycle
gonadotrophic hormones	glucocorticoids	ovarian follicles
(FSH and LH)	mineral corticoids	ovum
prolactin	sex corticoids	fallopian tubes
antidiuretic hormone (ADH)	Cushing's syndrome	fertilisation
oxytocin	Addison's disease	pregnancy
gigantism	adrenaline	trimester
acromegaly	noradrenaline	menopause

Revision summary of the endocrine system

- The endocrine system consists of ductless glands that secrete hormones into the bloodstream.
- Endocrine glands are concerned with the regulation of metabolic processes.
- A **hormone** is a chemical regulator secreted by an endocrine gland into the bloodstream and has the power to influence the activity of other organs.
- The main endocrine glands are the **pituitary** (attached to base of brain), **thyroid** (neck), **parathyroids** (posterior to the thyroid glands), **adrenals** (top of kidneys), **islets of Langerhans** (in the pancreas), **ovaries** (in the female) and **testes** (in the male).
- The principal hormones secreted by the **anterior lobe of the pituitary** include the **growth hormone, thyroid-stimulating hormone (TSH), adrenocorticotrophic hormone (ACTH), gonadotrophic hormones (FSH and LH), prolactin** and **melanocyte-stimulating hormone (MSH)**.

- The **growth hormone** controls the growth of long bone and muscle.
- **Thyroid-stimulating hormone (TSH)** controls the growth and activity of the **thyroid gland**.
- **Adrenocorticotrophic hormone (ACTH)** controls the growth and hormonal output of the **adrenal cortex**.
- **Gonadotrophic hormones (FSH and LH)** control the development and growth of the **ovaries** and **testes**.
- **Prolactin** stimulates the secretion of milk from the breasts following birth.
- **Melanocyte-stimulating hormone (MSH)** stimulates the production of melanin in the basal cell layer of the skin.
- **Hypersecretion** of the growth hormone from the pituitary gland can lead to **gigantism** in childhood and **acromegaly** in adulthood.

- **Hyposecretion** of the growth hormone from the pituitary gland during childhood leads to **dwarfism**.
- The posterior lobe of the pituitary secretes **anti-diuretic hormone (ADH)** and **oxytocin**.
- **Hyposecretion** of the anti-diuretic hormone (ADH) by the posterior lobe of the pituitary can lead to **diabetes insipidus**.
- The **pineal gland** is attached by a stalk in the central part of the brain and secretes a hormone called **melatonin** which is thought to regulate circadian rhythms and influence mood.
- The **thyroid gland**'s principal secretions are **triodothyronine (T3)** and **thyroxine (T4)** which regulate metabolism and influence growth and development.
- The thyroid gland also secretes **calcitonin** which controls the levels of calcium in the blood.
- **Hypersecretion** of the thyroid hormones leads to a condition called **thryrotoxicosis** or Graves' disease.
- **Hyposecretion** of the thyroid hormones leads to **cretinism** in childhood and **myxoedema** in adulthood.
- The **parathyroid glands** help regulate calcium metabolism.
- **Hypersecretion** of parathormone can lead to renal stones, kidney failure, softening of the bones, and tumours.
- **Hyposecretion** of parathormone can lead to a condition called **tetany**.
- The **adrenal glands** have two parts – an outer **cortex** and an inner **medulla**.
- The principal hormones secreted by the **adrenal cortex** include **glucocorticoids, mineral corticoids** and **sex corticoids**.
- **Glucocorticoids** influence the metabolism of protein, carbohydrates and utilisation of fats.
- **Mineral corticoids** are concerned with maintaining water and electrolyte balance.
- **Sex corticoids** control the development of the secondary sex characteristics and the function of the reproductive organs.
- **Hypersecretion** of the **mineral corticoids** can lead to kidney failure, high blood pressure and an excess of potassium in the blood.
- **Hypersecretion** of the **gluco corticoids** can lead to a condition called **Cushing's syndrome**.
- **Hypersecretion** of the **sex corticoids** can lead to **hirsutism** and **amenorrhea** in the female and muscle atrophy and development of breasts in the male.
- **Hyposecretion** of the corticosteroid hormones can lead to a condition called **Addison's disease**.
- The principal hormones secreted by the adrenal medulla include adrenaline and noradrenaline.
- **Adrenaline** and **noradrenaline** are under the control of the **sympathetic nervous system** and are released at times of stress.
- The **pancreas** is a dual organ as it has dual function – exocrine and endocrine.
- The exocrine function is the secretion of pancreatic juice to assist with digestion.
- The endocrine function is the secretion of **insulin** from the **islets of Langerhans** cells which helps regulate blood sugar levels.
- **Hypersecretion** can lead to **hypoglycaemia**.
- **Hyposecretion** can lead to a condition called **diabetes mellitus**.
- The **testes** (in the male) have two functions – the secretion of **testosterone** and the production of sperm.
- The **ovaries** (in the female) have two functions – the production of ova and production of the hormones **oestrogen** and **progesterone**.
- **Hypersecretion** of the hormone **testosterone** in women can lead to **virilism, hirsutism** and **amenorrhea**.
- **Hypersecretion** of **oestrogen** and **progesterone** in the male can lead to **gynaecomastia**.
- **Hyposecretion** of **oestrogen** and **progesterone** in the female can lead to **polycystic ovary syndrome**.
- **Puberty** is a natural glandular change due to stimulation of the ovaries and testes by the pituitary gonadotrophic hormones.
- Starting at **puberty**, the female reproductive system undergoes a regular sequence of monthly events, known as the **menstrual cycle**.
- The **ovaries** undergo cyclical changes, in which a certain number of **ovarian follicles** develop. When one **ovum** completes the development process, it is released into one of the **fallopian tubes**. If **fertilisation** does not occur, the developed ovum disintegrates and a new cycle begins.
- The **menstrual cycle** lasts approximately 28 days, although it can be longer or shorter than this.
- **Pregnancy** takes approximately nine calendar months and is divided into three trimesters.
- During the first **trimester** all of the body systems develop.
- The second **trimester** consists of rapid foetal growth and the completion of systemic development.
- The third **trimester** is mostly a weight-gaining and maturing process, preparing the baby for life outside of the womb.
- In the **menopause**, the **ovaries** cease responding to the follicle-stimulating hormone (FSH), resulting in lower levels of oestrogen and progesterone secretion.

1 The purpose of the endocrine system is to:
   a contribute to the reproductive process
   b produce and secrete hormones to regulate body activities
   c maintain the body during times of stress
   d all of the above

2 Which of the following secretes the adrenocorticotrophic hormone (ACTH)?
   a anterior lobe of pituitary
   b posterior lobe of pituitary
   c adrenal medulla
   d adrenal cortex

3 The endocrine gland responsible for secreting the thyroid-stimulating hormone (TSH) is:
   a anterior lobe of pituitary
   b posterior lobe of pituitary
   c thyroid
   d parathyroids

4 Which of the following hormones stimulates the uterus during labour?
   a prolactin
   b oestrogen
   c progesterone
   d oxytocin

5 The hormone parathormone regulates the metabolism of:
   a carbohydrates
   b calcium
   c protein
   d fats

6 Which of the following hormones increases blood circulation and heart rate?
   a noradrenaline
   b adrenaline
   c insulin
   d testosterone

7 The hormone responsible for increasing water reabsorption in the kidney tubules is:
   a luteinising hormone (LH)
   b aldosterone
   c anti-diuretic hormone (ADH)
   d oxytocin

8 The islets of Langerhans are situated in the:
   a liver
   b ovaries
   c kidneys
   d pancreas

9 Hyposecretion of the thyroid gland in an adult can lead to a condition called:
   a myxoedema
   b Cushing's syndrome
   c Addison's disease
   d cretinism

10 The hormone that is concerned with the development of the placenta is:
   a prolactin
   b progesterone
   c follicle-stimulating hormone (FSH)
   d oestrogen

11 The glucocorticoids are secreted by the:
   a adrenal medulla
   b pancreas
   c adrenal cortex
   d pineal gland

12 In puberty the ovaries are stimulated by:
   a growth hormone
   b prolactin
   c gonadotrophic hormones
   d oxytocin

13 Hyposecretion of oestrogen and progesterone in women can lead to the condition:
   a amenorrhea
   b polycystic ovary syndrome
   c gynaecomastia
   d menopause

14 Days 1 to 7 of the menstrual cycle are known as the:
   a proliferative phase
   b secretory phase
   c menstrual phase
   d pre-menstrual phase

15 The hormone responsible for helping to dilate the cervix and relax the ligaments and joints to assist labour is:
a relaxin
b progesterone
c human chorionic gonadotrophic hormone
d follicle-stimulating hormone

16 An increased metabolic rate, weight loss, sweating and restlessness are all symptoms of:
a Cushing's syndrome
b thyrotoxicosis
c myxoedema
d diabetes mellitus

17 Dwarfism is a result of:
a hyposecretion of the growth hormone
b hypersecretion of the growth hormone
c hyposecretion of thyroxine
d hypersecretion of thyroxine

18 Which of the following is **not** secreted by the thyroid gland?
a calcitonin
b triodothyronine
c melatonin
d thyroxine

19 Endocrine glands in the body have a feedback mechanism which is coordinated by which gland?
a pineal
b thyroid
c pituitary
d adrenals

20 Increased thirst, increased output of urine, weight loss, and thin skin with impaired healing capacity are all signs of:
a hypoglycaemia
b hyperglycaemia
c diabetes
d gynaecomastia

10 the reproductive system

Introduction

The reproductive systems are the only systems that are very different, both in terms of structure and function, for men and women. The sex organs (testes in men and ovaries in women) are also endocrine glands, therefore there are also sexual differences in the functioning of the endocrine system.

The reproductive system is also the only system that undergoes particular changes at certain times in an individual's life, maturing at puberty, and for women, ceasing to function in the same way after the menopause.

These systems are unique in that they are not vital to the survival of an individual, but they are essential to the continuation of the human species.

◉ Objectives

By the end of this chapter you will be able to recall and understand the following knowledge:

- Functions of the reproductive systems
- Structure and function/s of the parts of the female reproductive system
- Structure and function/s of the parts of the male reproductive system
- The interrelationships between the reproductive and other body systems
- Common pathologies of the reproductive system.

Functions of the reproductive systems

The male and female reproductive systems are specialised, in their dual function, to produce the sex hormones responsible for the male and female characteristics, and for producing the cells required for reproduction.

The female reproductive system

The function of the female reproductive system is the production of sex hormones and ova (egg cells), which, if fertilised, are supported and protected until birth. The female reproductive system consists of the following internal organs lying in the pelvic cavity:

- the ovaries
- the fallopian tubes
- the uterus
- the vagina.

The external genitalia is known collectively as the vulva and consists of:

- the labia major and minor, which are lip-like folds at the entrance of the vagina
- the clitoris, which is attached to the symphysis pubis by a suspensory ligament and contains erectile tissue
- the hymen, which is a thin layer of mucous membrane
- the greater vestibular glands, which lie in the labia majora, one on each side near the vaginal opening. These glands secrete mucus which lubricates the vulva.

The breasts are accessory glands to the female reproductive system.

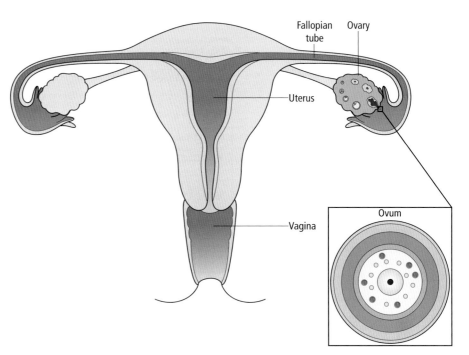

Fig 10.1 Female reproductive organs

Overview of the female reproductive organs

Female reproductive parts	Position	Function/s
Ovaries	Either side of uterus on lateral walls of pelvis	Production of ova Secretion of oestrogen and progesterone
Fallopian tubes	Extend from the sides of the uterus, passing upwards and outwards to end near each ovary	Convey the ovum from the ovary to the uterus
Uterus	Situated behind the bladder and in front of the rectum	Area in which an embryo grows
Vagina	Leads from the cervix to the vulva (connects internal sex organs with external genitalia)	Provides a passageway for menstruation and for childbirth

The ovaries

These are the female sex glands and they lie on the lateral walls of the pelvis. They are almond-shaped organs which are held in place, one on each side of the uterus, by several ligaments. The largest of the ligaments is the broad ligament which holds the ovaries in close proximity to the fallopian tubes.

The ovary contains numerous small masses of cells called ovarian follicles, within which the ova (egg cells) develop. At the time of birth there are about two million immature ova in the ovaries. Many of the ova degenerate, and at the time of puberty there are only about 400,000 left.

The immature ova (or oocytes) lie dormant in the ovary until they are stimulated by a sudden surge in the hormone FSH (follicle-stimulating hormone) at the time of puberty. Normally one egg (ovum) ripens and is released each month.

Functions

The ovaries have two distinct functions:

1 the production of ova
2 the secretion of the female hormones oestrogen and progesterone.

Oestrogen and progesterone regulate the changes in the uterus throughout the menstrual cycle and pregnancy. Oestrogen is responsible for the development of the female sexual characteristics, while progesterone, produced in the second phase of the menstrual cycle, supplements the action of oestrogen by thickening the lining of the uterus, ready for the possible implantation of a fertilised egg.

The fallopian tubes

The two fallopian tubes are each about 5 cm long, and extend from the sides of the uterus, passing upwards and outwards to end near each ovary. At the end of each fallopian tube are finger-like projections called fimbrae which encircle the ovaries.

Function

The function of the fallopian tubes is to convey the ovum from the ovary to the uterus. It is swept down the tube by peristaltic muscular contraction, assisted by the lining of ciliated epithelium.

Fertilisation of the ovum takes place within the fallopian tubes and it then passes to the uterus.

The uterus

The uterus is a small hollow, pear-shaped organ situated behind the bladder and in front of the rectum. It has thick muscular walls and is composed of three layers of tissue:

- The perimetrium: an outer covering which is part of the peritoneum (a serous membrane in the abdominal cavity). It covers the superior (top) part of the uterus.
- The myometrium: a middle layer of smooth muscle fibres. This layer forms 90 per cent of the uterine wall and is responsible for the powerful contractions that occur at the time of labour.
- The endometrium: a soft, spongy mucous membrane lining, the surface of which is shed each month during menstruation.

The uterus can be divided into three parts:`

1 The fundus is the dome-shaped part of the uterus above the openings of the uterine tubes.
2 The body is the largest and main part of the uterus and leads to the cervix.
3 The cervix of the uterus is a thick, fibrous muscular structure at the neck of the uterus which opens into the vagina.

Function

The uterus is part of the female reproductive tract which is specialised to receive an ovum and serves as the area in which an embryo grows and develops into a foetus. After puberty, the uterus goes through a regular cycle of changes which prepares it to receive, nourish and protect a fertilised ovum.

During pregnancy, the walls of the uterus relax to accommodate the growing foetus. If the ovum is not fertilised, the cycle ends with a short period of bleeding in which the endometrium undergoes periodic development and degeneration, known as the menstrual cycle.

The vagina

The vagina is a 10–15 cm muscular and elastic tube, lined with moist epithelium, which connects the internal organs of the female reproductive system with the external genitalia. It is made up of vascular and erectile tissue and extends from the cervix (internally) of the uterus above to the vulva (externally) below. During sexual stimulation, the erectile tissues become engorged with blood.

BODY FACT

The cervix of the uterus dilates during childbirth and the amount of dilation is used as a measurement to decide how soon the baby will be born.

Function

The function of the vagina is for the reception of the male sperm and to provide a passageway for menstruation and for childbirth. The wall of the vagina is sufficiently elastic to allow for expansion during childbirth. Between the phases of puberty and the menopause, the vagina also provides an acid environment, due to acid-secreting bacteria, in order to help prevent the growth of microbes that may infect the internal organs.

Stages of pregnancy

Pregnancy starts with fertilisation and ends with childbirth.

Fertilisation

This is the fusion of a spermatozoon with an ovum.

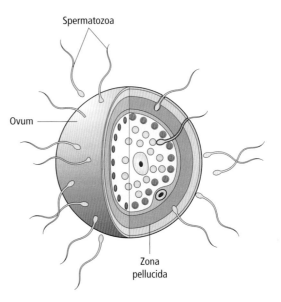

Spermatozoa

Ovum

Zona pellucida

Fig 10.2 Fertilisation

The spermatozoon approaches the ovum and penetrates the inner membrane of the ovum called the zona pellucida. This triggers the ovum's meiotic division, following meiosis, and makes the zona pellucida impenetrable to other spermatozoa. After the spermatozoon penetrates the ovum, its nucleus is released into the ovum, its tail degenerates, and its head enlarges amd fuses with the ovum's nucleus. This fusion provides the fertilised ovum, now called a zygote, with 46 chromosomes.

Pre-embryonic development

The pre-embryonic phase starts with ovum fertlisation and lasts for 2 weeks. As the zygote passes through the fallopian tube, it undergoes a series of mitotic divisions, forming daughter cells initially called blastomeres, that each contain the same number of chromosomes.

The first cell division ends about 30 hours after fertilisation; subsequent divisions occur rapidly. The zygote then develops into a small mass of cells called a morula, which reaches the uterus around the third day after fertilisation. Fluid then masses in the centre of the morula and forms a central cavity, which is then called a blastocyst. During the next phase, the blastocyst stays within the zona pellucida, unattached to the uterus. The zona pellucida degenerates and by the end of the first week of fertilisation, the blastocyst attaches to the endometrium.

Formation of embryo

By day 24 the blastocyst has formed an amniotic cavity containing an embryo. The developing zygote starts to take on a human shape. Each of the three germ layers (ectoderm, mesoderm and endoderm) forms specific tissues and organs in the developing embryo. Having reached its destination, the blastocyst attaches itself to the wall of the uterus (endometrium) where it will receive nutrients from the mother's blood vessels (via the placenta).

Foetal development

Significant growth and development takes place within the first 3 months following conception.

Month 1

At the end of the first month, the embryo has a definite form. The head, trunk and the tiny buds that will become the arms and legs are visible. The cardiovascular system has begun to function and the umbilical cord is visible in its most primitive form.

Month 2

During the second month the embryo grows to 2.5 cm in length. The head and facial features develop as the eyes, ears, nose, lips, tongue and tooth buds form. The arms and legs also take shape. Although the gender of the foetus is not yet visible, all external genitalia are present. Cardiovascular function is complete and the umbilical cord has a definite form. From the eighth week, the embryo is called a foetus.

Month 3

During the third month, the foetus grows to 7.5 cm in length. Teeth and bones begin to appear and the kidneys start to function. The foetus opens its mouth to swallow, grasps with its fully developed hands and prepares for breathing by inhaling and exhaling amniotic fluid (although its lungs are functioning properly). At the end of the 3 months, or trimester, the foetus's gender is distinguishable.

Months 4 to 9

Over the remaining 6 months, the foetal growth continues, as internal and external structures develop at a rapid rate. In the third trimester, the foetus stores the fats and minerals it will need to live outside of the womb.
At birth, the average full-term foetus measures 51 cm and weights 7–7½ lbs.

Birth

Childbirth is divided into three stages; the duration of each stage varies according to the size of the uterus, the woman's age and the number of previous pregnancies.

The first stage of labour is when the foetus begins its descent and the cervix begins to dilate to prepare to allow the foetus to pass from the uterus into the vagina. During this stage the amniotic sac ruptures as the uterine contractions increase in frequency and intensity (the amniotic sac can also rupture before the onset of labour).

The second stage of labour begins with full cervical dilation and ends with delivery of the foetus.

The third stage starts immediately after childbirth and ends with the placenta expulsion. After the neonate is delivered, the uterus continues to contract intermittently and grows smaller.

Female reproductive changes with ageing

Declining oestrogen and progesterone levels cause numerous physical changes in women with age. Ovulation usually stops 1–2 years before the menopause. As the ovaries reach the end of their productive cycle, they become unresponsive to gonadotrophic stimulation. With ageing, the ovaries atrophy and become thicker and smaller.

The vulva also atrophies with age and the tissue shrinks. Atrophy causes the vagina to shorten and the mucous lining to become thin, dry and less elastic.

After the menopause the uterus shrinks rapidly to half its pre-menstrual weight. The cervix atrophies and no longer produces mucus for lubrication and the endometrium and myometrium become thinner.

In the breasts the glandular, supporting and fatty tissues atrophy and as the Cooper's ligaments lose their elasticity, the breasts become pendulous.

Anatomy of the female breast

The female breasts are accessory organs to the female reproductive system and their function is to produce and secrete milk after pregnancy.

Position

The breasts lie on the pectoral region of the front of the chest. They are situated between the sternum and the axilla, extending from approximately the second to the sixth rib. The breasts lie over the pectoralis major and serratus anterior muscles and are attached to them by a layer of connective tissue.

Structure

The breasts consist of glandular tissue arranged in lobules, supported by connective, fibrous and adipose tissue. The lobes are divided into lobules which open up into milk ducts.

The milk ducts open into the surface of the breast at a projection called the nipple. Around each nipple, the skin is pigmented and forms the areola; this varies in colour from a deep pink to a light or dark brown colour. A considerable amount of fat or adipose tissue covers the surface of the gland and is found between the lobes. The skin on the breast is thinner and more translucent than the body skin.

Support

The breasts are supported and slung in powerful suspensory Cooper's ligaments, which go around the breast, both ends being attached to the chest wall. The pectoralis major and serratus anterior muscles help to support the ligaments.

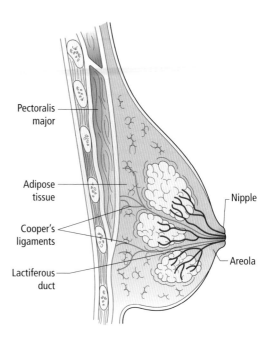

Pectoralis major

Adipose tissue

Cooper's ligaments

Lactiferous duct

Nipple

Areola

Fig 10.3 The structure of the female breast

If the breast grows large due to adolescence or pregnancy, the Cooper's ligaments may become irreparably stretched and the breast will then sag. With age, the supporting ligaments, along with the skin and the breast tissue, become thin and inelastic, and the breasts lose their support.

Physiology of the breast
Lymphatic drainage
The breasts contain many lymphatic vessels, and the lymph drainage is very extensive, draining mainly into the axillary nodes under the arms.

Blood supply
The blood vessels supplying blood to the breast include the subclavian and axillary arteries.

Nerve supply
There are numerous sensory nerve endings in the breast, especially around the nipple. When these touch, receptors are stimulated in lactation, the impulses pass to the hypothalamus, and the flow of the hormone oxytocin is increased from the posterior lobe of the pituitary. This promotes the constant flow of milk when required.

Hormones
The hormones responsible for developing the breast are:

- oestrogen: is responsible for the growth and development of the secondary sex characteristics
- progesterone: causes the mammary glands to increase in size if fertilisation and subsequent pregnancy occurs.

Development of the breasts

Puberty

The breast starts out as a nipple which projects from the surrounding ring of pigmented skin called the areola. Approximately two or three years before the onset of menstruation, the fat cells enlarge in response to the sex hormones (oestrogen and progesterone) released during adolescence.

Pregnancy

During pregnancy, the increased production of oestrogen and progesterone causes an increase in blood flow to the breast. This causes an enlargement of the ducts and lobules of the breast in preparation for lactation, and there is an increase in fluid retention. The areola and the nipple enlarge and become more pigmented.

Menopause

The reduction in the female hormones during the menopause causes the glandular tissue in the breast to shrink, and the supporting ligaments, along with the skin, become thinner and lose their elasticity. Therefore, during the menopause the breasts begin to lose their support and uplift, although the degree of loss is dependent on the original strength of the suspensory ligaments.

Factors determining size and shape

The size of the breast is largely determined by genetic factors, although there are other factors such as:

- amount of adipose tissue present
- fluid retention
- level of ovarian hormones in the blood and the sensitivity of the breasts to these hormones
- degree of ligamentary suspension
- exercise undertaken.

The male reproductive system

The male reproductive system consists of the:

- testes
- epididymis
- vas deferens
- urethra
- penis.

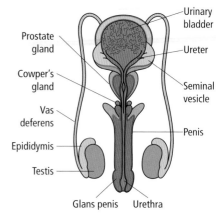

Fig 10.4 Male reproductive system

Student activity

Now complete Activity 10.2 in the resources for this book on Dynamic Learning Online.

Male reproductive parts	Position	Function/s
Testes	In the scrotum	Production of sperm
Epididymis	Lies along posterior border of each testis	Stores sperm until maturation
Vas deferens	Very long tubes leading from the seminiferous tubules of the testes to the urethra	Tubes through which sperm is released
Urethra	Extends from neck of bladder through the penis to outside of the body	Provides a common pathway for urine and semen
Penis	Male external sex organ	Excretes urine and ejaculates semen

The testes

The testes are the reproductive glands of the male, and lie in the scrotal sac. Each testis consists of approximately 200–300 lobules; these are separated by connective tissue and filled with seminiferous tubules, in which sperm cells are formed. Between the tubules are a group of secretory cells known as the interstitial cells which produce male sex hormones.

The testes are specialised to produce and maintain sperm cells, and to produce male sex hormones known collectively as androgens. Testosterone is the most important androgen as it stimulates the development of the male reproductive organs. It is also responsible for the development and maintenance of the male secondary sexual characteristics.

Epididymis

The epididymis are coiled tubes leading from the seminiferous tubules of the testis to the vas deferens. They store and nourish immature sperm cells and promote their maturation until ejaculation.

Vasa deferentia

The vasa deferentia (vas deferens, *singular*) are tubes leading from the epididymis to the urethra and through which the sperm are released.

Seminal vesicles

The seminal vesicles are pouches lying on the posterior aspect of the bladder attached to the vasa deferentia. They secrete an alkaline fluid which contains nutrients and is added to sperm cells during ejaculation.

Ejaculatory ducts

The two ejaculatory ducts are short tubes which join the seminal vesicles to the urethra.

Urethra

The urethra provides a common pathway for the flow of urine and the secretion of semen. A sphincter muscle prevents both functions occurring at the same time.

Penis

The penis is the main external sex organ of the male. It is composed of erectile tissue and is richly supplied with blood vessels. When stimulated by sexual activity the blood vessels become engorged with blood and the penis becomes erect. Its function is to convey urine and semen.

Accessory sex glands in the male

Cowper's glands

The Cowper's glands are a pair of small glands that open into the urethra at the base of the penis. These glands produce further secretions to contribute to the seminal fluid, but less than that of the prostate gland or seminal vesicles.

Prostate gland

The prostate gland is a male accessory gland about the size of a walnut. It lies in the pelvic cavity in front of the rectum and behind the symphysis pubis. During ejaculation it secretes a thin, milky fluid that enhances the mobility of sperm and neutralises semen and vaginal secretions.

Male reproductive changes with ageing

Physiological changes in older men include reduced testosterone production, with in turn may cause decreased libido. A reduced testosterone level also causes the testes to atrophy and soften and decreases sperm production by around 48–69 per cent between the ages of 60 and 80. Normally, the prostate glands enlarges with age and its secretions diminish. Seminal fluid also decreases in volume and becomes less viscous.

IN PRACTICE

In the case of a client with cancer, consult the client's GP/consultant regarding the extent of the disease; the spread of cancer is also determined by the type of breast cancer (some spread rapidly while others are slow growing). Avoid areas of radiation if client is on radiotherapy and remember that radio and chemotherapy can reduce the client's immunity and therefore you should avoid massaging if you have an infection.

Clients who have had surgery that involved removal of the axillary nodes are likely to have oedema of the arm. Provided permission has been granted by the client's GP/consultant, elevate the oedematous arm above heart level throughout the massage. Gently massage the arm with strokes directed towards the axilla. Advise client to open and close the hand tightly 6–8 times every few hours (the contraction of the muscles will help venous and lymphatic flow).

Common pathologies of the reproductive system

Female disorders

Amenorhhea

Amenorrhea is the absence or stopping of the menstrual periods. Causes may be associated with deficiency of ovarian, pituitary or thyroid hormones, mental disturbances, depression, radical weight loss, stress, excessive exercise or a major change in surroundings or circumstances.

Cancer of the breast

Most breast cancers are detected by the client noticing a breast or axillary lump; mammography screening can confirm these lumps. Breast cancer can present as redness and pain, discharge from or retraction of the nipple. Cancer can spread locally or to the axilla and neck lymph nodes causing oedema of the arm or by blood to the lung, bone and liver. The type of breast cancer can determine whether the spread is rapid or very slow.

Cancer of the cervix

It is asymptomatic in the early stages. Later there may be foul smelling, blood stained discharge through the vagina. Lower back pain, loss of weight, unexplained anaemia and pain during intercourse are other symptoms.

Cancer of the ovaries

It is asymptomatic. Diagnosis is usually made after the cancer has spread extensively. The symptoms are vague and are usually associated with gastrointestinal symptoms such as bloating of the abdomen, mild abdominal pain and excessive passage of gas. There may be fluid in the peritoneal cavity in late stages. Hormone changes may result in abnormal vaginal bleeding.

Dysmenorrhea

This condition is defined as painful and difficult menstruation. It presents with spasms and congestion of the uterus, resulting in cramping lower abdominal pains which start before or with the menstrual flow, and continue during menstruation. It is often associated with nausea, vomiting, headache and a feeling of faintness.

Ectopic pregnancy

The development of a foetus at a site other than in the uterus. An ectopic pregnancy may occur if the fertilised egg remains in the ovary, or in the fallopian tube, or if it lodges in the abdominal cavity.

The most common type of ectopic pregnancy occurs in the fallopian tube. There is a danger of haemorrhage and death as growth of the foetus may cause the tube to rupture and bleed.

Endometriosis

Inflammation of the endometrium (the inner lining of the uterus).
It presents with abnormal menstrual bleeding, lower abdominal pain and
a foul-smelling discharge. Fever and malaise may accompany this
condition.

Fibroid

An abnormal growth of fibrous and muscular tissue, one or more of which
may develop in the muscular wall of the uterus. Fibroids can cause pain
and excessive bleeding and become extremely large. Although they do not
threaten life, they render pregnancy unlikely.

Some fibroids may be removed surgically; in other cases a hysterectomy
may be necessary.

Polycystic ovary syndrome (as known as Stein-Leventhal syndrome)

A hormonal disorder in which there is inadequate secretion of the female
sex hormones. As a result the ovarian follicles fail to ovulate and remain
as multiple cysts, distending the ovary. Other associated symptoms include
obesity, hirsutism, acne and infertility.

Pre-menstrual syndrome

Pre-menstrual syndrome is a term for the physical and psychological
symptoms experienced 3–14 days prior to the onset of menstruation.
The condition presents with varying symptoms: headache, bloatedness,
water retention, backache, changes in coordination, abdominal pain,
swollen and painful breasts, depression, irritability and craving for
sweet things.

Infertility

Infertility is the inability in a woman to conceive or in a man to induce
conception. Female infertility may be due to a failure to ovulate, to
obstruction of the fallopian tubes, or endometriosis.

Male disorders

Cancer of the testis

Slight enlargement of the testis is the first symptom. It may be accompanied
by pain, discomfort and heaviness of the scrotum. Soon there is a rapid
enlargement of the testis which can become hot and red.

Cancer of the prostate

Usually no symptoms are seen. If the cancer is located close to the urethra,
there may be a frequency of micturition, urgency, difficulty in voiding, blood
in urine or blood in the ejaculate. Cancer of the prostate is often diagnosed
by rectal examination, where it feels nodular and hard. Prostate cancer
usually spreads to the bones and produces bony pain, or causes fractures in
the bone after trivial injury.

In the advanced stage, as in all cancers, the person loses weight and is
anaemic.

Prostatitis

Inflammation of the prostate gland, which is usually caused by bacteria. This condition presents with a frequency and urgency on passing urine (urine may be cloudy). High fever with chills, muscle and joint pain are common. A dull ache may be present in the lower back and pelvic area.

Infertility

Causes of male infertility can include decreased numbers or motility of sperm, or may be due to the total absence of sperm. In both male and female infertility, the cause may also be associated with stress.

Interrelationships with other systems

The reproductive system links to the following body systems:

Cells and tissues

Ova are the reproductive cells in the female and sperm cells are the reproductive cells in the male.

Skeletal

The pelvis offers protection for the uterus.

Muscular

Smooth muscle is responsible for the passage of ova from the ovaries to the vagina, and sperm from the testes to the urethra.

During orgasm in the female the muscles of the perineum, uterine wall and the uterine tubes contract rhythmically.

During orgasm in the male, motor impulses are transmitted to skeletal muscles at the base of the erectile penis causing them to contract rhythmically.

Circulatory

During erection of the penis the vascular spaces within the erectile tissue become engorged with blood as arteries dilate and veins are compressed.

During periods of sexual stimulation, the erectile tissues of the clitoris become engorged with blood.

Nervous

Orgasm is the culmination of sexual stimulation; the movement of semen occurs as a result of sympathetic reflexes.

Endocrine

The ovaries in women and the testes in the male are responsible for the development of the secondary sexual characteristics.

Key words associated with the reproductive system

ovaries	progesterone	Cowper's gland
fallopian tube	pregnancy	Cooper's ligament
uterus	menopause	penis
vagina	testes	scrotum
vulva	epididymides	sperm
genitalia	vasa deferentia	testosterone
breast/mammary gland	ejaculatory ducts	seminiferous tubules
ovum	urethra	ejaculation
ova	seminal vesicles	semen
oestrogen	prostate	

Revision summary of the reproductive system

- The male/female reproductive systems function to produce:
  a the sex hormones responsible for the male and female characteristics
  b the cells require for reproduction.
- The structures of the female reproductive system include: **ovaries, fallopian tubes, uterus, vagina** and **vulva.**
- The **breasts** or mammary glands are considered to be part of the female reproductive system.
- The **ovaries** lie on the lateral walls of the pelvis and have two distinct functions: the production of **ova** and the secretion of the female hormones **oestrogen** and **progesterone.**
- The **fallopian tubes** transport **ova** from the **ovaries** to the **uterus.**
- The **uterus** is situated behind the bladder and in front of the rectum and is designed to receive, nourish and protect a fertilised **ovum.**
- The **vagina** is a muscular and elastic tube designed for the reception of sperm and to provide a passageway for menstruation and childbirth.
- The **vulva** is a collective term for the female **genitalia.**
- In the female before the **menopause**, levels of **oestrogen** and **progesterone** decrease, ovaries atrophy and become thicker and smaller. The **vulva** atrophies and tissue shrinks. Atrophy causes the **vagina** to shorten and the mucous lining to become thin, dry and less elastic.

- After the **menopause** the **uterus** shrinks rapidly to half its pre-menstrual weight. The **breasts** atrophy and lose their elasticity and support.
- **Pregnancy** start with fertilisation and ends with childbirth and consists of the following stages: fertilisation, pre-embryonic development, formation of embryo, foetal development and birth.
- The structures of the male reproductive system include: **testes, epidydmides, vasa deferentia, ejaculatory ducts, urethra, seminal vesicles, prostate, Cowper's gland** and **penis.**
- The **testes** lie in a scrotal sac; they produce and maintain **sperm** cells, and produce the male sex hormone **testosterone.**
- Each **testis** is filled with **seminifereous tubules** in which **sperm** cells are formed.
- The **epididymides** are coiled tubes that lead from the **seminiferous tubules** of the **testis** to the **vas deferens.** They store and nourish immature **sperm** cells and promote their maturation until **ejaculation.**
- The **vasa deferentia** lead from the **epididymis** to the **urethra** and are tubes through which the **sperm** are released.
- The **seminal vesicles** are pouches lying on the posterior aspect of the bladder attached to the vas deferens. They secrete an alkaline fluid which contains nutrients and is added to **sperm** cells during **ejaculation.**

- The two **ejaculatory ducts** are short tubes which join the **seminal vesicles** to the **urethra**.
- The **Cowper's glands** are a pair of small glands that open into the **urethra** at the base of the **penis**. These glands produce further secretions to contribute to the **seminal fluid**.
- The **prostate** gland lies in the pelvic cavity in front of the rectum and behind the symphysis pubis. During ejaculation it secretes a thin, milky fluid that enhances the mobility of sperm and neutralises **semen** and vaginal secretions.

- The **urethra** provides a common pathway for the flow of urine and the secretion of **semen**.
- The **penis** is composed of erectile tissue and is richly supplied with blood vessels. Its function is to convey urine and **semen**.
- In the male, decreased levels of **testosterone** decreases sexual desire and viable **sperm**; testes also atrophy as muscle strength decreases.

1 The main function of the ovaries is to:
   a serve as a site for fertilisation
   b accommodate a growing foetus during pregnancy
   c receive male sperm
   d produce mature ova

2 Once an ovum has become fertilised it is known as a:
   a blastocyst
   b zygote
   c embryo
   d foetus

3 A foetus's gender is distinguishable at:
   a the end of the first trimester
   b the end of the first month
   c a month before birth
   d eight weeks

4 The function of the fallopian tubes is to:
   a convey ova from the ovary to the vulva
   b prepare for the implantation of a fertilised ovum
   c convey ova from the ovary to the uterus
   d secrete mucus

5 The uterus is situated:
   a behind the bladder and in front of the rectum
   b in front of the bladder and behind the rectum
   c on the lateral walls of the pelvis
   d at the entrance of the vulva

6 The cervix is:
   a an outer covering of the uterus
   b the largest and main part of the uterus
   c a thick muscular structure that opens into the vagina
   d the dome-shaped part of the uterus

7 The inner mucous membrane lining of the uterus is called the:
   a perimetrium
   b endometrium
   c myometrium
   d perineum

8 Where in the male reproductive system are sperm cells stored to maturation?
   a vasa deferentia
   b penis
   c epididymides
   d Cowper's glands

9 The collective term for male hormones is:
   a gonads
   b androgens
   c vesicles
   d interstitial secretions

10 Which of the following hormones prepares the lining of the uterus for the implantation of a fertilised egg?
   a oestrogen
   b follicle-stimulating hormone
   c luteinising hormone
   d progesterone

11 Where does fertilisation of the ovum take place?
   a ovaries
   b uterus
   c vagina
   d fallopian tubes

12 The absence or stopping of menstrual periods is known as:
   a dysmenorrhea
   b amenorrhea
   c endometriosis
   d fibroids

13 The ejaculatory ducts are:
   a two short tubes which join the seminal vesicle to the urethra
   b a pair of ducts that open into the urethra at the base of the penis
   c tubes leading from the epididymis to the urethra
   d composed of erectile tissue

14 Which of the following factors does **not** determine the size and shape of the breasts?
  a fluid retention
  b level of ovarian hormones
  c diet
  d exercise undertaken

15 The primary function of the testes is to:
  a store seminal fluid
  b produce and maintain sperm cells
  c development of the male secondary characteristics
  d nourish immature sperm cells

16 Progesterone is produced in which phase of the menstrual cycle?
  a first
  b second
  c between first and second
  d third

17 In a vasectomy which part of the male reproductive system is cut?
  a epididymis
  b seminal vesicle
  c urethra
  d vasa deferentia

18 A condition where there is an abnormal growth of fibrous and muscular tissue in the wall of the uterus is:
  a endometriosis
  b fibroids
  c ovarian cyst
  d ectopic pregnancy

19 The ovary contains numerous small masses of cells called:
  a oocytes
  b fimbrae
  c follicles
  d zygotes

20 The first stage of labour is when:
  a the cervix fully dilates
  b the placenta is expelled
  c the cervix begins to dilate
  d the foetus passes from uterus to vagina

the digestive system

Introduction

In the digestive system food is broken down and made soluble before it can be absorbed by the body for nutrition. Food is taken in through the mouth, broken into smaller particles and absorbed into the bloodstream where it is utilised by the body. Waste materials not required by the body are then passed through the body to be eliminated. Once food has been absorbed by the body, it is converted into energy to fuel the body's activities. This is known as metabolism.

◉ Objectives

By the end of this chapter you will be able to recall and understand the following knowledge:

- the functions of the digestive system
- the process of digestion from the ingestion of food to the elimination of waste
- the structure and functions of the organs associated with digestion
- the absorption of nutrients and their utilisation in the body
- the sources and functions of the main food groups required for good health
- the interrelationships between the digestive and other body systems
- common pathologies of the digestive system.

Functions of the digestive system

The digestive system serves two major functions:

- the breaking down of food and fluid into simple chemicals that can be absorbed into the bloodstream and transported throughout the body
- the elimination of waste products through excretion of faeces via the anal canal.

The structure and function of digestive organs

Digestion occurs in the alimentary canal, which is a long continuous muscular tube extending from the mouth to the anus. The process of breaking down food is called digestion. Digestion involves the following processes.

Ingestion

This is the act of taking food into the alimentary canal through the mouth.

Digestion

- **Mechanical digestion** – this is the breaking down of solid food into smaller pieces by the chewing action of the teeth, known as mastication, and the churning action of the stomach assisted by peristalsis.
- **Chemical digestion** – this involves the breakdown of large molecules of carbohydrates, proteins and fats into smaller ones by the action of digestive enzymes.

Absorption

This is the movement of soluble materials out through the walls of the small intestine. Nutrients are absorbed through the villi and pass out into the network of blood and lymph vessels to be delivered to various parts of the body.

Assimilation

This is the process by which digested food is used by the tissues after absorption.

Elimination/defecation

This is the expulsion of the semi-solid waste called faeces through the anal canal.

The digestive system consists of the following parts:

- **mouth**
- **pharynx**
- **oesophagus**
- **stomach**
- **small intestine** (consisting of the duodenum, jejunum and the ileum)
- **large intestine** (consisting of the caecum, appendix, colon and rectum)
- **anus**.

The **pancreas, gall bladder** and the **liver** are accessory organs to digestion.

Overview of the digestive organs

STUDY TIP

The digestive system is a process that has a start point (the mouth) and an end point (the anus). The table opposite should help you to break down the process for revision purposes.

Digestive organ	Function
Mouth	Commencement of digestion Food chewed and mixed with saliva
Pharynx	Swallowing/projects food down the oesophagus
Oesophagus	Pushes the food onwards to the stomach

Digestive organ	Function
Stomach	Mechanical breakdown of food
	Commences digestion of protein
Small intestine	Chemical breakdown of food
	Absorption of digested food
Large intestine	Formation and storage of faeces before defecation
Anus	Defecation (expulsion of faeces)

Student activity

Now complete Activity 11.1 in the resources for this book on Dynamic Learning Online.

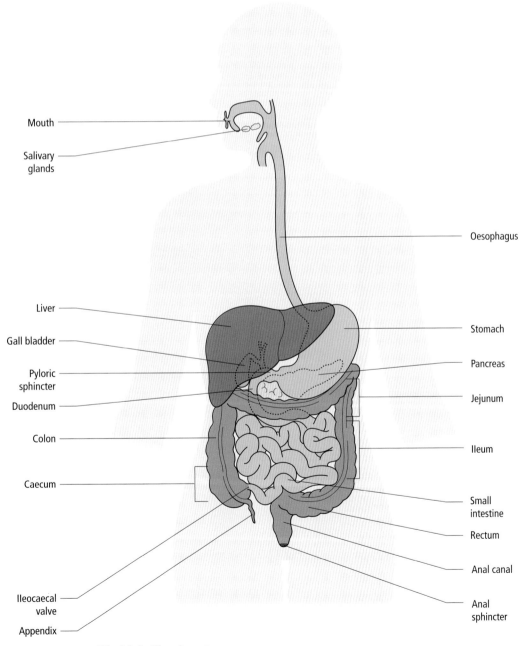

Fig 11.1 The digestive organs

Mouth

The digestive system commences in the mouth. Food is broken up into smaller pieces by the action of the jaws and the teeth and shaped into a ball by the tongue. Mastication renders the food small enough to be swallowed and allows saliva to be thoroughly mixed with it.

The smell and sight of food triggers the reflex action of the secretion of saliva in the mouth. Saliva enters the mouth from three pairs of salivary glands. These are the:

- **sublingual glands** – located in the lower part of the mouth on either side of the tongue
- **submandibular glands** – located inside the arch of the mandible
- **parotid glands** – located superficial to the masseter muscle.

Saliva, containing the enzyme salivary amylase, commences the digestion of starch, or carbohydrates, in the mouth.

> **KEY FACT**
>
> An enzyme is a chemical catalyst which activates and speeds up a chemical reaction without any change to itself. Enzymes are highly specific in that each enzyme catalyses only one type of metabolic action. An example is salivary amylase which will only act on starch but has no effect on protein.

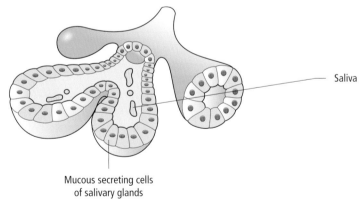

Mucous secreting cells of salivary glands

Fig 11.2 The salivary glands

> **KEY FACT**
>
> Peristalsis is the coordinated rhythmical contractions of the circular and oblique muscles in the wall of the alimentary tract. These muscles work in opposition to one another to break food down and move it along the alimentary canal. Peristalsis is an automatic action stimulated by the presence of food and occurs in all sections of the alimentary tract.

Pharynx and oesophagus

The ball of food is projected to the back of the mouth. The muscles of the pharynx force the food down the oesophagus which is a long narrow tube linking the pharynx to the stomach. A lubricative substance called mucus, secreted from the lining of the oesophagus, makes the food easier to swallow. The food is then conveyed by peristalsis down the oesophagus to the stomach.

Stomach

The stomach is a curved J-shaped muscular organ, positioned in the left-hand side of the abdominal cavity below the diaphragm.

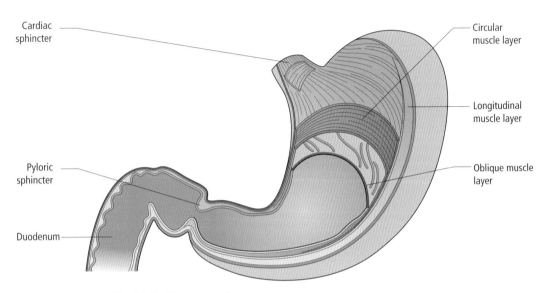

Fig 11.3 The stomach

Food enters the stomach via the cardiac sphincter which is a strong circular muscle at the junction of the stomach and the oesophagus. Its function is to control the entry of food into the stomach.

The layers of the stomach are as follows:

Stomach layer	Description
Peritoneum	Serous membrane that lines the abdominal cavity, supporting the alimentary canal and secretes a serous fluid which prevents friction
Muscular coat	Consists of longitudinal, circular and oblique fibres which assist the mechanical breakdown of food
Sub-mucous coat	Made up of areolar tissue containing blood vessels and lymphatics
Mucous coat	Secretes mucous to protect the stomach lining from the damaging effects of the acidic gastric juice
Surface epithelium	Infolded into numerous tubular gastric glands which secrete gastric juice

The main constituents of gastric juice, produced and secreted by cells in the stomach wall are as follows:

Pepsin	An enzyme which starts the breakdown of proteins
Hydrochloric acid	Provides the acidic conditions needed for pepsin to become active, kill germs present in food and prepares it for intestinal digestion
Mucus	Secreted by the neck cells in the stomach wall. It protects the stomach lining from the damaging effects of the acidic gastric juice
Rennin	An enzyme found in the gastric juices of infants that curdles milk protein.
Gastrin	A hormone released by endocrine cells in the stomach wall and is stimulated by the presence of food. This hormone circulates in the blood stream, stimulating the further release of gastric juice

The functions of the stomach are to:

- churn and break up large particles of food mechanically
- mix food with gastric juice to begin the chemical breakdown of food
- commence the digestion of protein
- absorb alcohol.

Food stays in the stomach for approximately five hours until it has been churned down to a liquid state called chyme. Chyme is then released at intervals into the first part of the small intestine. The exit from the stomach is controlled by the pyloric sphincter which sits at the junction of the stomach and the duodenum. Its function is to relax and release chyme at intervals into the small intestine.

Small intestine

The small intestine is approximately 3 m long and consists of three parts:

Duodenum	The first and shortest part of the small intestine
Jejunum	Lies between the duodenum and the ileum
Ileum	The longest segment of the small intestine where the main absorption of food takes place

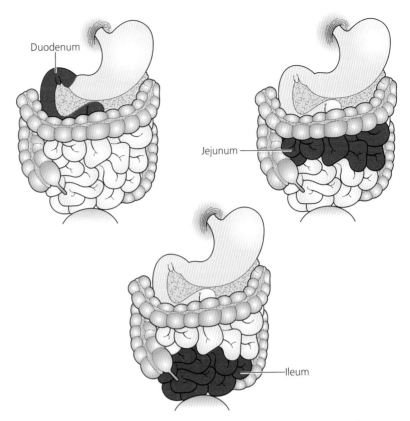

Duodenum

Jejunum

Ileum

Fig 11.4 The small intestine (showing duodenum, jejunum and ileum)

The small intestine consists of the same four layers as the stomach:

- peritoneum
- muscular coat excluding the oblique fibres
- sub-mucous layer containing numerous blood and lymph vessels and nerves
- circular folds of mucosa which protect the intestine from bacteria.

The special features of the small intestine are the thousands of minute projections called villi, each containing a lymph vessel called a lacteal. The villi have a network of capillaries into which the nutrients pass to be absorbed into the bloodstream.

Chemical breakdown of food

The muscles in the wall of the small intestine continue the mechanical breakdown of food by peristaltic movements, while the chemical digestion is brought about by the following juices which prepare the food to be absorbed into the bloodstream:

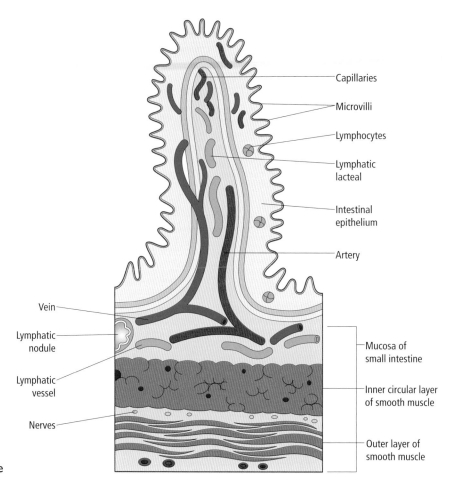

Labels (top to bottom, right side): Capillaries, Microvilli, Lymphocytes, Lymphatic lacteal, Intestinal epithelium, Artery, Mucosa of small intestine, Inner circular layer of smooth muscle, Outer layer of smooth muscle

Labels (left side): Vein, Lymphatic nodule, Lymphatic vessel, Nerves

Fig 11.5 The villi of the small intestine

Bile (green alkaline liquid) Consists of water, mucus, bile pigments, bile salts and cholesterol	Produced in the liver and stored in the gall bladder	Neutralises the chyme and breaks up any fat droplets in a process called emulsification
Pancreatic juice	Pancreas	Enzymes contained within pancreatic juice continue the digestion of protein, carbohydrates and fats **Trypsin** Continues the breakdown of proteins which was started by pepsin in the stomach **Pancreatic amylase** Continues the breakdown of starch and has the same effects as salivary amylase **Pancreatic lipase** Breaks down lipids into fatty acids and glycerol. The pancreas also has an endocrine function in that it secretes insulin from the islet of Langerhans cells in the pancreas. Insulin is important to digestion because it regulates blood sugar levels
Intestinal juice	Released by the glands of the small intestine	Completes the final breakdown of nutrients, including simple sugars to glucose and protein to amino acids

Carbohydrate digestion is completed by the following enzymes:

- **maltase** – this splits maltose into glucose
- **sucrase** – this splits sucrose into glucose and fructose
- **lactase** – this splits lactose into glucose and galactose.

Protein digestion is completed by peptidases which split short chain **polypeptides** into **amino acids**.

Absorption of the digested food

The absorption of the digested food takes place in the jejunum and mainly in the ileum. It occurs by diffusion through the villi of the small intestine which are well supplied with blood capillaries to allow the digested food to enter. Each villus contains a lymph vessel called a **lacteal** into which **fatty acids** and **glycerol** can pass.

Simple sugars from carbohydrate digestion and amino acids from protein digestion pass into the bloodstream via the villi and are then carried to the liver via the hepatic portal vein to be processed. The products of fat digestion pass into the intestinal lymphatics which absorb the fat molecules and carry them through the lymphatic system before they reach the blood circulation. Vitamins and minerals travel across to the blood capillaries of the villi and are absorbed into the bloodstream to assist in normal body functioning and cell metabolism.

How the body's nutrients are assimilated

Once all the nutrients have been absorbed into the bloodstream they are transported to the body's cells for metabolism:

Glucose	End product of carbohydrate digestion	Used to provide energy for the cells to function
Amino acids	End products of protein digestion	Used to produce new tissues, repair damaged cell parts and formulate enzymes, plasma proteins and hormones
Fatty acids and glycerol	End products of fat digestion	Used primarily to provide heat and energy in addition to glucose Those fats which are not required immediately by the body are used to build cell membranes and some are stored under the skin or around vital organs such as the kidneys and the heart

When all the body's nutrients have been assimilated by the body, the fate of the undigested food is to pass into the large intestine where it is eventually eliminated from the body.

Large intestine

The large intestine is formed of the **caecum, appendix, colon** and **rectum**. It coils around the small intestine and is characterised by:

- three bands of longitudinal muscle
- deep, longitudinal folds of mucosa which increase in the rectum
- numerous tubular glands which secrete mucus from their goblet cells.

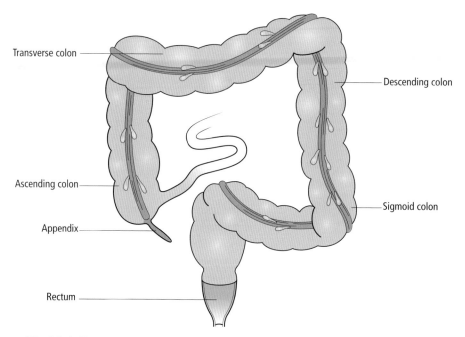

Fig 11.6 The large intestine

Parts of the large intestine:

Caecum	Small pouch to which the appendix is attached and into which the ileum opens through the ileo-caecal valve
Appendix	Sac attached to caecum of large intestine No known function in humans
Colon	Main part of the large intestine and is divided into four sections – ascending, transverse, descending and sigmoid colons **Ascending colon** – this is the part that passes upwards on the right side of the abdomen from the caecum (a pouch at the junction of the small and large intestines) to the lower edge of the liver **Transverse colon** – this is the longest and most mobile part and extends across the abdomen from right to left below the stomach **Descending colon** – this is the part that passes downwards along the left side of the abdominal cavity to the brim of the pelvis **Sigmoid colon** – this is the S-shaped part of the large intestine between the descending colon and the rectum
Rectum	Last part of the large intestine extending from the sigmoid colon to the anal canal. It is firmly attached to the sacrum and ends about 5 cm below the tip of the coccyx where it becomes the anal canal. Faeces are stored in the rectum before defecation
Anus	An opening at the lower end of the alimentary canal. It is the anal canal through which faeces are discharged. The anus is guarded by two sphincter muscles: ● **internal sphincter** – this is composed of smooth muscle under involuntary control ● **external sphincter** – this is composed of skeletal muscle under voluntary control The anus remains closed except during defecation

The functions of the large intestine are:

- absorption of most of the water from the faeces in order to conserve moisture in the body
- formation and storage of faeces which consists of undigested food, dead cells and bacteria
- production of mucus to lubricate the passage of faeces
- the expulsion of faeces out of the body through the anus.

Overview of the accessory organs to digestion

Liver	Has many important functions in the metabolism of food
	Regulates the nutrients absorbed from the small intestine to make them suitable for use in the body's tissues
Gall bladder	Stores bile and releases it when needed
Pancreas	Secretes pancreatic juice which contains enzymes to continue the digestion of protein, carbohydrates and fats
	Secretes the hormone insulin which is important to carbohydrate metabolism

Liver

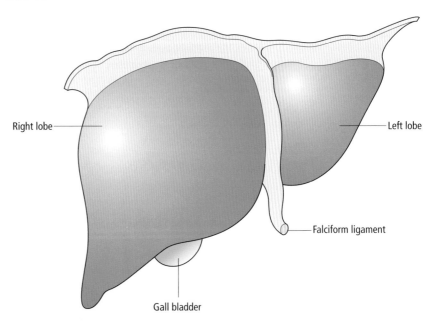

Fig 11.7 The liver

The liver is the largest gland in the body and is situated in the upper right-hand side of the abdominal cavity under the diaphragm. It has a soft reddish-brown colour and four lobes. Its internal structure is made up of cells called hepatocytes. The liver receives oxygenated blood from the hepatic artery and deoxygenated blood from the hepatic portal vein. Blood from the digestive tract, which is carried in the portal veins, brings newly absorbed nutrients into the sinusoids and nourishes the liver cells.

The liver is a vital organ and, therefore, has many important functions in the metabolism of food. It regulates the nutrients absorbed from the small intestine to make them suitable for use in the body's tissues.

Functions of the liver

Function	Significance
Secretion of bile	Bile is manufactured by the liver but is stored and released by the gall bladder to assist the body in the breakdown of fats
Regulation of blood sugar levels	When the blood sugar levels rise after a meal, the liver cells store excess glucose as glycogen. Some glucose may be stored in the muscle cells as muscle glycogen. When both these stores are full, surplus glucose is converted into fat by the liver cells
Regulation of amino acid levels	As our bodies cannot store excess protein and amino acids they are processed by the liver. Some are removed by the liver cells and are used to make plasma proteins. Some are left for the body cells tissues' use, while the rest are deaminated and excreted as urea in the kidneys
Regulation of the fat content of blood	The liver is involved in the processing and transporting of fats. Those already absorbed in the diet are used for energy and excess fats are stored in the tissues
Regulation of plasma proteins	The liver is active in the breakdown of worn-out red blood cells
Detoxification	The liver detoxifies harmful toxic waste and drugs and excretes them in bile or through the kidneys
Storage	The liver stores vitamins A, D, E, K and B12 and the minerals iron, potassium and copper. The liver can also hold up to a litre of blood. During exercise the liver supplies extra blood and increases oxygen transport to the muscles
The production of heat	Due to its many functions, the liver generates heat

Gall bladder

The gall bladder is a pear-shaped organ attached to the posterior and inferior surface of the liver by the cystic and bile ducts.

Bile is a thick alkaline liquid that is produced in the liver as a result of the breakdown of red blood cells. Bile is partially an excretory product and partially a digestive secretion. Bile salts (sodium and potassium) play a role in emulsification and the breakdown of large fat globules.

When worn-out red blood cells are broken down substances such as iron and globin are recycled but some of the bilirubin is excreted into the bile ducts. Bilirubin is eventually broken down in the intestines and one of its breakdown products gives the faeces the normal brown colour.

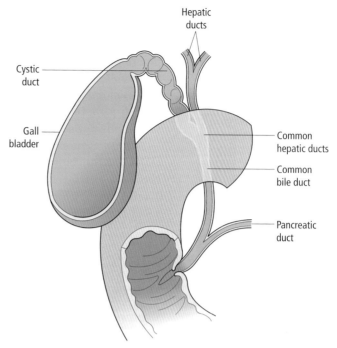

Fig 11.8 The gall bladder

Functions of the gall bladder

The gall bladder stores and concentrates bile produced by the liver until it is needed. It releases bile into the common bile duct for delivery to the duodenum.

Pancreas

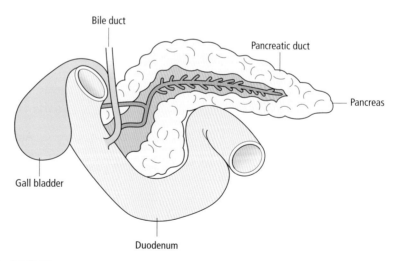

Fig 11.9 The pancreas

The pancreas is situated behind the stomach between the duodenum and the spleen. It is divided into a head, body and tail. The head is the expanded portion that fits into the C-shaped curve of the duodenum. The pancreas is composed of numerous lobules, each containing secretory alveoli (small sac-like cavities) which contain cells that produce pancreatic juice. In between the network of alveoli are the islets of Langerhans which produce insulin.

Functions of the pancreas

The pancreas has two functions – exocrine and endocrine.

Exocrine function

The pancreas secretes pancreatic juice which contains water, alkaline salts, the enzymes lipase, pancreatic amylase, trypsinogen and chymotrypsinogen. The alkalinity of pancreatic juice helps to neutralise the acidity of chyme from the stomach and allows the pancreatic and intestinal enzymes to work.

Endocrine function

The islets of Langerhans are endocrine glands which secrete the hormone **insulin** into the bloodstream. The insulin circulates around the body in the blood and is important to carbohydrate metabolism.

Nutrition

Nutrition is the utilisation of food to facilitate growth and maintain the normal working of the body. Poor nutrition can have a dramatic effect on our general health, energy levels, sleep patterns and stress response.

Food group	Dietary sources	Main functions
Carbohydrates also known as starches and sugars	Bread, cereals, potatoes, fruit and sugars	Body's main source of energy, required for the metabolism of other nutrients such as proteins and fats
Proteins	First-class proteins such as fish, milk, egg and meat. Second-class proteins include pulses, beans and peas	Necessary for the growth and repair of the body tissues which are used in the production of hormones and enzymes
Fats classified as saturated or unsaturated, depending on whether they are solid (saturated) or liquid (unsaturated) at room temperature	Meat, milk, cheese, butter and eggs	Source of stored energy Offer support and protection for the body and are used to build cell structures
Water (although not usually considered as food, it is nevertheless an essential nutrient needed by every part of the body)	Fresh water, fruit and vegetables	Aids digestion and elimination Essential to maintaining the body's fluid balance and aids in the transport of substances around the body
Fibre Although fibre is not broken down into nutrients, it is a very necessary component for effective digestion	Pulses, peas, beans, brown rice, wholemeal bread, jacket potatoes and green leafy vegetables	Aids digestion and bowel functioning Provides the bulk in food to satisfy the appetite
Vitamins (divided into two groups according to whether they are soluble in water or fat)	Essential for normal physiological and metabolic functioning of the body Regulate the body's processes and contribute to its resistance to disease	

Food group	Dietary sources	Main functions
Vitamin A (fat soluble)	Carotene in carrots, liver, kidney, eggs, dairy products, fish and liver oils	Essential for healthy vision, healthy skin and mucous membrane
Vitamin D (fat soluble)	Fish liver oils, fatty fish, margarine and eggs. Is also synthesised from ultra-violet light	Essential for healthy teeth and bones Maintains the blood calcium level by increasing calcium absorption from food
Vitamin E (fat soluble)	Peanuts, wheatgerm, milk, butter and eggs	Inhibits the oxidation of fatty acids that help form cell membranes
Vitamin K (fat soluble)	Green leafy vegetables, cereals, liver and fruit	Essential for blood clotting
Vitamin B1 (water soluble)	Egg yolk, liver, milk, wholegrain cereals, vegetables and fruit	Necessary for the steady release of energy from glucose
Vitamin B2 (water soluble)	Milk, liver, eggs and yeast	Essential for using energy released from food
Vitamin B5 (water soluble)	Wholegrain cereals, yeast extract, liver, beans, nuts and meat	Involved in the breakdown of glucose to release energy
Vitamin B6 (water soluble)	Wholegrain cereals, yeast extract, liver, meat, nuts, bananas, salmon and tomatoes	Necessary for the metabolism of protein and fat
Vitamin B12 (water soluble)	Liver, kidney, milk, eggs and cheese	Necessary for the formation of red blood cells in bone marrow Also involved in protein metabolism
Folic acid (water soluble)	Liver, kidney, fresh leafy vegetables, oranges and bananas	Essential for the normal production of red and white blood cells
Vitamin C (water soluble)	Citrus fruits and blackcurrants	Assists in the formation of connective tissue and collagen Helps prevent bleeding and aids healing
Minerals		Provide the body with materials for growth and repair and for the regulation of body processes Needed in trace amounts and are used to build bone, work muscles, support various organs and transport oxygen and carbon dioxide
Calcium	Milk, egg yolk, cheese and green leafy vegetables	Essential for the formation of healthy bones and teeth, blood coagulation and the normal function of muscles and nerves
Iron	Liver, kidney, red meats, egg yolk, nuts and green vegetables	Essential for the production of haemoglobin in red blood cells

(Continued)

Food group	Dietary sources	Main functions
Phosphorus	Cheese, eggs, white fish, wholemeal bread, peanuts and yeast extract	Important in the formation of bones and teeth, muscle contraction and the transmission of nerve impulses
Sulphur	Egg yolk, fish, red meat and liver	Main component of structural proteins (those in the skin and hair)
Sodium and chlorine	Table salt, bacon, kippers and is found in all body fluids	Maintains fluid balance in the body. Necessary for the transmission of nerve impulses and contraction of muscle
Magnesium	Green vegetables and salad	Important for the formation of bone and is required for the normal functioning of muscles and nerves

Common pathologies of the digestive system

Anorexia nervosa

This is a psychological illness in which clients starve themselves or use other techniques such as vomiting or laxatives to induce weight loss. They are motivated by a false perception of their body image and a phobia of becoming fat. The result is a severe loss of weight with amenorrhea and even death from starvation.

Appendicitis

This is an acute inflammation of the appendix. The main symptom is abdominal pain centrally and in the right lower abdomen over the appendix. It is usually treated by surgical removal known as an appendectomy.

Bulimia

This is a psychological illness which is characterised by overeating (bingeing), followed by self-induced vomiting.

Cancer of the colon

In the early stages the signs and symptoms are vague and related to the location of the cancer. A dull abdominal pain may or may not be present. General symptoms include loss of weight, fatigue, anaemia and weakness. If the tumour is on the right side of the abdomen (caecum or ascending colon) symptoms of obstruction appear slowly, as tumours in this region generally tend to spread along the walls of the gut without narrowing the lumen of the gut. If on the left side (descending colon, sigmoid colon or rectum), the signs of obstruction appear early in the disease. There is constipation or diarrhoea with passage of pencil-shaped or ribbon-like stools. The blood in the stools may be red or dark in colour.

Cancer of the gall bladder

Indigestion and colicky pain may be present especially after a fatty meal. The pain is located in the upper right quadrant of the abdomen and may be referred to the back, right shoulder, right scapula or between the scapula.

Cancer of the liver

The more common type of cancer is that which has spread from other areas of the body – a metastatic carcinoma. Spread is common from those areas from which blood flows through the liver. Cancer can also arise from the liver tissue – primary cancer. Commonly, liver cancer is due to secondary spread from the stomach, intestine or pancreas. Liver cancer may be present as a swelling in the upper right quadrant associated with jaundice or fluid in the abdomen. Other general symptoms may include weight loss, weakness and loss of appetite. Usually, this type of cancer is well advanced when diagnosed, whether arising from the liver or secondary to cancer elsewhere in the body.

Cancer – oral

This may be caused by chronic irritation of the mucosa of the oral cavity as in tobacco chewing. A recurrence of chronic ulcers of the mouth can lead to this type of cancer. Oral cancer may appear as a non-healing, slow-growing red ulcer or as a growth. Usually it is painful and firm to touch.

Cancer of the pancreas

The person presents with severe weight loss and pain in the lower back. The pain increases a few hours after taking food and is worsened on lying down. If the tumour is growing around the bile duct obstruction may result in jaundice and diarrhoea. The accumulation of bilirubin under the skin causes severe itching. The jaundice may be so severe that the skin may turn green or black as the bilirubin changes in structure. The reduction in bile slows down the absorption and digestion of fat causing clay-coloured, foul-smelling stools and diarrhoea. The cancer spreads directly and rapidly to the surrounding tissues, including the lymph nodes and liver. The kidneys, spleen and blood vessels may also be involved. The symptoms may vary according to the tissues affected.

Cancer of the stomach

In the early stages the person has chronic pain or discomfort in the upper part of the abdomen. Since the symptoms are vague, this cancer is often not diagnosed until it has spread considerably. There is weight loss, anaemia, loss of appetite and the person will feel easily fatigued. Vomiting is common and often the content has blood in it. A mass may be felt in the upper abdomen. Indigestion and acidity is not relieved by medication.

Cirrhosis of the liver

Cirrhosis refers to a distorted or scarred liver as a result of chronic inflammation. The functional liver cells are replaced by fibrous or adipose connective tissue. The symptoms of cirrhosis include jaundice, oedema in the legs, uncontrolled bleeding and sensitivity to drugs. Cirrhosis may be caused by hepatitis, alcoholism, certain chemicals that destroy the liver cells or parasites that infect the liver.

Colitis

This is inflammation of the colon. The usual symptoms are diarrhoea, sometimes with blood and mucus and lower abdominal pain.

Constipation

This condition presents as a difficulty in passing stools or where there is infrequent evacuation of the bowels. The causes may be dietary due to reduced fibre and fluid intake, certain medications or intestinal obstruction.

Diabetes mellitus

This is a carbohydrate metabolism disorder in which sugars are not oxidised to produce enough energy due to lack of the pancreatic hormone insulin. The accumulation of sugar leads to its appearance in the blood then in the urine. Symptoms of diabetes mellitus include thirst, loss of weight and excessive production of urine.

Diabetes insipidus

This is a rare metabolic disorder in which a person produces large quantities of dilute urine and is constantly thirsty. It is due to the deficiency of the hormone ADH which regulates reabsorption of water in the kidneys. It is treated by administration of the hormone.

Diarrhoea

This condition presents with frequent bowel evacuation or the passage of abnormally soft or liquid faeces. It may be caused by intestinal infections or other forms of intestinal inflammation such as colitis or irritable bowel syndrome.

Gallstones

This is a hard pebble-like mass which is formed within the gall bladder. The condition may be asymptomatic or indigestion and colicky pain may be present. Changes in the composition of bile cause cholesterol and/or bile pigment bilirubin to form stones. Stagnation of bile and inflammation of the gall bladder increase the concentration of bile and promote stone formation.

Haemorrhoids

This condition presents with abnormal dilatation of veins in the rectum. It is caused by increased pressure in the venous network of the rectum. If the haemorrhoids are chronic they may be seen or felt as soft swellings in the anus.

Heartburn

This is a burning sensation felt behind the sternum and often appears to rise from the abdomen up the oesophagus towards or into the throat. It is caused by regurgitation of the acidic stomach contents.

IN PRACTICE

In the case of a client with gallstones, avoid massage to the upper right quadrant of the abdomen.

Hepatitis

This is an inflammation of the liver caused by viruses, toxic substances or immunological abnormalities.

- **Hepatitis A** – this is highly contagious and is transmitted by the faecal/oral route. It is transmitted by ingestion of contaminated food, water or milk. The incubation period is 15 to 45 days.
- **Hepatitis B** – this is also known as serum hepatitis and is more serious than Hepatitis A. It lasts longer and can lead to cirrhosis, cancer of the liver and a carrier state. It has a long incubation period of one and a half to two months. The symptoms may last from weeks to months. The virus is usually transmitted through infected blood, serum or plasma. However, it can spread by oral or sexual contact as it is present in most body secretions.
- **Hepatitis C** – this can cause acute or chronic hepatitis and can also lead to a carrier state and liver cancer. It is transmitted through blood transfusions or exposure to blood products. Most clients with hepatitis are jaundiced but they can appear to be entirely healthy. Hepatitis as a side-effect of drugs and alcohol intake is not infective.

Hernia

This is an abnormal protrusion of an organ or part of an organ through the wall of the body cavity in which it normally lies.

Hiatus hernia

This is the most common type of hernia and occurs when part of the stomach is protruding into the chest. This sometimes causes no symptoms at all but it can cause acid reflux when acid from the stomach passes to the oesophagus, causing pain and heartburn.

Jaundice

This is a yellowing of the skin or whites of the eyes caused by excessive bilirubin (bile pigment) in the blood. It is caused by a malfunctioning gall bladder or obstructed bile duct.

Irritable bowel syndrome

This is a common condition in which there is recurrent abdominal pain with constipation and/or diarrhoea and bloating. Clients with stress and hectic lifestyles are more vulnerable to this illness. They usually defecate infrequently, usually in the morning, but may feel that their bowel is not empty or they may pass stool-like pellets.

Stress

Stress can be defined as any factor that affects physical or emotional well-being. Signs of stress affecting the digestive system include the development of ulcers, irritable bowel syndrome and indigestion.

Ulcers

This is a break in the skin or a break in the lining of the alimentary tract which fails to heal and is accompanied by inflammation. Peptic, duodenal

IN PRACTICE

In the case of a client with IBS remember that the lower abdomen in particular can be painful and tender. Clients with this condition may need easy/quick access to the toilet. Advise the client to avoid wind-producing foods, e.g. onion, dry beans. Relaxation through any form of therapy is helpful.

and gastric ulcers can present with increased acidity, epigastric pain and heartburn. This may be worst when hungry or after consumption of irritating foods and alcohol such as spicy or fatty foods, mayonnaise, wines and spirits. It can present with similar symptoms of a hiatus hernia and reflux.

Interrelationships with other systems

The digestive system links to the following body systems.

Cells and tissues

In areas of the digestive system, such as the small intestine where absorption of nutrients is required, there is a thin lining of simple epithelium to allow for speedy absorption.

Integumentary

One of the skin's functions is in vitamin D production which helps in the absorption of calcium in the small intestine.

Skeletal

The maxilla and mandible, the larger bones in the face, support the jaw and teeth when food in ingested in the mouth.

Muscular

The action of peristalsis is due to the involuntary contraction of the smooth muscle in the alimentary canal that propels the food through the digestive tract. Skeletal facial muscles, such as masseter and buccinator, assist in chewing.

Circulatory

Nutrients are carried in the body to nourish the cells and tissues and waste products are carried away by the blood to be eliminated.

Lymphatic

Lymphatic vessels called lacteals (in the villi of the small intestine) assist digestion by absorbing the products of fat digestion.

Respiratory

Oxygen absorbed from the lungs activates glycogen from the digestive system to produce energy for cell metabolism.

Nervous

All the organs of the digestive system are stimulated by nerve impulses.

Endocrine

The pancreas secretes insulin from cells called the islets of Langerhans which help control blood sugar levels.

Key words associated with the digestive system

digestion	chyme	lacteal
ingestion	small intestine	fatty acids
absorption	duodenum	glycerol
assimilation	jejunum	liver
elimination	ileum	hepatic portal vein
alimentary tract	villi	large intestine
peristalsis	gall bladder	caecum
mouth	bile	appendix
pharynx	pancreas	colon
oesophagus	pancreatic juice	ascending colon
saliva	intestinal juice	transverse colon
salivary amylase	emulsification	descending colon
starch	trypsin	sigmoid colon
stomach	pancreatic amylase	rectum
gastric juice	pancreatic lipase	faeces
enzyme	glucose	defecation
pepsin	peptidases	anus
hydrochloric acid	polypeptides	
mucus	amino acids	

Revision summary of the digestive system

- **Digestion** is the process of breaking down food and involves **ingestion, mechanical** and **chemical digestion, absorption, assimilation** and **elimination.**
- Digestion occurs in the **alimentary tract** which extends from the mouth to the anus.
- **Peristalsis** is the coordinated rhythmical contraction of the muscles in the wall of the alimentary tract.
- The digestive system consists of the **mouth, pharynx, oesophagus, stomach, small intestine, large intestine** and **anus.**
- The accessory organs to digestion are the **pancreas, gall bladder** and **liver.**
- The digestive system commences in the **mouth** where food is broken down by mastication and mixed with **saliva.**
- **Saliva** contains the enzyme **salivary amylase** which commences the digestion of **starch** in the mouth.
- The muscles of the **pharynx** force the food down the **oesophagus** to the **stomach.**
- In the **stomach** food is mixed with **gastric juice** containing the enzyme **pepsin** which starts the

breakdown of proteins, **hydrochloric acid**, to kill germs present in food and to prepare it for intestinal digestion, and **mucus** which protects the stomach lining from the damaging effects of the acidic gastric juice.
- The functions of the **stomach** are to churn and break up large particles of food mechanically, mix food with gastric juice to begin the chemical breakdown of food, commence the digestion of protein and absorb alcohol.
- Food stays in the stomach for approximately five hours until it has been churned down to a liquid state called **chyme.**
- **Chyme** is then released at intervals into the first part of the **small intestine.**
- The **small intestine** consists of three parts – **duodenum** (the first part), **jejunum** and **ileum** (where absorption of food mainly takes place).
- Special features of the small intestine are the thousands of minute projections called **villi**, a network of capillaries, into which the nutrients pass to be absorbed into the bloodstream.

- The **small intestine** continues the mechanical breakdown of food by **peristalsis**, whilst the chemical digestion is brought about by **bile** (released by the gall bladder), enzymes in **pancreatic juice** (released by the pancreas) and **intestinal juice** (released by the walls of the small intestine which prepare the food to be absorbed into the bloodstream).
- The function of **bile** is to neutralise the **chyme** and break up any fat droplets by **emulsification**.
- The enzymes contained within **pancreatic juice** continue the digestion of protein (**trypsin**), carbohydrates (**pancreatic amyalse**) and fats (**pancreatic lipase**).
- **Intestinal juice** is released by the glands of the small intestine and completes the final breakdown of nutrients, including **simple sugars** to **glucose** and **protein** to **amino acids**.
- Protein digestion is completed by **peptidases** which split short chain **polypeptides** into **amino acids**.
- The absorption of the digested food takes place in the **jejunum** and mainly in the **ileum**.
- Each villus contains a lymph vessel called a **lacteal** into which fatty acids and glycerol can pass.
- Simple sugars from carbohydrate digestion and amino acids from protein digestion pass into the bloodstream via the **villi** and are then carried to the **liver** via the **hepatic portal vein** to be processed.
- Products of fat digestion pass into the **lacteals** (intestinal lymphatics) which absorb the fat molecules and carry them through the lymphatic system before they reach the blood circulation.
- Vitamins and minerals travel across to the blood capillaries of the villi and are absorbed into the bloodstream to assist in normal body functioning and cell metabolism.
- **Glucose**, the end product of carbohydrate digestion, is used to provide energy for the cells to function.
- **Amino acids**, the end products of protein digestion, are used to produce new tissues, repair damaged cell parts and formulate enzymes, plasma proteins and hormones.

- **Fatty acids** and **glycerol** are the end products of fat digestion.
- Fats are used primarily to provide heat and energy in addition to glucose. Those fats which are not required immediately by the body are used to build cell membranes and some are stored under the skin or around vital organs such as the kidneys and the heart.
- When all the body's nutrients have been assimilated by the body, the undigested food is passed into the large intestine where it is eventually eliminated from the body.
- The **large intestine** is made up of the **cacecum**, **appendix**, **colon** and **rectum**.
- The **colon** is the main part of the large intestine and is divided into **ascending**, **transverse**, **descending** and **sigmoid** colons.
- The **rectum** is the last part of the large intestine where **faeces** are stored before **defecation**.
- The functions of the large intestine are the absorbtion of most of the water from the faeces, formation and storage of faeces, production of mucus to lubricate the passage of faeces and the expulsion of faeces out of the body.
- The **anus** is an opening at the lower end of the alimentary canal (the anal canal), through which faeces are discharged.
- The **liver** is the largest gland in the body and is an accessory organ to digestion with many metabolic functions.
- The functions of the **liver** include the secretion of bile, regulation of blood sugar levels, regulation of amino acid levels, regulation of the fat content of blood, regulation of plasma proteins, detoxification, storage and the production of heat.
- The **pancreas** is also an accessory organ to digestion. Its exocrine function is the secretion of pancreatic juice.
- The **gall bladder** is attached to the posterior and inferior surface of the liver and its function is to store bile produced by the liver until it is needed.

The digestive system
Multiple-choice questions

1 The alimentary tract is a long continuous muscular tube extending from the:
 a mouth to anus
 b stomach to anus
 c small intestine to anus
 d large intestine to anus

2 Which of the following completes digestion?
 a large intestine
 b gall bladder
 c small intestine
 d stomach

3 Which of the following is produced in the stomach?
 a bile
 b pancreatic juice
 c pepsin
 d maltase

4 The commencement of protein digestion occurs in the:
 a mouth
 b small intestine
 c pancreas
 d stomach

5 Food stays in the stomach for approximately how long before it is churned to a liquid state?
 a one hour
 b two hours
 c three hours
 d five hours

6 Which of the following is responsible for the chemical reactions of digestion?
 a enzymes
 b absorption
 c peristalsis
 d homeostasis

7 Salivary amylase commences:
 a protein digestion
 b carbohydrate digestion
 c fat digestion
 d breakdown of roughage

8 The main constituents of gastric juice are:
 a gastrin and pepsin
 b gastrin and pepsinogen
 c gastric amylase
 d pepsin, hydrochloric acid and mucus

9 Trypsin is an enzyme produced by the:
 a liver
 b duodenum
 c gall bladder
 d pancreas

10 Where does peristalsis occur?
 a in all sections of the alimentary canal
 b only in the mouth
 c only in the small intestine
 d only in the stomach

11 Which of the following does the liver **not** regulate?
 a blood sugar levels
 b amino acid levels
 c fatty acid levels
 d plasma proteins

12 Vitamins and minerals are absorbed into the bloodstream:
 a via the liver cells
 b via the villi in the small intestine
 c via the lacteals in the small intestine
 d via the hepatic portal vein

13 The main part of the large intestine is the:
 a duodenum
 b caecum
 c colon
 d ileum

14 Which of the following is responsible for producing bile?
 a gall bladder
 b pancreas
 c liver
 d duodenum

15 In which part of the large intestine is faeces stored before defecation?
   a rectum
   b caecum
   c descending colon
   d appendix

16 The three sections of the small intestine from beginning to end are:
   a ascending, transverse and descending
   b jejunum, ileum and duodenum
   c duodenum, jejunum and ileum
   d duodenum, ileum and jejunum

17 The colon primarily absorbs:
   a proteins
   b carbohydrates
   c fats and lipids
   d water

18 The digestive disorder which presents as a burning sensation behind the sternum is:
   a hernia
   b hepatitis
   c haemorrhoids
   d heartburn

19 Glucose, the end product of carbohydrate digestion is used to:
   a produce new tissues
   b repair damaged cell parts
   c provide energy for cells to function
   d all of the above

20 Saliva is secreted by how many pairs of salivary glands?
   a two
   b three
   c four
   d five

12 the urinary system

Introduction

The kidneys and its associated structures are all part of the excretory system along with the skin, lungs and the intestines which also contribute to the job of waste elimination in the body.

The urinary system is made up the kidneys, ureters, bladder and urethra which are involved in the processing and elimination of normal metabolic waste from the body and can be likened to the body's 'plumbing system'.

◎ Objectives

By the end of this chapter you will be able to recall and understand the following knowledge:

- the functions of the urinary system
- the structure and functions of the individual parts of the urinary system (kidneys, ureters, urinary bladder and urethra)
- the interrelationships between the urinary and other body systems
- common pathologies of the urinary system.

Functions of the urinary system

Maintaining homeostasis

The prime function of the urinary system is to help maintain homeostasis by controlling the composition, volume and pressure of blood. It does this by removing and restoring selected amounts of water and dissolved substances.

Regulation of the composition and volume of body fluids

Waste products, such as urea and uric acid, along with excess water and mineral salts must be removed from the body in order to maintain good health. If these waste materials were allowed to accumulate in the body they would cause ill health. The primary function of the urinary system, therefore, is to regulate the composition and the volume of body fluids in order to provide a constant internal environment for the body.

Structures of the urinary system

The urinary system consists of the following parts:

Part of urinary system	Location	Function
Kidneys × 2	Posterior wall of the abdomen on either side of the spine (between twelfth thoracic vertebra and third lumbar vertebra)	Main functional organs of the urinary system Site where blood is filtered and urine is processed
Ureters × 2	Long, thin tubes that lead from each kidney down to the bladder	Transport urine from the kidneys to the bladder
Urinary bladder × 1	Lies in the pelvic cavity behind the symphysis pubis	Collects and temporarily stores urine
Urethra × 1	Extends from the neck of the bladder to the outside of the body	Tube through which urine is discharged from the bladder and out of the body In men also acts as conducting channel for semen

Student activity

Now complete Activity 12.1 in the resources for this book on Dynamic Learning Online.

Kidneys

The kidneys are bean-shaped organs lying on the posterior wall of the abdomen on either side of the spine between the level of the twelfth thoracic vertebra and the third lumbar vertebra. Due to the presence of the liver, the kidney on the right side of the body is slightly lower than the one on the left.

Structure of the kidney

A kidney has an outer fibrous renal capsule and is supported by adipose tissue. It has two main parts:

- **Outer cortex** – this is reddish-brown and is the part where fluid is filtered from blood.
- **Inner medulla** – this is paler in colour and is made up of conical-shaped sections called **renal pyramids**. This is the area where some materials are selectively reabsorbed back into the bloodstream.

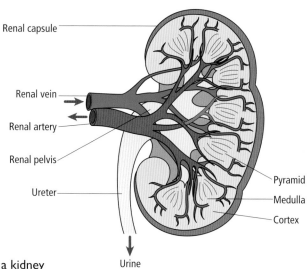

Fig 12.1 Structure of a kidney

When studying the functional unit of a nephron, it may be helpful to liken it to a household recycling station. The blood is like a vehicle that transports the waste to the recycling site (your kidneys). Inside your kidneys the toxic waste is removed and any substances that the body can reuse are recycled. What is left is transported out of the recycling station and deposited as waste (urine).

BODY FACT

Each day the kidneys process and filter gallons of blood through more than 2 million nephrons. Due to the filtering ability of a nephron, around 99 per cent of blood is recycled by the body.

BODY FACT

Urine is the body's primary waste product and so the release of urine is the final step of all metabolism.

There is a large area in the centre of the kidney called the **renal pelvis** which is a funnel-shaped cavity that collects urine from the renal pyramids in the medulla and drains it into the ureter. The medial border of the kidney is called the **hilus** and is the area where the renal blood vessels leave and enter the kidney.

Nephron

The cortex and the medulla contain tiny blood filtration units called nephrons. Nephrons are the functional units of the kidney and they extend from the renal capsule through the cortex and medulla to the cup-shaped renal pelvis. Nephrons are approximately 2 to 4 cm long and a single kidney has more than a million nephrons.

Urine production

Urine is produced by three processes:

- filtration
- selective reabsorption
- collection.

Filtration

The blood that needs to be processed enters the medulla of the kidney from the renal artery. Inside the kidney the renal artery splits into a network of capillaries called the glomerulus which filter the waste. Almost encasing the glomerulus lies a sac called the Bowman's capsule.

The blood pressure in the glomerulus is maintained at a high level, assisted by the fact that the arteriole feeding into the glomerulus has a larger diameter than the arteriole leaving it. This pressure forces fluid out through the walls of the glomerulus together with some of the substances of small molecular size able to pass through the capillary walls into the Bowman's capsule. This process constitutes simple filtration.

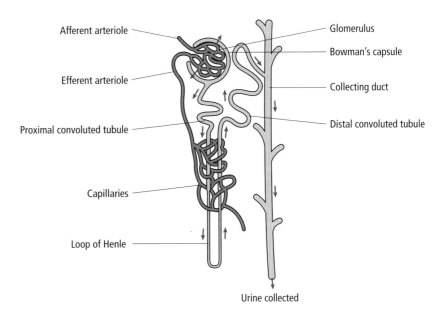

Afferent arteriole

Efferent arteriole

Proximal convoluted tubule

Capillaries

Loop of Henle

Glomerulus

Bowman's capsule

Collecting duct

Distal convoluted tubule

Urine collected

Fig 12.2 Nephron

Selective reabsorption

The filtered liquid continues through a series of twisted tubes called the convoluted tubules which are surrounded by capillaries. The tubules of the nephron that lead away from the Bowman's capsule are known as the proximal convoluted tubules and they straighten out to form a long loop called the loop of Henle. There are then another series of twists called the distal convoluted tubules which lead to a straightened collecting duct which leads to the pelvis of the kidney and on to the ureter.

The composition of the filtered liquid alters as it flows through the convoluted tubules. Some substances contained within the waste, such as glucose, amino acids, mineral salts and vitamins, are reabsorbed back into the bloodstream as the body cannot afford to lose them.

This reabsorption process is selective as the amounts of these substances which pass back in the bloodstream depend on the level already present in the bloodstream and within the body. The reabsorption of salts and water is variable and is associated with the maintenance of a stable condition of acidity/alkalinity and electrolyte (sodium and potassium) balance of body fluids. Excess water, salts and the waste product urea are all filtered and processed through the kidneys and the treated blood leaves the kidney via the renal vein.

Some substances are not removed from the blood completely in the glomerular filtrate such as the residue of medicinal drugs. These substances are passed from the blood, in particular, into the distal convoluted tubule by secretion in order that they may be excreted in the urine.

Collection

The wastes remaining in the distal convoluted tubule (now known as urine) then flow on via a collecting tubule to the renal pelvis of the kidney. From here it passes into the ureter to be passed to the bladder and urethra to be excreted.

Composition of urine

Urine is the concentrated filtrate from the kidneys.
Its composition is:

- 96 per cent water
- 2 per cent urea
- 2 per cent other substances such as uric acid, creatinine, sodium, potassium, phosphates, chlorides, sulphates, excess vitamins and drug residues.

Urine is a pale watery fluid varying in colour according to its composition and quantity. Urine is usually acidic and its pH varies between 4.5 and 7.4 depending on the blood pH.

The salts, chiefly sodium chloride, must be reabsorbed in the kidney tubules or at least removed in sufficient quantities necessary to keep the blood at its normal pH (7.4) and to maintain the water and electrolyte balance. As the pH and salt concentration are both essential to the life of the blood and tissue cells, the functions of the kidneys are of paramount importance.

Functions of the kidney

The function of the kidney is the:

- filtration of impurities and metabolic waste from blood and preventing poisons from fatally accumulating in the body
- regulation of water and salt balance in the body

BODY FACT

How much you have of certain substances in your urine is a good indication of the state of health of your body. Urine tests are often used to diagnose a disorder. If urine contains glucose it could indicate that a person has diabetes. Protein in the urine could indicate that the kidneys are failing. Urine can be used to confirm a pregnancy. A fertilised ovum releases a hormone which the mother excretes in the urine. This can usually be detected from about 14 days after fertilisation and is the basis of most pregnancy tests.

- maintenance of the normal pH balance of blood
- formation of urine
- regulation of blood pressure and blood volume.

Role of the kidneys in fluid balance

The amount of fluid taken into the body must equal the amount of fluid excreted from it in order for the body to maintain a constant internal environment. The balance between water intake and water output is controlled by the kidneys.

Water intake

Water is mainly taken into the body as liquid through the process of digestion. However, some is also released through the cells' metabolic activities.

Water output

Water is lost from the body in the following ways:

- through the kidneys as urine
- through the alimentary tract as faeces
- through the skin as sweat
- through the lungs as saturated exhaled breath.

The kidneys are responsible for regulating the amount of water contained within the blood. The amount of water reabsorbed into the blood is controlled by the anti-diuretic hormone (ADH) which is stored and released into the blood by the posterior lobe of the pituitary gland.

The release of ADH is triggered by dehydration. The hypothalamus detects when the water concentration of blood is low and triggers the release of ADH. An increase in the level of ADH increases the amount of water that is reabsorbed from the nephron back into the blood.

The reabsorption of water reabsorbed from the nephron into the blood decreases the volume of urine expelled from the kidneys and increases the hydration level of the blood. This mechanism reduces the amount of water in the blood back to an acceptable level.

Factors affecting fluid balance

Factors affecting fluid balance in the body include:

> **KEY FACT**
>
> This important negative feedback mechanism between the nervous and endocrine systems maintains the blood concentration within normal limits and is the means by which fluid balance is controlled in the body.

Body temperature	If the body temperature increases, more water is lost from the body in sweat
Diet	A high salt intake can result in increased water reabsorption, which reduces the volume of urine produced. Diuretics, such as alcohol, tea and coffee, can also increase the volume of urine
Emotions	Nervousness can result in an increased production of urine
Blood pressure	When the blood pressure inside the kidney tubules rises, less water is reabsorbed and the volume of urine will be increased (but not decreased) When the blood pressure inside the kidney tubules falls, more water is reabsorbed into the blood and the volume of urine will be decreased

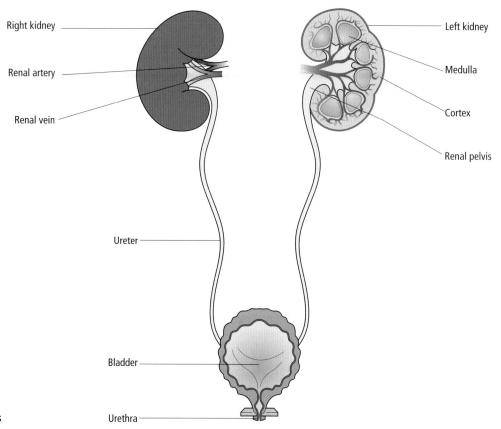

Fig 12.3 The urinary organs

Labels: Right kidney, Renal artery, Renal vein, Ureter, Bladder, Urethra, Left kidney, Medulla, Cortex, Renal pelvis

Ureters

The ureters are two very fine muscular tubes which transport urine from the renal pelvis of the kidney to the urinary bladder. They consist of three layers of tissue:

- an outer layer of fibrous tissue
- a middle layer of smooth muscles
- an inner layer of mucous membrane.

Function of the ureters

Their function is to propel urine from the kidneys into the bladder by the peristaltic contraction of their muscular walls.

Urinary bladder

This is a pear-shaped sac which lies in the pelvic cavity behind the symphysis pubis. The size of the bladder varies according to the amount of urine it contains. The bladder is composed of four layers of tissue:

- a serous membrane which covers the upper surface
- a layer of smooth muscular fibres
- a layer of adipose tissue
- an inner lining of mucous membrane.

Functions of the urinary bladder

The urinary bladder stores urine. It expels urine out of the body assisted by the muscular wall of the bladder, the lowering of the diaphragm and the contraction of the abdominal cavity.

The expelling of urine from the bladder is called micturition and is a reflex over which there is voluntary control. When the volume of urine in the bladder causes it to expand, stretch receptors in the bladder wall are stimulated to trigger urination. The micturition reflex causes the detrusor muscle in the wall of the bladder to contract and the internal urethral sphincter to relax. It is the combination of both the micturition reflex and voluntary relaxation of the urethral sphincter that allows urination to occur.

Urethra

This is a canal which extends from the neck of the bladder to the outside of the body. The length of the urethra differs in males and females. The female urethra is approximately only 4 cm in length, whereas the male urethra is longer at approximately 18 to 20 cm in length. The exit from the bladder is guarded by a round sphincter of muscles which must relax before urine can be expelled from the body. The urethra is composed of three layers of tissue:

- a muscular coat continuous with that of the bladder
- a thin spongy coat which contains a large number of blood vessels
- a lining of mucous membrane.

Function of the urethra

The urethra serves as a tube through which urine is discharged from the bladder to the exterior. As the urethra is longer in a male it also serves as a conducting channel for semen.

Common pathologies of the urinary system

Cancer of the bladder

This usually presents with blood in the urine and urgency and pain on passing urine. Secondary symptoms may arise if it has spread to the lungs, liver, lymph nodes and neighbouring tissues.

Cystitis

This is an inflammation of the urinary bladder, usually caused by infection of the bladder lining. Common symptoms are pain just above the pubic bone, lower back or inner thigh, blood in the urine and frequent, urgent and painful urination with a burning sensation. This condition is very common in women due to the shorter length of the female urethra.

Incontinence

This is a condition in which the individual is unable to control urination voluntarily. Loss of muscle tone and problems with innervation are associated with this condition.

Kidney stones

These are deposits of substances found in the urine which form solid stones in the renal pelvis of the kidney, ureter or bladder. This condition can be extremely painful. Stones are usually removed by surgery.

IN PRACTICE

In the case of a client with cystitis it is important to encourage a client to increase their intake of fluids (water and cranberry juice). If symptoms persist, they may need GP advice and assessment.

Massage over the lower abdomen is better avoided to reduce chances of pain and spasm induction.

Nephritis

A general non-specific term used to describe inflammation of the kidney. Glomerulonephritis (also known as Bright's disease) is an inflammation of the glomeruli in the kidneys. This condition is characterised by blood in the urine, fluid retention and hypertension.

Pyelonenephritis

This is a bacterial infection of the kidney. In acute pyelonenephritis there is pain in the back, high temperature and shivering fits. Treatment is usually with antibiotics.

Urinary tract infection

This is a bacterial infection of one or more of the structures of the urinary system. Symptoms include fever, lower back pain, frequency of urination, a burning sensation on passing urine (urine may be blood stained and cloudy). If the infection is severe there may be blood and pus in the urine.

Interrelationships with other systems

The urinary system links to the following body systems.

Cells and tissues
Transitional epithelium lines urinary organs such as the bladder which change shape when stretched.

Skin
Like the urinary system the skin is also an excretory organ. When the skin loses excess water through sweating, the kidneys release less water in the urine to help maintain the body's fluid balance.

Skeletal
The kidneys and the bones of the skeleton help to control the amount of calcium in the blood by storing some in the bones and excreting some from the body in urine.

Muscular
Smooth muscle is responsible for the passage of urine through the urinary tract.

Circulatory
The kidneys filter the blood to avoid poisons from fatally accumulating in the body.

Nervous
The relaxation and contraction of the bladder and closing and opening of the sphincter muscles is under the control of the autonomic nervous system (sympathetic and parasympathetic nervous systems).

Digestive
Water is an essential nutrient which is needed by every part of the body and is taken in through the process of digestion to aid the metabolic process. The colon absorbs most of the water from the faeces in order to conserve mositure in the body.

IN PRACTICE

In the case of a client with a urinary tract infection, all forms of therapeutic treatment should be avoided until the infection has run its course.

Key words associated with the urinary system

kidney
renal artery
renal vein
cortex
medulla
nephron

glomerulus
Bowman's capsule
proximal convoluted
    tubule
loop of Henle
distal convoluted tubule

collecting duct
renal pelvis
urine
ureter
urinary bladder
urethra

Revision summary of the urinary system

- The organs that contribute to the elimination of wastes in the body are the kidneys, lungs, skin and the digestive system.
- The organs of the urinary system are the **kidneys, ureters, urinary bladder** and **urethra**.
- The **kidneys** are bean-shaped organs lying on the posterior wall of the abdomen.
- The **kidney** has two main parts – the outer **cortex** where fluid is filtered from blood and the inner **medulla** which is the area where some materials are selectively reabsorbed back into the bloodstream.
- The **cortex** and the **medulla** contain tiny blood filtration units called **nephrons**.
- Urine is produced by three processes – **filtration, selective reabsorption** and **collection**.
- Blood to be processed enters the kidneys via the **renal artery**.
- **Filtration** takes place inside a network of capillaries in the **nephron** called the **glomerulus**.
- The sac encasing the **glomerulus** is called the **Bowman's capsule**.
- The filtered liquid then continues through a series of twisted tubes called the **convoluted tubules**, to the **loop of Henle** and the **distal convoluted tubule** before passing to the **collecting duct** and to the **renal pelvis**.
- The composition of the filtered liquid alters as it flows through the **convoluted tubules**.

- Some substances in the filtrate like glucose, amino acids, mineral salts and vitamins are reabsorbed back into the bloodstream via the **renal vein**.
- From the **distal convoluted tubule** the filtrate then flows into the **collecting duct** (as urine) and passes to the pelvis of the kidney to be passed to the **ureter** and **bladder**.
- The composition of urine is 96 per cent water, 2 per cent urea and 2 per cent other substances (uric acid, creatinine, sodium, potassium, phosphates, chlorides, sulphates, excess vitamins and drug residues).
- Functions of the kidneys include filtration of impurities and metabolic waste from blood, regulation of water and salt balance, formation of urine and regulation of blood pressure and volume.
- The **ureters** are muscular tubes that transport urine from the pelvis of the kidney to the urinary bladder.
- The **urinary bladder** is a pear-shaped sac which lies in the pelvic cavity behind the symphysis pubis.
- It functions as a storage organ for urine.
- The **urethra** is a canal which extends from the neck of the bladder to the outside of the body.
- The urethra serves as a tube through which urine is discharged from the bladder to the exterior and as a conducting channel for semen in men.

The urinary system
Multiple-choice questions

1 The function of the kidneys is the:
   a filtering of impurities from the blood
   b regulation of water and salt balance
   c formation of urine
   d all of the above

2 Which of the following is not considered an excretory organ?
   a muscular system
   b digestive system
   c respiratory system
   d skin

3 Blood is filtered inside what section of the kidney?
   a Bowman's capsule
   b loop of Henle
   c glomerulus
   d proximal convoluted tubule

4 The blood filtration unit inside a kidney is known as the:
   a hilus
   b medulla
   c nephron
   d renal pyramid

5 The hormone responsible for controlling water reabsorption in the kidneys is:
   a insulin
   b oxytocin
   c anti-diuretic hormone (ADH)
   d adrenocorticotrophic hormone (ACTH)

6 The function of the ureter is to:
   a store urine
   b filter impurities
   c propel urine from the bladder to the exterior
   d propel urine from the kidneys to the bladder

7 The bladder is situated:
   a in the pelvic cavity behind the symphysis pubis
   b in the abdominal cavity behind the intestines
   c on the posterior of the abdominal cavity
   d behind the urethra

8 The condition cystitis commonly affects females as:
   a women tend to have a weaker bladder than men
   b women have a shorter urethra
   c women have smaller kidneys
   d all of the above

9 Which of the following factors does **not** affect fluid balance?
   a diet
   b body temperature
   c time of day
   d blood pressure

10 Which of the following also serves as a conducting channel for semen in the male?
   a ureter
   b urethra
   c bladder
   d penis

11 Inside the kidney, the renal artery splits into a network of capillaries called the:
   a afferent arteriole
   b glomerulus
   c efferent arteriole
   d hilus

12 The part of the kidney where the fluid is filtered from blood is the:
   a medulla
   b cortex
   c hilus
   d renal pyramid

13 The composition of the filtered liquid alters as it flows through the:
   a convoluted tubules
   b glomerulus
   c renal pelvis
   d collecting duct

14 As well as being lost through the kidneys as urine, water is also lost from the body through:
   a faeces
   b skin
   c lungs
   d all of the above

15 Which muscle contracts to allow micturition?
  a detrusor
  b external urethral sphincter
  c internal urethral sphincter
  d anal sphincter

16 You are feeling dehydrated due to failing to drink enough fluids. How do your kidneys respond?
  a release aldosterone
  b increase urine output
  c release ADH
  d inhibit the release of ADH

17 Kidney stones may be deposited in:
  a renal pelvis
  b ureter
  c bladder
  d all of the above

18 Which of the following best describes the position of the kidneys on the posterior of the abdomen?
  a between 12th thoracic and 3rd lumbar vertebrae
  b between 10th thoracic and 5th lumbar vertebrae
  c between 12th thoracic and 5th lumbar vertebrae
  d between 10th thoracic and 3rd lumbar vertebrae

19 Which vessels drain the filtered blood away from the kidneys?
  a renal arteries
  b renal veins
  c hepatic arteries
  d hepatic veins

20 Nephrons are approximately:
  a 2 to 4 cm long
  b 12 to 14 cm long
  c 5 to 10 cm long
  d 15 to 20 cm long

Glossary

Abdominal nodes: lymph nodes located within the abdominal cavity along the branches of the abdominal aorta. They drain lymph from organs within the abdominal cavity.

Abducens nerve: mixed nerve that innervates only the lateral rectus muscle of the eye.

Abduction: movement of a limb away from the midline.

Absorption: movement of soluble materials out through the walls of the small intestine to be delivered to various parts of the body.

Accessory nerve: functions primarily as a motor nerve, innervating muscles in the neck and upper back, as well as muscles of the palate, pharynx and larynx.

Acetylcholine: neurotransmitter substance which diffuses across the junction and stimulates the muscles fibre to contract.

Acne vulgaris: common inflammatory disorder of the sebaceous glands which leads to the overproduction of sebum. It involves the face, back and chest and is characterised by the presence of comedones, papules and, in more severe cases, cysts and scars.

Acromegaly: increase in the size of the hands, feet and face due to excessive production of the growth hormone.

Actin: protein found in muscle that plays an important role in muscle contraction.

Active transport: energy-dependent process in which certain substances with larger molecules are able to cross cell membranes against a concentration gradient.

Addison's disease: condition caused by undersecretion of corticosteroid hormones. Symptoms include loss of appetite, weight loss, brown pigmentation around joints, low blood sugar, low blood pressure, tiredness and muscular weakness.

Adduction: movement of a limb towards the midline.

Adductors: group of four muscles on the medial aspect of the thigh.

Adipose tissue: type of tissue containing fat cells, found in the subcutaneous layer of skin.

ADP (adenosine diphosphate): compound that releases the energy needed for processes such as muscle contraction.

Adrenal: one of two triangular-shaped glands which lie on top of each kidney. They consist of two parts, an outer cortex and an inner medulla.

Adrenaline: hormone secreted by the medulla of the adrenal glands. It prepares the body for 'fright, fight or flight' response (sympathetic nervous system) having widespread effects on the circulation, muscles and glucose metabolism.

Adrenocorticotrophic hormone (ACTH): secreted from the anterior lobe of the pituitary gland, it stimulates and controls the growth and hormonal output of the adrenal cortex.

Agonist/prime mover: main activating muscle.

AIDS (Acquired Immune Deficiency Syndrome): condition contracted as a result of the Human Immunodeficiency Virus (HIV) which progressively destroys the immunity of the individual.

Albinism: inherited absence of pigmentation in the skin, hair and eyes, resulting in white hair, pink skin and eyes. The pink colour is produced by underlying blood vessels which are normally masked by pigment. Other clinical signs of this condition include poor eyesight and sensitivity to light.

Alimentary tract: long, continuous muscular tube, extending from the mouth to the anus.

Allergic reaction: disorder in which the body becomes hypersensitive to a particular allergen. The body produces histamine in the skin, as part of the body's defence or immune system.

Alveoli: tiny air sacs inside the lungs.

Amenorrhea: absence or stopping of the menstrual period.

Amino acids: end products of protein digestion.

Anaemia: condition where the haemoglobin level in the blood is below normal.

Anagen: active, growing phase of hair.

Androgens: collective term for male hormones.

Aneurysm: abnormal balloon-like swelling in the wall of an artery.

Angina: pain in the left side of the chest and usually radiating to the left arm. It is caused by insufficient blood to the heart muscle and usually on exertion or excitement.

Ankylosing spondylitis: systemic joint disease characterised by inflammation of the intervertebral disc spaces, costo-vertebral and sacroiliac joints.

Anorexia nervosa: psychological illness in which clients starve themselves or use other techniques, such as vomiting or laxatives, to induce weight loss.

Antagonists: two muscles or sets of muscles which pull in opposite directions to each other.

Antibody: specific protein produced to destroy or suppress antigens.

Anti-diuretic hormone (ADH): hormone secreted from the posterior lobe of the pituitary. It increases water reabsorption in the renal tubules of the kidneys.

Antigen: any substance that the body regards as foreign or potentially dangerous and against which it produces an antibody.

Anus: opening at the lower end of the alimentary tract through which faeces are discharged.

Anxiety: psychological condition which can be defined as fear of the unknown. As an illness it can vary from a mild form to panic attacks and severe phobias that can be disabling socially, psychologically and at times physically.

Aorta: main artery of the systemic circulation.

Apocrine gland: type of sweat gland found in the genital and underarm regions.

Appendicitis: acute inflammation of the appendix.

Appendicular skeleton: part of skeleton consisting of the shoulder girdle, bones of the upper and lower limbs and bones of the pelvic girdle.

Appendix: short, thin blind-end tube that is attached to the end of the caecum and has no known function in humans.

Arteriosclerosis: circulatory disorder characterised by a thickening, narrowing, hardening and loss of elasticity of the walls of the arteries.

Artery: type of blood vessel with thick muscular and elastic walls. It carries blood away from the heart.

Arthritis – gout: joint disorder due to deposition of excessive uric acid crystals accumulating in the joint cavity.

Arthritis – osteoarthritis: joint disease characterised by the breakdown of articular cartilage, growth of bony spikes, swelling of the surrounding synovial membrane and stiffness and tenderness of the joint.

Arthritis – rheumatoid: chronic inflammation of peripheral joints resulting in pain, stiffness and potential damage to joints.

Assimilation: process by which digested food is used by the tissues after absorption.

Asthma: attacks of shortness of breath and difficulty in breathing due to spasm or swelling of the bronchial tubes.

Atony: state in which the muscles are floppy and lacking their normal degree of elasticity.

ATP (adenosine triphosphate): compound that stores the energy needed for processes such as muscle contraction.

Atrium: upper chamber of heart.

Atrophy: wasting of muscle tissue due to undernourishment or lack of use.

Autonomic nervous system: part of the nervous system which supplies impulses to smooth muscles, cardiac muscle, skin, special senses and proprioceptors. It consists of a sympathetic and parasympathetic division.

Axial skeleton: forms the main axis or central core of the body and consists of the skull, vertebral column, sternum and ribs.

Axillary nodes: lymph nodes located in the underarm region. They drain lymph from the upper limbs, wall of the thorax, breasts and upper wall of the abdomen.

Axon: long single nerve fibre extending from the cell body. Its function is to transmit impulses away from the cell body.

Ball-and-socket joint: type of synovial joint formed when the rounded head of one bone fits into a cup-shaped cavity of another bone. Movement is possible in several directions.

Basal cell layer (stratum germinativum): deepest and innermost of the five layers of epidermis.

Basilar artery: artery in the base of the brain, formed by the joining together of the two vertebral arteries.

Bell's palsy: disorder of the seventh cranial nerve (facial nerve) that results in paralysis on one side of the face.

Benign: term used to describe a tumour that does not invade and destroy the tissue in which it originates or spread to distant sites in the body.

Biceps: muscle on the anterior of the upper arm.

Bile: green alkaline liquid, produced in the liver and stored in the gall bladder.

Blood: fluid tissue or medium in which all materials are transported to and from individual cells in the body.

Blood pressure: amount of pressure exerted by blood on an arterial wall due to the contraction of the left ventricle.

Boil: begins as a small inflamed nodule which forms a pocket of bacteria around the base of a hair follicle, or a break in the skin.

Bone: hardest type of connective tissue in the body.

Bowman's capsule: cup-shaped end of a nephron and site of primary filtration of the blood into the kidney tubule.

Brachialis: muscle attaching to the distal half of the anterior surface of the humerus at one end and the ulna at the other.

Brachial plexuses: spinal nerves at the top of the shoulder supplying the skin and muscles of the arm, shoulder and upper chest.

Brachioradialis: anterior muscle of the forearm, connecting the humerus to the radius.

Brain: highly developed mass of nervous tissue that forms the upper part of the central nervous system.

Brain stem: enlarged extension upwards within the skull of the spinal cord, consisting of the medulla oblongata, the pons and the midbrain.

Breast/mammary gland: accessory female sex gland that produces milk following childbirth.

Bronchi: two short tubes which lead to and carry air into each lung.

Bronchiole: subdivision of the bronchial tree.

Bronchitis: chronic or acute inflammation of the bronchial tubes.

Buccinator: main muscle of the cheek. It is attached to both the upper and lower jaw..

Bulimia: psychological illness which is characterised by overeating (bingeing), followed by self-induced vomiting.

Bunion: swelling of the joint between the big toe and the first metatarsal.

Bursitis: inflammation of a bursa (small sac of fibrous tissue that is lined with synovial membrane and filled with synovial fluid).

Caecum: small pouch to which the appendix is attached and into which the ileum opens.

Calcaneum: bone at the end of the metatarsals.

Calcitonin: hormone secreted by the thyroid gland which controls the level of calcium in the blood.

Cancellous bone: open spongy bone tissue found at the ends of long bones or at the centre of other bones.

Cancer: any malignant tumour. It arises from the abnormal and uncontrolled division of cells that invade and destroy the surrounding tissues.

Capillary: smallest blood vessels with a single layer of cells. It is responsible for supplying the cells and tissues with nutrients.

Carcinoma: malignant tumour that arises from epithelial cells.

Cardiac cycle: sequence of events between one heartbeat and the next, normally less than a second in duration.

Cardiac muscle: special type of involuntary muscle found only in the heart.

Carotid artery: either of the two main arteries of the neck whose branches supply the head and neck.

Carpal tunnel syndrome: condition characterised by pain and numbness in the thumb or hand, resulting from pressure on the median nerve of the wrist.

Carpals: eight small bones forming the wrist.

Cartilage: dense connective tissue that consists of collagen and elastin fibres embedded in a strong gel-like substance.

Cartilaginous joint: slightly movable joints which have a pad of fibrocartilage between the end of the bones making the joint.

Catagen: transitional stage of hair growth from active to resting.

Cell: basic unit of all living organisms.

Cell membrane: fine membrane that encloses the cell and protects its contents.

Cell regeneration: process by which the cells of the epidermis regenerate themselves by the process of mitosis.

Cell respiration: controlled exchange of nutrients for waste by the cell to activate the energy needed for the cell to function.

Central nervous system (CNS): part of the nervous system consisting of the brain and spinal cord.

Centrioles: small spherical structures associated with cell division, contained within the centrosome.

Centromere: portion of a chromosome where the two chromatids are joined.

Centrosome: area of clear cytoplasm found next to the nucleus, containing the centrioles.

Cerebellum: cauliflower-shaped structure located at the posterior of the cranium and below the cerebrum.

Cerebral palsy: condition caused by damage to the central nervous system of a baby during pregnancy, delivery or soon after birth. The damage could be due to bleeding, lack of oxygen or other injuries to the brain.

Cerebrum: largest portion of the brain which makes up the front and top part of the brain.

Cervical plexuses: spinal nerves supplying the skin and muscles of the head, neck and upper region of the shoulders.

Cervical vertebrae: seven vertebrae of the neck.

Chloasma: pigmentation disorder which presents with irregular areas of increased pigmentation, usually on the face.

Cholesterol: fat-like material present in the blood and most tissues.

Chondrocyte: cartilage-forming cell.

Chromatid: pair of identical strands that are joined at the centromere and separate during cell division.

Chromatin: substance inside the nucleus that contains the genetic material.

Chromosome: thread-like structure in the cell nucleus that carries the genetic information.

Chyme: semi-liquid, acid mass in which food passes from the stomach to the small intestine.

Cilia: microscopic hair-like processes on the exposed surfaces of certain epithelial tissue.

Circumduction: circular movement of a joint (360 degrees).

Cirrhosis of the liver: distorted or scarred liver as a result of chronic inflammation.

Clavicle: bone forming anterior of shoulder girdle.

Clear layer (stratum lucidum): epidermal layer below the most superficial layer (horny), consisting of small, tightly packed transparent cells which permit light to pass through.

Coccygeal plexus: supplies the skin in the area of the coccyx and the muscles of the pelvic floor.

Coccygeal vertebrae (coccyx): four fused vertebrae at the base of spine forming the tail bone.

Coccygeus: muscle forming the pelvic floor.

Colitis: inflammation of the colon.

Collagen: protein in the dermis which gives the skin its strength and resilience.

Collecting duct: vessel that leads to the pelvis of the kidney and on to the ureter.

Colon: main part of the large intestine, consisting of four sections – ascending, transverse, descending and sigmoid colons.

Comedone: collection of sebum, keratinised cells and wastes which accumulate in the entrance of a hair follicle. It may be open or closed.

Comminuted fracture: where a bone has splintered at the site of impact and smaller fragments of bone lie between the two main fragments.

Compact bone: hard portion of bone that makes up the main shaft of the long bones and the outer layer of other bones.

Complicated fracture: when a broken bone damages tissues and/or organs around it.

Compound fracture: open fracture where the broken ends of the bone protrude through the skin.

Concentric contraction: type of contraction when a muscle shortens to move the attachments closer.

Condyloid joint: type of synovial joint that is shaped so that the concave surface of one bone can slide over the convex surface of another bone in two directions.

Congenital heart disease: defect in the formation of the heart which usually decreases its efficiency.

Conjunctivitis: bacterial infection following irritation of the conjunctiva of the eye. The inner eyelid and eyeball appear red and sore and there may be a pus-like discharge from the eye.

Connective tissue sheath: surrounds both the follicle and sebaceous gland. Its function is to supply the follicle with nerves and blood.

Constipation: difficulty in passing stools or infrequent evacuation of the bowel.

Contact dermatitis: inflammation of the skin caused by a primary irritant which causes the skin to become red, dry and inflamed.

Coracobrachialis: muscle that extends from the scapula to the middle of the humerus along its medial surface.

Corrugator: muscle located on the inner edge of the eyebrow.

Cortex: middle layer of hair; outer reddish-brown part of kidney where fluid is filtered from blood.

Cowper's glands: pair of small glands that open into the urethra at the base of the penis. Their secretion contributes to the seminal fluid.

Cramp: prolonged painful contraction of a muscle.

Cranial nerves: set of 12 pairs of nerves originating from the brain.

Cretinism: syndrome of dwarfism, mental retardation and coarseness of skin and facial features due to lack of thyroid hormones.

Crow's feet: fine lines around the eyes caused by habitual facial expressions and daily movement.

Cushing's syndrome: caused by the hypersecretion of the glucocorticoids. Symptoms include weight gain, reddening of the face and neck, excess growth of facial and body hair, raised blood pressure, loss of mineral from bone and sometimes mental disturbances.

Cuticle: fold of overlapping skin that surrounds the base of the nail, providing a protective seal against bacteria; outer layer of hair.

Cyst: abnormal sac containing liquid or a semi-solid substance.

Cystitis: inflammation of the urinary bladder, usually caused by infection of the bladder lining.

Cytoplasm: gel-like substance enclosed by the cell membrane.

Deep cervical nodes: lymph nodes located deep within the neck, they drain lymph from the larynx, oesophagus, posterior of the scalp and neck, and superficial part of chest and arm.

Defecation: elimination of faeces through the anal canal.

Deltoid: thick triangular muscle that caps the top of the humerus and shoulder.

Dendrites: highly branched extensions of the nerve cell that receive and transmit stimuli towards the cell body.

Depression: psychological condition which combines symptoms of lowered mood, loss of appetite, poor sleep, lack of concentration and interest, lack of sense of enjoyment, occasional constipation and loss of libido.

Depressor anguli oris: muscle extending from the mandible (lower jaw) to the angle of the mouth.

Depressor labii inferioris: muscle extending from the mandible to the midline of the lower lip.

Dermal papilla: elevation at the base of the bulb which contains a rich blood supply to provide the hair with food and oxygen.

Dermatosis papulosa nigra (DPN): benign cutaneous condition that is common among black skins. It is characterised by multiple, small, hyperpigmented, asymptomatic papules.

Dermis: deeper layer of the skin found below the epidermis.

Desquamation: shedding of dead skin cells from the horny layer (stratum corneum).

Diabetes insipidus: rare metabolic disorder in which a person produces large quantities of dilute urine and is constantly thirsty.

Diabetes mellitus: carbohydrate metabolism disorder in which sugars are not oxidised to produce enough energy due to lack of the pancreatic hormone insulin.

Diaphragm: dome-shaped muscle of respiration that separates the thorax from the abdomen.

Diarrhoea: condition where there is frequent bowel evacuation or the passage of abnormally soft or liquid faeces.

Diastolic: static pressure against the arterial wall during rest or pause between heart contractions.

Diffusion: process in which small molecules move from areas of high concentration to those of lower concentration.

Digestion: process of breaking down food.

Distal convoluted tubule: tube with a series of twists leading to a straightened collecting duct which leads to the pelvis of the kidney and onto the ureter.

Dorsiflexion: upward movement of the foot so that feet point upwards.

Duodenum: first of the three parts of the small intestine.

Dupuytren's contracture: forward curvature of the fingers (usually the ring and little fingers) caused by contracture of the fibrous tissue in the palm and fingers.

Dwarfism: hyposecretion of the growth hormone during childhood.

Dysmenorrhoea: painful and difficult menstruation.

Eccentric contraction: type of contraction when a muscle is stretched as it tries to resist a force pulling the bones of attachment away from one another.

Eccrine gland: simple coiled tubular sweat gland that opens directly onto the surface of the skin.

Ectopic pregnancy: development of a foetus at a site other than in the uterus. The most common type of ectopic pregnancy occurs in the fallopian tube.

Eczema: mild-to-chronic inflammatory skin condition characterised by itchiness, redness and the presence of small blisters that may be dry or weep if the surface is scratched. Eczema is non contagious but its cause may be genetic or due to internal and external influences.

Ejaculation: discharge of semen from the erect penis at the moment of sexual climax in the male.

Ejaculatory ducts: short tubes which join the seminal vesicles to the urethra.

Elastin: protein in the dermis which gives the skin its elasticity.

Emphysema: chronic obstructive pulmonary disease in which the alveoli of the lungs become enlarged and damaged, reducing the surface area for the exchange of oxygen and carbon dioxide.

Emulsification: process by which fat globules are broken up into smaller droplets by the action of bile salts.

Endocardium: inner layer of the heart.

Endocrine gland: ductless gland that manufactures one or more hormones and secretes them directly into the bloodstream.

Endometriosis: condition in which tissue resembling the lining of the uterus (endometrium) is abnormally present in the pelvic cavity.

Endomysium: fine connective tissue sheath that surrounds a single muscle fibre.

Endoplasmic reticulum: series of membranes continuous with the cell membrane. Cell's intracellular transport system, allowing movement of materials from one part of the cell to another.

Enzyme: chemical catalyst.

Ephelides: also known as freckles, these present as small pigmented areas of skin and appear where there is excessive production of the pigment melanin (after exposure to sunlight).

Epidermis: outermost, superficial layer of the skin.

Epidydmides: highly convoluted tubes that connect the testes to the vasa deferentia.

Epilepsy: neurological disorder which makes the individual susceptible to recurrent and temporary seizures.

Epimysium: fibrous elastic tissue surrounding a muscle.

Erector pili muscle: small, smooth, weak muscle attached at an angle to the base of a hair follicle which makes the hair stand erect in response to cold.

Erector spinae: long postural muscle in three bands either side of spine, attaching to the spine, ribcage and head.

Erythema: deadening of the skin due to the dilation of blood capillaries just below the epidermis.

Erythrocyte: red blood cells that transport the gases of respiration.

Ethmoid: skull bone forming part of the wall of the orbit, roof of the nasal cavity and part of the nasal septum.

Eversion: soles of the feet face outwards.

Expiration: act of breathing out air from the lungs.

Extension: straightening of a body part at a joint so that the angle between the bones is increased.

Extensor carpi radialis: muscle extending along the radial side of the posterior of the forearm.

Extensor carpi ulnaris: muscle extending along the ulnar side of the posterior of the forearm.

Extensor digitorum: muscle extending along the lateral side of the posterior of the forearm.

Extensor digitorum longus: long muscle of the lower leg that extends the toes.

Extensor hallicus longus: long muscle of the lower leg that extends the big toe.

Facial nerve: mixed nerve that conducts impulses to and from several areas in the face and neck. The sensory branches are associated with the taste receptors on the tongue and the motor fibres transmit impulses to the muscles of facial expression.

Faeces: solid or semi-solid mass of undigested food that is eliminated through the anus.

Fallopian tubes: tubes extending on the sides of the uterus, passing upwards and outwards to end near each ovary. Their function is to convey the ovum from the ovary to the uterus.

Fascia: fibrous connective tissue that envelops muscles and organs.

Fasciculi: bundle of muscle fibres.

Fatty acids: end product of fat digestion.

Femur: long bone of the thigh.

Fertilisation: fusion of a spermatozoon and an ovum.

Fibrin: insoluble fibrous protein formed from fibrinogen during blood coagulation.

Fibrinogen: plasma protein that is converted into fibrin during blood cogulation.

Fibroblast: cell found in reticular layer of dermis that forms new fibrous tissue.

Fibroid: abnormal growth of fibrous and muscular tissue, one or more of which may develop in the muscular wall of the uterus.

Fibromyalgia: chronic condition that produces musculo-skeletal pain.

Fibrositis: inflammatory condition of the fibrous connective tissues, especially in the muscle fascia (also known as muscular rheumatism).

Fibrous joint: immovable joint with tough fibrous tissue between the bones.

Fibrous joint capsule: part of synovial joint reinforced by connective tissue to hold the bones together and enclose the joint.

Fibula: long bone situated on lateral side of tibia in lower leg.

Filtration: movement of water and dissolved substances across the cell membrane due to differences in pressure.

Fissure: crack in the epidermis exposing the dermis.

Fixator: muscles that stabilise a bone to give a steady base from which the agonist works.

Flexion: bending of a body part at a joint so that the angle between the bones is decreased.

Flexor carpi digitorum: anterior muscle of the forearm extending from the medial end of the humerus, the anterior of the ulna and radius to the anterior surfaces of the second to fifth fingers.

Flexor carpi radialis: muscle of the forearm extending along the radial side of the anterior of the forearm.

Flexor carpi ulnaris: anterior muscle of the forearm extending along the ulnar side of the anterior of the forearm.

Flexor digitorum longus: long muscle of the lower leg that flexes the toes.

Flexor hallicus longus: long muscle of the lower leg that flexes the big toe.

Follicle-stimulating hormone: in women stimulates the development of the graafian follicle in the ovary which secretes the hormone oestrogen. In men it stimulates the testes to produce sperm.

Folliculitis: bacterial infection which occurs in the hair follicles of the skin and appears as a small pustule at the base of a hair follicle. There is redness, swelling and pain around the hair follicle.

Fracture: breakage of a bone, either complete or incomplete.

Free edge: part of the nail plate that extends beyond the nail bed.

Frontal: skull bone forming the forehead.

Frontalis: muscle that extends over the front of the skull and the width of the forehead.

Frozen shoulder (adhesive capsulitis): chronic condition in which there is pain and stiffness and reduced mobility, or locking, of the shoulder joint.

Gall bladder: pear-shaped sac lying underneath the right lobe of the liver, where bile is stored.

Gallstone: hard pebble-like mass which is formed within the gall bladder.

Gastric juice: liquid secreted by the gastric glands of the stomach (main constituents are hydrochloric acid, mucus, rennin and pepsinogen).

Gastrin: hormone released by endocrine cells in the stomach wall and stimulated by the presence of food.

Gastrocnemius: large superficial calf muscle with two bellies.

Genitalia: external reproductive organs.

Gigantism: abnormal growth causing excessive height, most commonly due to oversecretion of the growth hormone during childhood.

Gliding joint: type of synovial joint where two flat bones slide over one another.

Glomerulus: network of blood capillaries contained within the cuplike end (Bowman's capsule) of a nephron.

Glossopharyngeal nerve: mixed nerve that innervates structures in the mouth and throat.

Glucocorticoids: group of steroid hormones synthesised by the adrenal cortex, essential for the utilisation of carbohydrate, fat and protein by the body and for a normal response to stress.

Glucose: single sugar that serves as the primary source of cellular energy, the end product of carbohydrate digestion.

Gluteus maximus: large muscle covering the buttock.

Gluteus medius: medium-sized muscle of the buttock.

Gluteus mimimus: smallest of the buttock muscles.

Glycerol: clear viscous liquid obtained by the breakdown of fats, and the end product of fat digestion.

Glycogen: carbohydrate consisting of branched chains of glucose units, the principal form in which carbohydrate is stored in the body.

Golgi body: collection of flattened sacs within the cytoplasm near the nucleus and attached to the endoplasmic reticulum. It is the 'packaging and storage' department of the cell.

Gonadotrophic hormones: secreted from the anterior lobe of the pituitary gland, these hormones control the development and growth of the ovaries and testes.

Gracilis: long strap-like muscle that adducts the thigh.

Granular layer: (stratum granulosum) layer of epidermis linking the living cells of the epidermis (basal and prickle cell layers) to the dead cells above.

Greenstick fracture: partial fracture in which one side of the bone is broken and the other side bends (only occurs in children).

Growth hormone: secreted from the anterior lobe of the pituitary gland, controls the growth of long bones and muscles.

Gynaecomastia: enlargement of the breasts in the male due to either a hormone imbalance or hormone therapy.

Haemophilia: hereditary disorder in which the blood clots very slowly due to deficiency of either of two coagulation factors – Factor VIII (the antihaemophiliac factor) or Factor IX (the Christmas factor).

Haemorrhoids: condition with abnormal dilatation of veins in the rectum.

Hair: appendage of the skin which grows from a sac-like depression in the epidermis, called a hair follicle.

Hair bulb: enlarged part of hair at the base of the hair root.

Hair root: part of hair found below the surface of the skin.

Hair shaft: part of hair lying above the surface of the skin.

Hamstrings: group of three muscles situated on the posterior of the thigh.

Hay fever: allergic reaction involving the mucous passages of the upper respiratory tract and the conjunctiva of the eyes, caused by pollen or other allergens.

Headache: pain felt deep within the skull but excluding facial pain.

Heart: hollow organ made up of cardiac muscle tissue which lies in the thorax above the diaphragm and between the lungs. Its function is to maintain a constant circulation of blood throughout the body.

Heart attack (myocardial infarction): damage to the heart muscles which results from blockage of the coronary arteries.

Heartburn: burning sensation felt behind the sternum and often appearing to rise from the abdomen, up the oesophagus, towards or into the throat.

Hepatic arteries: blood vessels supplying blood to the liver.

Hepatic portal vein: blood vessels that drain blood from the liver.

Hepatitis: inflammation of the liver caused by viruses, toxic substances or immunological abnormalities.

Hepatitis A: highly contagious and transmitted by the faecal-oral route. It is transmitted by ingestion of contaminated food, water or milk.

Hepatitis B: also known as serum hepatitis. It lasts longer and is more serious than hepatitis A and can lead to cirrhosis, cancer of the liver and a carrier state.

Hepatitis C: can cause acute or chronic hepatitis. It can also lead to a carrier state and liver cancer. It is transmitted through blood transfusions or exposure to blood products.

Hernia: abnormal protrusion of an organ or part of an organ through the wall of the body cavity in which it normally lies.

Herpes simplex (cold sores): normally found on the face and around the lips. It begins as an itching sensation, followed by erythema and a group of small blisters which then weep and form crusts.

Herpes zoster (shingles): painful infection along the sensory nerves by the virus that causes chickenpox.

Hiatus hernia: most common type of hernia, occuring when part of the stomach is protruding into the chest.

High blood pressure: when the resting blood pressure is above normal, as consistently exceeding 160 mmHg systolic and 95 mmHg diastolic.

Hilus: medial border of the kidney where the renal blood vessels leave and enter the kidney.

Hinge joint: type of synovial joint where the rounded surface of one bone fits the hollow surface of another bone. Movement is only possible in one direction.

Hirsutism: presence of coarse, pigmented hair on the face, chest and upper back or abdomen in a female due to excessive production of androgens.

Hodgkin's disease: malignant disease of the lymphatic tissues, usually characterised by painless enlargement of one or more groups of lymph nodes in the neck, armpit, groin, chest, or abdomen.

Homeostasis: process by which the body maintains a stable internal environment for its cells and tissues.

Hormone: chemical messenger or regulator, secreted by an endocrine gland, which reaches its destination by the bloodstream and has the power of influencing the activity of other organs.

Horny layer (stratum corneum): most superficial, outer layer of the skin consisting of dead, flattened, keratinised cells.

Humerus: long bone of the upper arm.

Hydrochloric acid: strong acid present in a very dilute form in gastric juice.

Hyperhidrosis: excessive production of sweat affecting the hands, feet and underarms.

Hypertrophic disorders: refer to conditions which have resulted in an increase of size of a tissue or organ. This is caused by an enlargement of the cells.

Hypoglossal nerve: motor nerve that innervates the muscles of the tongue.

Hypoglycaemia: deficiency of glucose in the bloodstream, causing muscular weakness and incoordination, mental confusion and sweating. If severe it can lead to a hypoglycaemic coma.

Hypothalamus: small structure lying beneath the thalamus which governs many important homeostatic functions.

Hypothenar eminence: projection of soft tissue located on the ulnar side of the palm of the hand. It consists of three muscles – abductor digiti minimi manus, flexor digiti minimi manus and opponens digiti minimi.

Ileum: lowest part of the three portions of the small intestine.

Iliacus large, fan-shaped muscle deeply situated in the pelvic girdle.

Ilium: largest and most superior pelvic bone.

Immunisation: artificial stimulation of the body into producing antibodies.

Immunity: body's ability to resist infection.

Impacted fracture: where one fragment of bone is driven into the other.

Impetigo: superficial, contagious inflammatory disease caused by streptococcal and staphylococcal bacteria. It is commonly seen on the face and around the ears and features include weeping blisters which dry to form honey-coloured crusts.

Incontinence: condition in which the individual is unable to control urination voluntarily.

Inferior vena cava: main vein receiving blood from the lower parts of the body, below the diaphragm.

Infertility: inability in a woman to conceive or in a man to induce conception.

Infraspinatus: muscle that attaches to the middle two-thirds of the scapula, below the spine of the scapula at one end and the top of the humerus at the other.

Ingestion: act of taking food into the alimentary canal through the mouth.

Inginual nodes: lymph nodes located in the groin. They drain lymph from the lower limbs, the external genitalia and the lower abdominal wall.

Inner root sheath: originates from the dermal papilla at the base of the follicle and grows upwards with the hair, shaping and contouring.

Innominate artery (brachiocephalic): short artery originating as the first large branch of the aortic arch.

Innominate vein (brachiocephalic): either of the two veins, one on each side of the neck, formed by the junction of the external jugular and subclavian veins.

Insertion: most movable part of a muscle.

Inspiration: act of breathing air into the lungs through the mouth and nose.

Insulin: hormone produced in the pancreas by the islets of Langerhans cells. It is important for regulating the amount of glucose in the blood.

Intercostal muscles: muscles that occupy the spaces between the ribs and are responsible for controlling some of the movements of the ribs.

Intestinal juice: released by the glands of the small intestine and completes the final breakdown of nutrients, including simple sugars to glucose and protein to amino acids.

Inversion: soles of the feet face inwards.

Irritable bowel syndrome: common condition in which there is recurrent abdominal pain with constipation and/or diarrhoea and bloating.

Ischium: bone forming the posterior part of the pelvic girdle.

Islets of Langerhans: small groups of cells scattered through the pancreas. They secrete the hormones insulin and glucagon.

Isometric contraction: when a muscle works without actual movements or changing length.

Isotonic contraction: when a muscles force is considered to be constant but the muscle length changes.

Jaundice: yellowing of the skin or whites of the eyes, caused by excessive bilirubin (bile pigment) in the blood.

Jejunum: middle part of the small intestine, connecting the duodenum to the ileum.

Joint: point where two or more bones or cartilage meet.

Jugular vein: major vein draining blood from the head and neck (divides into internal and external branches).

Keloid: overgrowth of an existing scar which grows much larger than the original wound.

Keratin: tough fibrous protein found in the epidermis, hair and nails.

Keratinisation: process that cells undergo when they change from living cells with a nucleus to dead, horny cells without a nucleus.

Kidney: pair of organs responsible for excretion of waste from blood, situated at the back of abdomen, one on each side of spine.

Kidney stones: deposits of substances found in the urine which form solid stones with the renal pelvis of the kidney, the ureter or the bladder.

Kyphosis: abnormally increased outward curvature of the thoracic spine.

Lacrimal: smallest of the facial bones located close to the medial part of the orbital cavity.

Lacteal: intestinal lymphatic vessel.

Lactic acid: compound that forms in the cells as an end product of glucose metabolism in the absence of oxygen.

Lanugo hair: fine, soft hair found on a foetus.

Large intestine: part of the digestive system concerned with absorption of water from the material passed from the small intestine. It consists of the caecum, appendix, colon and rectum.

Larynx (voice box): short passage connecting the pharynx to the trachea.

Lateral longitudinal arch: arch of the foot which runs along the lateral side of the foot from the calcaneum bone to the end of the metatarsals.

Latissimus dorsi: wide muscle of the back extending across the back of the thorax.

Lentigo: also known as 'liver spots', these are flat dark patches of pigmentation which are found mainly in the elderly, on skin exposed to light.

Lesion: zone of tissue with impaired function as a result of damage by disease or wounding.

Leucocyte: white blood cells that aid the body's defence mechanism.

Leukaemia: cancer of blood-forming organs characterised by rapid growth and distorted development of leucocytes; refers to any of a group of malignant diseases in which the bone marrow and other blood-forming organs produce an increased number of certain types of white blood cells.

Levator anguli oris: muscle extending from the maxilla (upper jaw) to the angle of the mouth.

Levator ani: muscle forming the pelvic floor.

Levator labii superioris: muscle located towards the inner cheek beside the nose and extending from the upper jaw to the skin of the corners of the mouth and the upper lip.

Levator scapula: strap-like muscle that runs almost vertically through the neck, connecting the cervical vertebrae to the scapula.

Ligament: tough band of white fibrous connective tissue that links tow bone together at a joint.

Liver: largest gland in the body, occupying the top right portion of the abdominal cavity. It is concerned with regulation of blood sugar and amino acid levels, secretion of bile and detoxification of waste.

Loop of Henle: part of the kidney tubule that forms a loop extending towards the centre of the kidney. It absorbs water and selected soluble substances back into the bloodstream.

Lordosis: abnormally increased inward curvature of the lumbar spine.

Low blood pressure: when the blood pressure is below normal, a systolic blood pressure of 99 mmHg or less and a diastolic of less than 59 mmHg.

Lower limb: part of the skeleton containing the femur, patella, tibia, fibula, tarsals, metatarsals and phalanges.

Lumbar plexuses: spinal nerves located between the waist and the hip. They supply the front and sides of the abdominal wall and part of the thigh.

Lumbar vertebrae: five vertebrae of the lower back.

Lungs: cone-shaped spongy organs situated in the thoracic cavity on either side of the heart. Their function is to facilitate the exchange of the gases oxygen and carbon dioxide.

Lunula: light-coloured semicircular area of the nail, commonly called the half moon, lying between the matrix and the nail plate.

Lupus erythematosus: chronic inflammatory disease of connective tissue affecting the skin and various internal organs. It is an auto-immune disease and can be diagnosed by the presence of abnormal antibodies in the bloodstream.

Luteinizing hormone: in women it helps to prepare the uterus for the fertilised ovum. In men it acts on the testes to produce testosterone.

Lymph: transparent, colourless, watery liquid derived from tissue fluid.

Lymphatic capillaries: minute, blind-end tubes that commence in the tissue spaces of the body.

Lymphatic node: oval or bean-shaped structure that filters lymph.

Lymphatic vessels: tubes similar in structure to veins, with thin collapsible walls and valves; responsible for transporting lymph through its circulatory pathway.

Lymphoma: malignant tumour of the lymph nodes.

Lysosome: round sacs present in the cytoplasm, containing powerful enzymes to destroy any part of the cell that is worn out.

Macule: small flat patch of increased pigmentation or discolouration such as a freckle.

Malignant: term used to describe a tumour that invades and destroys the tissue in which it originates and can spread to other sites in the body via the bloodstream and lymphatic system.

Malignant melanoma: deeply pigmented mole which is life-threatening if it is not recognised and treated promptly. Its main characteristic is a blue-black module which increases in size, shape and colour and is most commonly found on the head, neck and trunk.

Mandible: only moveable bone of the skull forming the lower jaw.

Masseter: thick muscle in the cheek extending from the zygomatic arch to the outer corner of the mandible.

Mast cells: cells found in reticular layer of dermis which secrete histamine during an allergic reaction.

Mastication: process of chewing food.

Mastoid nodes: lymph nodes located behind the ear; they drain lymph from the skin of the ear and the temporal region of the scalp.

Matrix: substance of a tissue or organ in which specialised structures are embedded.

Matrix (hair): area of mitotic activity of the hair cells located at the lower part of the hair bulb.

Matrix (nail): area of nail situated immediately below the cuticle, the area where the living cells are produced.

Maxilla: largest bone of the face forming the upper jaw.

Medial longitudinal arch: arch of the foot running along the medial side of the foot from the calcaneum bone to the end of the metatarsals.

Medulla: inner layer of hair; inner part of kidney made up of conical-shaped sections called renal pyramids.

Meiosis: type of cell division that produces four daughter cells, each having half the number of chromosomes of the original cell.

Melanocyte-stimulating hormone (MSH): hormone synthesised and released by the pituitary gland. It stimulates the production of melanin in the basal cell layer of the skin.

Melanoma: cancerous growth of melanocytes.

Melatonin: hormone produced by the pineal gland. It is involved in the regulation of circadian rhythms, sleep/wake rhythms and is thought to influence the mood.

Meninges: special type of connective tissue with three layers that protects the brain and spinal cord.

Meningitis: inflammation of the meninges due to infection by viruses or bacteria.

Menopause: time when a women ceases to menstruate and is no longer able to bear children.

Menstrual cycle: periodic sequence of events in women in which an egg cell (ovum) is released from the ovary at four weekly intervals until the change of life.

Mentalis: muscle radiating from the lower lip over the centre of the chin.

Metabolism: physiological processes to convert the food we eat and the air we breathe into the energy the body needs to function.

Metacarpals: five long bones in the palm of the hand.

Metastasis: spread of cancerous cells to other parts of the body.

Metatarsals: five long bones forming the dorsal surface of the foot.

Migraine: specific form of headache, usually unilateral (one side of the head), associated with nausea or vomiting and visual disturbances such as scintillating or zigzag light waves.

Milia: sebum trapped in a blind duct with no surface opening. They appear as pearly, white, hard nodules under the skin.

Mineral corticoid: hormone secreted by the adrenal cortex, acting on the kidney tubules, retaining salts in the body, excreting excess potassium and maintaining the water and electrolyte balance.

Mitochondria: oval shaped organelles that lie within the cytoplasm. It is the site of the cell's energy production.

Mitosis: type of cell division when a single cell produces two genetically identical daughter cells.

Mixed/association neurone: type of nerve cell that links sensory and motor neurones, helping to form the complex pathways that enable the brain to interpret incoming sensory messages, decide on what should be done and send out instructions along motor pathways in response.

Mole: also known as a pigmented naevus. They appear as round, smooth lumps on the surface of the skin. They may be flat or raised and vary in size and colour from pink to brown or black.

Motor/efferent neurone: type of nerve cell that conducts impulses away from the brain and spinal cord to muscles and glands.

Motor nerve: type of nerve that carries impulses outwards from the central nervous system to bring about an activity in a muscle or gland.

Motor neurone disease: progressive degenerative disease of the motor neurones of the nervous system. It tends to occur in middle age and causes muscle weakness and wasting.

Motor point: point where the nerve supply enters the muscle.

Mucus: viscous fluid secreted by mucous membrane, acting as a protective barrier and lubricant.

Multiple sclerosis: disease of the central nervous system in which the myelin (fatty) sheath covering the nerve fibres is destroyed and various functions become impaired, including movement and sensations.

Muscle cramp: acute painful contraction of a single muscle or group of muscles.

Muscle fatigue: loss of the ability of a muscle to contract efficiently due to insufficient oxygen, exhaustion of energy supply and the accumulation of lactic acid.

Muscle spasm: increase in muscle tension due to excessive motor nerve activity, resulting in a knot in the muscle.

Muscle tone: state of partial contraction of a muscle.

Muscular atrophy: wasting away of muscles due to poor nutrition, lack of use or a dysfunction of the motor nerve impulses.

Muscular dystrophy: progressively crippling disease in which the muscles gradually weaken and atrophy.

Myelin sheath: fatty insulating sheath that covers the axon. Its function is to insulate the nerve and accelerate the conduction of nerve impulses along the length of the axon.

Myocardium: middle layer of heart.

Myofibrils: contractile filaments found within skeletal/voluntary muscle cells.

Myosin: most abundant protein found in muscle, plays an important role in muscle contraction.

Myositis: inflammation of a skeletal muscle.

Myxoedema: hypothyroidism in adult life, symptoms include coarsening of the skin, intolerance to cold, weight gain and mental dullness.

Naevus: birthmark and clearly defined malformation of the skin; mass of dilated capillaries.

Nail bed: area of the nail below the nail plate that provides nourishment and protection for the nail.

Nail groove: deep ridges under the sides of the nail which guide it and help it to grow straight.

Nail plate: main visible part of the nail which rests on the nail bed and ends at the free edge.

Nail wall: fold of skin overlapping the sides of the nails to protect the edges of the nail plate from external damage.

Nasal: small facial bone forming bridge of nose.

Nasalis: muscle located at the sides of the nose.

Naso-pharynx: upper part of the nasal cavity behind the nose.

Neoplasm: any new or abnormal growth (any benign or malignant tumour).

Nephritis: general non-specific term used to describe inflammation of the kidney.

Nephron: tiny blood filtration unit inside kidney.

Neuralgia: attacks of pain along the entire course or branch of a peripheral sensory nerve. A common example is trigeminal neuralgia affecting the trigeminal nerve in the face.

Neuritis: inflammation/disease of a single or several nerves, caused by infection, injury or poison.

Neuroglia: also known as glial cells, a special type of connective tissue of the central nervous system designed to support, nourish and protect the neurones.

Neurone: specialised nerve cell, designed to receive stimuli and conduct impulses.

Neurotransmitter: chemical substance released from nerve endings across synapses to other nerves.

Noradrenaline: hormone secreted by the medulla of the adrenal glands. It is closely related to adrenalin and helps the body create the conditions needed for rest through the parasympathetic nervous system.

Nose: organ which moistens, warms and filters the air and senses smell.

Nuclear membrane: perforated outer membrane enclosing the nucleus.

Nucleolus: dense, spherical structure inside nucleus, containing ribonucleic acid (RNA) to form of ribosomes.

Nucleus: control centre of the cell. It regulates the cell's functions and contains genetic information (DNA).

Obliques (external and internal): muscles located at the sides of the waist (external obliques are superficial to the internal obliques).

Occipital: skull bone forming the back of the skull.

Occipitalis: muscle found at the back of the head. It is attached to the occipital bone and the skin of the scalp.

Occipital nodes: lymph nodes located at the base of the skull. They drain lymph from the back of scalp and the upper part of the neck.

Oculomotor nerve: mixed nerve that innervates both internal and external muscles of the eye and a muscle of the upper eyelid.

Oedema: abnormal swelling of body tissues due to an accumulation of tissue fluid.

Oestrogen: hormone controlling female sexual development.

Olfactory: pertaining to the sense of smell.

Olfactory nerve: sensory nerve of olfaction (smell).

Oncologist: physician who specialises in the study and practice of treating tumours.

Oncology: study and practice of treating tumours.

Optic nerve: sensory nerve of vision.

Orbicularis oculi: circular muscle that surrounds the eye.

Orbicularis oris: circular muscle that surrounds the mouth.

Organ: part of the body, composed of more than one tissue that forms a structural unit responsible for a particular function.

Origin: most fixed point of a muscle.

Osmosis: process of the movement of water through the cell membrane from areas of low chemical concentration to areas of high chemical concentration.

Ossification: process of bone formation.

Osteoblast: bone-building cell.

Osteoclast: cartilage-destroying cell.

Osteocyte: mature bone cells.

Osteoporosis: brittle bones due to ageing and the lack of the hormone oestrogen which affects the ability to deposit calcium in the matrix of bone.

Outer root sheath: forms the follicle wall and provides a permanent source of growing cells (hair germ cells).

Ova: egg cells (plural of ovum).

Ovarian follicle: cavity in which an ovum is formed.

Ovaries: female sex glands lying on the lateral walls of the pelvis. They are concerned with the production of ova (eggs).

Ovum: egg cell.

Oxytocin: hormone secreted from the posterior lobe of pituitary. It stimulates the uterus during labour and stimulates the breasts to produce milk.

Palatine: L-shaped bones which form the anterior part of the roof of the mouth.

Pancreas: gland extending from the loop of the duodenum to behind the stomach and secretes pancreatic juice.

Pancreatic amylase: enzyme that continues the breakdown of starch and has the same effects as salivary amylase.

Pancreatic juice: secretes by the pancreas into the duodenum and contains enzymes that continue the digestion of protein, carbohydrates and fats.

Pancreatic lipase: enzyme that breaks down lipids into fatty acids and glycerol.

Papillary layer: most superficial layer of the dermis, situated above reticular layer.

Papule: small raised elevation on the skin, less than 1 cm in diameter, which may be red in colour. It often develops into a pustule.

Parasympathetic nervous system: one of the two divisions of the autonomic nervous system. It balances the action of the sympathetic division by working to conserve energy and create the conditions needed for rest and sleep.

Parietal: forms the upper sides of the skull and the back of the roof of the skull.

Parkinson's disease: damage to grey matter of brain known as basal ganglia. It causes involuntary tremors of limbs, with stiffness, rigidity and shuffling gait.

Parotid nodes: lymph nodes located at the angle of the jaw. They drain lymph from the nose, eyelids and ear.

Patella: kneecap.

Pectoralis major: thick, fan-shaped muscle covering the anterior surface of the upper chest.

Pectoralis minor: thin muscle that lies beneath the pectoralis major.

Pediculosis (lice): a contagious parasitic infection where the lice live off the blood sucked from the skin. With head lice, nits may be found in the hair. They are pearl-grey or brown, oval structures found on the hair shaft close to the scalp. The scalp may appear red and raw due to scratching.

Pelvic girdle: bony structure to which bones of lower limb are attached (consists of ilium, ischium and pubis bones).

Pelvic nodes: lymph nodes located within the pelvic cavity, along the paths of the iliac blood vessels. They drain lymph from organs within the pelvic cavity.

Penis: male organ made of erectile tissue that carries the urethra, through which urine and semen are discharged.

Pepsin: enzyme in the stomach that begins the digestion of proteins.

Peptidases: group of digestive enzymes that split proteins in the stomach and intestine into their constituent amino acids.

Pericardium: outer layer of heart.

Perimysium: fibrous sheath that surrounds each bundle of muscle fibres.

Periosteum: thin membrane of connective tissue covering bone.

Peripheral nervous system (PNS): part of the nervous system containing all the nerves outside of the central nervous system. It consists of cable-like nerves that link the central nervous system to the rest of the body.

Peristalsis: coordinated, rhythmical contractions of the circular and oblique muscles in the wall of the alimentary tract to break down food and move it along the alimentary canal.

Peroneus longus/brevis: muscles situated on the lateral aspect of the lower leg. They attach to the fibula and are plantar flexors of the foot.

Phalanges: finger and toes bones.

Pharynx: throat, serving as an air and food passage.

Phlebitis: inflammation of the wall of a vein, most commonly seen in the legs as a complication of varicose veins.

Pineal gland: pea-sized mass of nerve tissue attached by a stalk in the central part of the brain. It secretes a hormone called melatonin and is involved in the regulation of circadian rhythms.

Piriformis: deeply seated, pelvic girdle muscle that is a deep lateral rotator of the thigh.

Pituitary: lobed structure attached by a stalk to the hypothalamus of the brain.

Pivot joint: type of synovial joint where a process of bone rotates in a socket.

Plantar flexion: downward movement of the foot so that feet face downwards towards the ground.

Platysma: superficial neck muscle that extends from the chest up either side of the neck to the chin.

Pleurisy: inflammation of the pleura of the lung. It presents as an intense stabbing pain over the chest on breathing deeply.

Plexuses: network of nerves or blood vessels.

Pneumonia: inflammation of the lung caused by bacteria, in which the alveoli become filled with inflammatory cells and the lung becomes solid. Symptoms include fever, malaise and headache together with a cough and chest pain.

Polycystic ovary syndrome: condition caused by hyposecretion of the hormones oestrogen and progesterone in the female. It is characterised by cysts on the ovaries, cessation of periods, obesity, atrophy of the breasts, hirsutism and sterility.

Polypeptide: molecule consisting of three or more amino acids linked together by peptide bonds.

Popliteal nodes: lymph nodes located behind the knee. They drain lymph from the lower limbs through deep and superficial nodes.

Portal circulation: special branch of the systemic circulation which collects blood from the digestive organs and delivers it to the liver for processing, via the hepatic portal vein.

Port wine stain: also known as a 'deep capillary naevus'. It is present at birth and may vary in colour from pale pink to deep purple. It has an irregular shape but is not raised above the skin's surface and is usually found on the face but may also appear on other areas of the body.

Pregnancy: period in which a woman carries a developing foetus.

Pre-menstrual syndrome: term for the physical and psychological symptoms experienced from three to 14 days prior to the onset of menstruation.

Prickle cell layer (stratum spinosum): binding and transitional layer between the stratum granulosum and the stratum germinativum.

Procerus: muscle located in between the eyebrows.

Progesterone: hormone responsible for preparing the uterus for pregnancy.

Prolactin: hormone secreted by the anterior lobe of the pituitary. It stimulates the secretion of milk from the breasts following birth.

Pronation: turning the hand so that the palm is facing downwards.

Pronator teres: anterior muscle of the forearm, crossing the anterior aspect of the elbow.

Proprioceptors: sensory nerve endings located in muscles and tendons that transmit information to coordinate muscular activity, organs and glands.

Prostate: male accessory sex gland situated just below the bladder. During ejaculation it secretes an alkaline fluid that forms part of semen.

Prostatitis: inflammation of the prostate gland which is usually caused by bacteria.

Proximal convoluted tubule: highly coiled, twisted tube that leads away from the Bowman's capsule of a nephron and into the loop of Henle.

Psoas: long, thick, deep pelvic muscle.

Psoriasis: chronic, inflammatory skin condition. Psoriasis may be recognised as the development of well-defined red plaques, varying in size and shape and covered by white or silvery scales.

Pterygoids: facial muscles extending from the sphenoid bone in the skull to the mandible in the jaw.

Puberty: time at which the onset of sexual maturity occurs and the reproductive organs become functional.

Pubis: bone forming anterior of pelvic girdle.

Pulmonary arteries: two blood vessels (right and left) carrying deoxygenated blood from the right ventricle of the heart to the lungs.

Pulmonary circulation: circulatory system between the heart and lungs.

Pulmonary embolism: blood clot carried into the lungs.

Pulmonary veins: four blood vessels that carry oxygenated blood from the lungs and returns it to the left atrium of the heart.

Pulse: pressure wave that can be felt in the arteries, which corresponds to the beating of the heart.

Pustule: small raised elevation on the skin containing pus.

Quadratus lumborum: muscle located in the lower back/lumbar region.

Quadriceps: group of four muscles on the anterior aspect of the thigh.

Radius: long bone of the forearm (on thumb side of forearm).

Rectum: end part of large intestine where faeces are stored before defecation.

Rectus abdominis: long, flat muscle that extends bilaterally along the entire length of the front of the abdomen.

Reflex action/arc: rapid and automatic response to a stimulus without any conscious thought of the brain.

Renal artery: either of the two large arteries arising from the abdominal aorta and supplying the kidneys.

Renal pelvis: funnel-shaped cavity that collects urine from the renal pyramids in the medulla and drains it into the ureter.

Renal vein: blood vessels via which treated blood leaves the kidney.

Reticular fibres: fibres found in the reticular layer of dermis which help to maintain the skin's tone, strength and elasticity.

Reticular layer: deepest layer of the dermis situated below the papillary layer.

Rhinitis: inflammation of the mucous membrane of the nose, causing a blocked, runny and stuffy nose.

Rhomboids: either of the two muscles situated in the upper part of the back between the thoracic vertebrae and the scapula.

Ribosome: tiny organelles made up of ribonucleic acid (RNA) and protein. Its function is to manufacture proteins for use within the cell.

Right lymphatic duct: short duct that lies in the root of the neck and collects lymph from the right.

Ringworm: fungal infection of the skin which begins as small red papules that gradually increase in size to form a ring. Affected areas on the body vary in severity from mild scaling to inflamed itchy areas.

Risorius: triangular-shaped muscle that lies horizontally on the cheek, joining at the corners of the mouth.

Rodent ulcer: malignant tumour which starts off as a slow-growing pearly nodule, often at the site of a previous skin injury.

Rosacea: chronic inflammatory disease of the face in which the skin appears abnormally red. The condition is gradual, and begins with flushing of the cheeks and nose. As the condition progresses it can become pustular.

Rotation: movement of a bone around an axis (180 degrees).

Rupture: tearing of a muscle fascia or tendon.

Sacral plexuses: spinal nerves located at the base of the abdomen supplying the skin and muscles and organs of the pelvis.

Sacral vertebrae (sacrum): five fused vertebrae forming a flat, triangular-shaped bone between the pelvic bones.

Saddle joint: type of synovial joint where the articulating surfaces of bone have both rounded and hollow surfaces so that the surface of one bone fits the complementary surface of the other.

Saliva: alkaline liquid secreted by the salivary glands and by mucous membrane of the mouth.

Salivary amylase: enzyme that commences the digestion of starch or carbohydrates in the mouth.

Sarcoma: general term for any cancer arising from muscle cells or connective tissues.

Sarcomere: basic contractile unit of which skeletal/voluntary muscle fibres are composed.

Sartorius: narrow ribbon-like muscles which cross the anterior of the thigh.

Scabies: contagious parasitic skin condition caused by the female mite who burrows into the horny layer of the skin where she lays her eggs.

Scapula: bone forming posterior of shoulder girdle.

Scar: mark left on the skin after a wound has healed.

Sciatica: lower back pain which can affect the buttock and thigh.

Scoliosis: lateral curvature of the vertebral column which may be to the left or right side.

Scrotum: paired sac that holds the testes and epididymides.

Sebaceous cyst: round, nodular lesion with a smooth shiny surface which develops from a sebaceous gland.

Sebaceous gland: small sac-like pouches found all over the body, except for the soles of the feet and the palms of the hands. They produce an oily substance called sebum.

Seborrhoea: excessive secretion of sebum by the sebaceous glands. The glands are enlarged and the skin appears greasy, especially on the nose and the centre zone of the face. The condition may develop into acne vulgaris and is common at puberty, lasting for a few years.

Seborrhoeic dermatitis: mild-to-chronic inflammatory disease of hairy areas well supplied with sebaceous glands. Common sites are the scalp, face, axilla and in the groin.

Semen: fluid ejaculated from the penis at sexual climax.

Seminal vesicles: pair of male accessory sex glands that open into the vas deferens before it joins the urethra. They secrete most of the liquid component of semen.

Seminiferous tubules: long convoluted tubules that make up the bulk of the testes.

Sensory/afferent neurone: type of nerve cell that receives stimuli from sensory organs and receptors and transmits the impulse to the spinal cord and brain.

Septum: partition dividing an anatomical structure such as the heart.

Serratus anterior: broad curved muscle located on the side of the chest/rib cage below the axilla.

Sex corticoids: hormones secreted by the adrenal cortex, controlling the development of the secondary sex characteristics and the function of the reproductive organs, including testosterone, oestrogen and progesterone.

Shin splints: soreness in the front of the lower leg due to straining of the flexor muscles used in walking.

Shoulder girdle: part of skeleton that connects the upper limbs with the thorax and consists of two scapulae and clavicles.

Simple fracture: clean break with little damage to surrounding tissues and no break in the overlying skin (also known as a closed fracture).

Sinoatrial (SA) node: built-in electrical system which sets the pace of the heart rate.

Sinusitis: condition involving inflammation of the paranasal sinuses. It is usually caused by a viral or bacterial infection or may be associated with a common cold or allergy.

Skeletal/voluntary muscle: striped in appearance, this type of muscle tissue is attached to the skeleton. It is responsible for the movement of bones.

Skin tag: small growths of fibrous tissue which stand up from the skin and sometimes are pigmented.

Small intestine: part of the digestive system where most of the processes of digestion and absorption of food take place. It consists of three parts – duodenum, jejunum and ileum.

Smooth/involuntary muscle: type of muscle tissue found in the walls of hollow organs such as the stomach, intestines, bladder, uterus and blood vessels.

Soleus: large, flat calf muscle situated deep in gastrocnemius.

Somatic nervous system: division of the peripheral nervous system that consists of 31 pairs of spinal nerves and 12 pairs of cranial nerves.

Spasticity: increase in muscle tone and stiffness.

Specific immunity: type of immunity programmed genetically in the human body from birth. It includes mechanical barriers, chemicals, inflammation, phagocytosis and fever.

Sperm (spermatozoa): mature, male sex cells.

Sphenoid: skull bone located in front of the temporal bone.

Sphygmomanometer: instrument used to measure blood pressure.

Spider naevi: collection of dilated capillaries which radiate from a central papule.

Spina bifida: congenital defect of the vertebral column in which the halves of the neural arch of a vertebra fail to fuse in the midline.

Spinal cord: portion of the central nervous system enclosed in the vertebral column which extends from an opening at the base of the skull down to the second lumbar vertebra. Its function is to relay impulses to and from the brain.

Spinal nerves: set of 12 pairs of nerves originating from the spinal cord.

Spleen: largest of the lymphatic organs, located in left hand side of the abdominal cavity between the diaphragm and the stomach. It is concerned with protection from disease and the manufacture of antibodies.

Splenius capitis: long, posterior neck muscle that extends from the spinous processes of C7–T3 to the mastoid process of the temporal bone and the occipital bone.

Splenius cervicus: long, posterior neck muscle that extends from the spinous processes of T3–T6 to the transverse processes of C1–C3.

Sprain: injury to a ligament caused by overstretching or tearing.

Squamous cell carcinoma: malignant tumour which arises from the prickle cell layer of the epidermis.

Sternocleidomastoid: long muscle that lies obliquely across each side of the neck. Its fibres extend upwards from the sternum and clavicle at one end to the mastoid process of the temporal bone (at the back of the ear).

Stomach: muscular, J-shaped organ located between the oesophagus and the small intestine. It is concerned with the mechanical breakdown of food.

Strain: injury caused by excessive stretching or working of a muscle or tendon that results in a partial or complete tear.

Strawberry naevus: raised, red lump usually appearing on the face and growing rapidly in the first month of life. It usually disappears spontaneously before the child reaches the age of ten.

Stress: factor which affects physical or emotional health.

Stroke: blocking of blood flow to the brain by an embolus in a cerebral blood vessel.

Stye: acute inflammation of a gland at the base of an eyelash caused by bacterial infection. The gland becomes hard and tender and a pus-filled cyst develops at the centre.

Subclavian artery: either of the two arteries supplying blood to the neck and arms.

Subclavian veins: two main veins at the base of the neck into which the jugular veins empty blood.

Subcutaneous layer: thick layer of connective and adipose tissue found below the dermis.

Submandibular nodes: lymph nodes located beneath the jaw. They drain lymph from the chin, lips, nose, cheeks and tongue.

Subscapularis: muscle that attaches the inside surface of the scapula to the anterior of the top of the humerus.

Superficial cervical nodes: lymph nodes located at the side of the neck, they drain lymph from the lower part of the ear and the cheek region.

Superior vena cava: main vein draining blood from the upper parts of the body (head, neck, thorax and arms).

Supination: turning the hand so that the palm is facing upwards.

Supinator: muscle that attaches to the lateral aspect of the lower humerus and the radius and supinates the forearm.

Supraspinatus: muscle located in the depression above the spine of the scapula.

Suptratrochlear nodes: lymph nodes located in the elbow region. They drain lymph from the upper limbs and pass through to the axillary nodes.

Sympathetic nervous system: one of the two divisions of the autonomic nervous system. It prepares the body for expending energy and dealing with emergency situations.

Synapse: minute gap across which nerve impulses pass from one neurone to the next at the end of a nerve fibre.

Synergyst: muscles on the same side of a joint, that work together to perform the same movements.

Synovial cavity: space between the articulating bones of a synovial joint.

Synovial fluid: thick lubricating fluid secreted by the synovial membrane.

Synovial joint: freely moveable joint.

Synovial membrane: membrane that forms the sac enclosing a freely movable joint.

Synovitis: inflammation of a synovial membrane in a joint.

System: group of organs that work together to perform a specific function.

Systemic circulation: largest circulatory system that carries oxygenated blood from the left ventricle of the heart through to the aorta.

Systolic: pressure exerted on the arterial wall during active ventricular contraction.

Tarsals: seven irregular bones in the foot.

Telangiecstasia: term for dilated capillaries where there is persistent vasodilation of capillaries in the skin.

Telogen: short, resting stage of hair.

Temporal: skull bone forming the sides of the skull below the parietal bones and above and around the ears.

Temporalis: fan-shaped muscle situated on the side of the skull above and in front of the ear.

Temporomandibular joint tension (TMJ syndrome): collection of symptoms and signs produced by disorders of the temporomandibular joint (hinge joint between the mandible of the jaw and the temporal bone of the skull).

Tendinitis: inflammation of a tendon accompanied by pain and swelling.

Tendon: white fibrous cords of connective tissue that attach muscles to a bone.

Tennis elbow: inflammation of the tendons that attach the extensor muscles of the forearm at the elbow joint.

Tensor fascia lata: leg muscle attached to the outer edge of the ilium of the pelvis which runs via the long fascia lata tendon to the lateral aspect of the top of the tibia.

Teres major: muscle that attaches to the bottom lateral edge of the scapula at one end and the back of the humerus (just below the shoulder joint) at the other.

Teres minor: muscle that attaches to the lateral edge of the scapula, above teres major at one end and into the top of the posterior of the humerus at the other.

Terminal hair: longer, coarser hairs, mostly pigmented hairs found on the scalp, under the arms, eyebrows, pubic regions, arms and legs.

Testes: pair of male sex organs that produce sperm.

Testosterone: principal male sex hormone.

Tetany: condition caused by a reduction in the blood calcium level. It presents as spasm and twitching of the muscles, particularly those of the face, hands and feet.

Thalamus: positioned on each side of the forebrain, the thalami are relay and interpretation stations for the sensory messages (except olfaction) that enter the brain before they are transmitted to the cortex.

Thenar eminence: eminence of soft tissue located on the radial side of the palm of the hand.

Thoracic cavity: collective group of body parts (sternum, ribs and thoracic vertebrae) which offer protection for the heart and lungs.

Thoracic duct: main collecting duct of the lymphatic system that collects lymph from the left side of the head and neck, left arm, lower limbs and abdomen. It drains into the left subclavian vein to return it to the bloodstream.

Thoracic nodes: lymph nodes located within the thoracic cavity and along the trachea and bronchi. They drain lymph from the organs of the thoracic cavity and from the internal wall of the thorax.

Thoracic vertebrae: 12 vertebrae of the mid spine.

Thrombocyte: smallest cellular elements of blood cells, significant in the blood clotting process, otherwise known as platelets.

Thrombosis: condition in which the blood changes from a liquid to a solid state and produces a blood clot.

Thymus: gland composed of lymphatic tissue located in the upper chest. It is important in the newborn baby in promoting the development and maturation of lymphocytes.

Thyroid: gland in the neck situated on either side of the trachea. The principal role is in regulating metabolism.

Thyroid-stimulating hormone (TSH): secreted from the anterior lobe of the pituitary gland, it controls the growth and activity of the thyroid gland.

Thyrotoxicosis: excessive amounts of thyroid hormones in the bloodstream, causing rapid heartbeat, sweating, tremors, anxiety, increased appetite, loss of weight and intolerance to heat.

Thyroxine (T4): one of the hormones synthesised and secreted by the thyroid gland.

Tibia: long bone situated on anterior and medial side of lower leg.

Tibialis anterior: muscle on the anterior and lateral side of the lower leg extending from the tibia to the metatarsals.

Tibialis posterior: muscle on the posterior of the lower leg extending from the tibia to the metatarsals.

Tinea capitis: type of ringworm and a fungal infection of the scalp. It appears as painless, round, hairless patches on the scalp. Itching may be present and the lesion may appear red and scaly.

Tinea pedis (athlete's foot): highly contagious fungal condition which is easily transmitted in damp, moist conditions such as swimming pools, saunas and showers. It appears as flaking skin between the toes which becomes soft and soggy.

Tissue: group of similar cells that perform a certain function.

Tissue (interstitial) fluid: intercellular fluid located between cells other than blood cells.

Tonsils: lymphatic tissue located in the oral cavity and the pharynx.

Torticollis: condition in which the neck muscles (sternomastoids) contract involuntarily. It is commonly called 'wryneck'.

Trachea: windpipe that passes down into the thorax and connects the larynx with the bronchi.

Transverse arch: arch of the foot which runs between the medial and lateral aspect of the foot and is formed by the navicular, three cuneiforms and the bases of the five metatarsals.

Transversus abdominus: deep abdominal muscle that runs transversely across the abdomen.

Trapezius: large triangular-shaped muscle in the upper back that extends horizontally from the base of the skull (occipital bone) and the cervical and thoracic vertebrae to the scapula.

Triangularis: triangular-shaped muscle located below the corners of the mouth.

Triceps: muscle on the posterior of the upper arm.

Trigemenal nerve: mixed nerve (containing motor and sensory nerves).

Trimester: any one of the three successive three-month periods (first, second and third) into which a pregnancy may be divided.

Triodothyronine (T3): one of the hormones synthesised and secreted by the thyroid gland.

Trochlear nerve: smallest of the cranial nerves. It is a motor nerve that innervates the superior oblique muscle of the eyeball which helps you look upwards.

Trypsin: enzyme that continues the digestion of proteins by breaking down peptones into smaller peptide chains and is secreted by the pancreas.

Tuberculosis (TB): infectious disease caused by the bacillus (bacteria) Mycobacterium tuberculosis. Main transportation is via droplet infection and most common site for the bacilli to be spread to is the lungs.

Tumour: abnormal growth of tissue which may be benign or malignant. Tumours may be cancerous and sometimes fatal or they may be quite harmless.

Turbinate: layers of bone located either side of the outer walls of the nasal cavities.

Ulcer: break or open sore in the skin extending to all its layers.

Ulcer (peptic, duodenal or gastric): break in the lining of the alimentary tract which fails to heal and is accompanied by inflammation. This condition can present with increased acidity, epigastric pain and heartburn.

Ulna: long bone of the forearm on little finger side of forearm.

Upper limb: part of the skeleton containing the humerus, radius, ulna, carpals, metacarpals and phalanges.

Ureter: either of a pair of muscular tubes that convey urine from the pelvis of kidney to the bladder.

Urethra: tube that conducts urine from the bladder to the exterior. In the male it also serves as a conducting channel for semen.

Urinary bladder: pear-shaped sac which lies in the pelvic cavity where urine is collected and temporarily stored.

Urinary tract infection: bacterial infection of one or more of the structures of the urinary system.

Urine: fluid excreted by the kidneys containing water, urea, uric acid and creatinine.

Urticaria: also known as 'hives'. It is an itchy rash resulting from the release of histamine by mast cells.

Uterus: small, hollow, pear-shaped organ situated behind the bladder and in front of the rectum. It is the area in which an embryo grows and develops into a foetus.

Vacuole: empty space within the cytoplasm containing waste materials or secretions formed by the cytoplasm.

Vagina: lower part of female reproductive tract. It is a muscular tube lined with mucous membrane connecting the cervix of uterus to the exterior.

Vagus nerve: unlike the other cranial nerves, it has branches to numerous organs in the thorax and abdomen as well as the neck.

Varicose veins: veins which have become distended, lengthened and swollen.

Vasa deferentia: pair of ducts that conduct sperm from the epididymis to the urethra on ejaculation.

Vein: type of blood vessels with thinner muscular, elastic walls and valves. They carry blood towards the heart.

Vellus hair: soft, downy hair found all over the face and body, except for the palms of the hands, soles of the feet, eyelids and lips.

Ventricle: lower chamber of heart.

Vertebral arteries: main division of the subclavian artery, arising from the subclavian arteries in the base of the neck and pass upwards where they unite to form a single basilar artery.

Vertebral veins: main veins descending from the transverse openings (or foramina) of the cervical vertebrae and entering deep structures of the neck such as the vertebrae and muscles.

Vesicle: small, sac-like blister.

Vestibulocochlear nerve: sensory nerve that transmits impulses generated by auditory stimuli and stimuli related to equilibrium, balance and movement.

Villi: short finger-like processes that project from membranous surfaces such as from the wall of the small intestine.

Virilism: masculinisation in the female from the development of a combination of increased body hair, muscle bulk, deepening of the voice and male psychological characteristics.

Vitiligo: areas of the skin lacking pigmentation due to the basal cell layer of the epidermis no longer producing melanin. The cause of vitiligo is unknown.

Vomer: single bone at the back of the nasal septum.

Vulva: female external genitalia.

Wart: benign growth on the skin caused by infection with the human papilloma virus.

Weal: raised area of skin containing fluid, which is white in the centre with a red edge.

Whiplash: condition produced by damage to the muscles, ligaments, intervertebral discs or nerve tissues of the cervical region by sudden hyperextension and/or flexion of the neck.

Zygomatic: facial bone forming the cheeks.

Zygomatic major and minor/zygomaticus: muscles lying in the cheek area, extending from the zygomatic bone to the angle of the mouth.

Index